"Jorge Cruise gets it right by eliminating excessive sugar and processed carbohydrates. His recipes make eating smart easy. I recommend them highly."

— **Andrew Weil, M.D.,** Director of the Arizona Center for Integrative Medicine, University of Arizona, and author of *Why Our Health Matters*

"**The Belly Fat Cure** makes a solid case for healthful eating based on sound science. This way of eating will increase your energy, help you slow the aging process, and reduce your risk for major killers like heart disease and cancer. I strongly advise you to listen to Jorge's recommendations."

— **Terry Grossman, M.D.,** co-author of *Transcend: Nine Steps to Living Well Forever*

"When it comes to your health, forward thinking will allow you to avoid obesity and disease and achieve longevity. Jorge's program springs from progressive science that can truly change your body—and it all starts with controlling your consumption of sugar and processed carbs."

— **Ray Kurzweil,** world-renowned scientist and author of *The Singularity Is Near: When Humans Transcend Biology,* and *Fantastic Voyage: Live Long Enough to Live Forever*

"Jorge, again, is on to something; belly fat is surely an indicator of poor health. This book will turn your life around."

— **Suzanne Somers,** actress, and best-selling author of *Breakthrough: Eight Steps to Wellness*

The
BELLY FAT
CURE
SUGAR & CARB
COUNTER

ALSO BY JORGE CRUISE

The Belly Fat Cure™

Body at Home™

The 12-Second Sequence™

The 3-Hour Diet™

The 3-Hour Diet™ Cookbook

The 3-Hour Diet™ for Teens

The 3-Hour Diet™ On-The-Go

8 Minutes in the Morning®

8 Minutes in the Morning®: Extra-Easy Weight Loss

8 Minutes in the Morning®: Flat Belly

8 Minutes in the Morning®: Lean Hips and Thin Thighs

• •

Please visit:

Hay House USA: **www.hayhouse.com**®
Hay House Australia: **www.hayhouse.com.au**
Hay House UK: **www.hayhouse.co.uk**
Hay House South Africa: **www.hayhouse.co.za**
Hay House India: **www.hayhouse.co.in**

The
BELLY FAT
CURE
SUGAR & CARB
COUNTER

Discover which foods will melt up to 9 lbs. this week

JORGE CRUISE

HAY HOUSE, INC.
Carlsbad, California • New York City
London • Sydney • Johannesburg
Vancouver • Hong Kong • New Delhi

Published and distributed in the United States by: Hay House, Inc.: www.hayhouse.com • **Published and distributed in Australia by:** Hay House Australia Pty. Ltd.: www.hay house.com.au • **Published and distributed in the United Kingdom by:** Hay House UK, Ltd.: www.hayhouse.co.uk • **Published and distributed in the Republic of South Africa by:** Hay House SA (Pty), Ltd.: www.hayhouse.co.za • **Distributed in Canada by:** Raincoast: www .raincoast.com • **Published in India by:** Hay House Publishers India: www.hayhouse.co.in

Design: Tricia Breidenthal

Notice: The information given here is designed to help you make informed decisions about your body and health. The suggestions for specific foods in this program are not intended to replace appropriate or necessary medical care. Before starting any diet or exercise program, always see your physician. If you have specific medical symptoms, consult your physician immediately. If any recommendations given in this program contradict your physician's advice, be sure to consult him or her before proceeding. Mention of specific products, companies, organizations, or authorities in this book does not imply endorsement by the author or the publisher; nor does mention of specific companies, organizations, or authorities in the book imply that they endorse this book. The author and the publisher disclaim any liability or loss, personal or otherwise, resulting from the procedures in this program.

Product trademark names are used throughout this book to describe and inform the reader about various proprietary products that are owned by others. The presentation of such information is intended to benefit the owner of the products and trademarks and is not intended to infringe upon trademark, copyright, or other rights; nor to imply any claim to the mark other than that made by the owner. No endorsement of the information contained in this book has been given by the owners of such products and trademarks, and no such endorsement is implied by the inclusion of product trademarks in this book.

The reference material in this book was compiled using a number of sources, and all information was accurate at the time of printing. Internet addresses given in this book were accurate at the time the book went to press.

TRADEMARKS

The Belly Fat Cure	12-Second Sequence	Controlled Tension
TheBellyFatCure.com	12Second.com	Jorge Cruise
Carb Swap System	3-Hour Diet	JorgeCruise.com
S/C Value	3HourDiet.com	Time-Based Nutrition
Body at Home	8 Minutes in the Morning	Jorge's Packs
	Be in Control	

Library of Congress Control Number: 2010925403

ISBN: 978-1-4019-2912-1
Digital ISBN: 978-1-4019-2913-8

14 13 12 11   10 9 8 7
1st edition, August 2010
7th edition, May 2011

Printed in the United States of America

I'd like to dedicate this book to my friends and fans on Facebook, whose success and encouragement continue to inspire me every day to do what I do. Join the revolution at: **Facebook.com/JorgeCruiseFan**.

Contents

Welcome!

You have just picked up the *only* food list that singles out the true cause of belly fat: hidden sugar! Whether you are new to this groundbreaking revelation or are a seasoned veteran of the Belly Fat Cure, this book contains all you need to banish belly fat forever!

Before we can empower ourselves with the solution, we must fully understand the problem. First, we are very unhealthy as a nation: 68 percent of Americans are overweight. And not only are Americans overweight, but the vast majority of us carry excess belly fat, which is the most dangerous type of fat to have. A large waistline is a clear indicator that someone is at risk for the three biggest killers in this country: heart disease, cancer, and type 2 diabetes.

Read just the first chapter and you will join the ranks of hundreds of thousands of Americans who are standing up for the truth about weight loss and disease. Did you know that heart disease and cancer are the two leading causes of death in the U.S.? Or that the number one cause of bankruptcy is medical bills? In that respect, curing belly fat isn't just an exercise in looking better—this book contains the dietary principle that will save our country! That is, if you help me spread the word.

This book will reveal what to eat (and what *not* to eat) in order to flatten your belly, but the food list included in these pages is useless unless you discover my secret first! Commit to this program for just two weeks and you will be a believer, guaranteed. Turn the page now, and kiss dieting good-bye forever!

To looking and feeling your best,

Jorge

• •

Note: I have had many clients lose anywhere between 2 and 13 pounds in the first week following the Belly Fat Cure program, largely determined by the amount of weight they needed to lose in order to reach a healthy weight. As you approach your own goal weight, fat loss will naturally slow down. This should not discourage you, as even a modest decrease in dangerous belly fat is a step in the right direction. Because this program is not a restrictive diet, your body will safely and naturally choose its own pace . . . trust your body, and cherish each pound lost as a gift to your health!

• • • •

How This Book Will Help You
Melt Up to 9 lbs. a Week

When combined with the wealth of information found in the rest of this book, the tools you're being given in this single chapter make up the ultimate resource for weight loss and true empowerment. You're about to discover the _one critical element_ that gives you the power to come up with fat-melting meals that will destroy your hunger and banish your belly fat forever!

Take a few short minutes to read this chapter, learn how to create your own Belly Good Menu™, and lose up to 9 pounds this week.

What Is the Belly Fat Cure?

The first thing you must awaken to is the truth about what causes belly fat and obesity, and let go of the misguided effort to count calories or fat grams. It is critical you understand that the foods you eat are packed with hidden sugars. The latest breakthrough research has proven that losing and gaining fat isn't determined by how many calories you eat, but by the *kind* of calories you eat. That's why the focus of the Belly Fat Cure is about eating the right amount of sugar and carbohydrates to maximize fat loss while still satisfying your sweet tooth. The reason we single out the sugar and carbohydrates, not the calories and fat, has to do with the science of a naturally occurring hormone we all have: insulin.

Why Insulin?

You may be thinking, *I'm not diabetic; my insulin is fine!* or *I've always known that it's bad to eat sugar, so I hardly ever have candy.* That's where the breakthrough research about insulin and the huge amounts of hidden sugar in our everyday "healthy" foods comes into play. It is absolutely vital that you know that insulin is the hormone controlling your body's ability to push fat into fat cells. Without lowering insulin levels, it's impossible to lose weight, regardless of calorie intake or exercise intensity.

If you control your insulin, you'll have your foot on the brake pedal of your body's ability to store fat. This method of weight loss is the car that will drive you to the destination of your ultimate self.

How Do You Control Your Insulin?

The only way to control your insulin level is to eat the right amount of sugar and carbohydrates—a ratio I call the Sugar/Carb Value, or S/C Value™. The ideal S/C Value is less than or equal to 15/6: 15 grams of sugar and 6 servings of carbohydrates. It's sugar and carbs, not fat or protein, that lead to weight gain and belly fat. Allow me to explain how this process works.

First, let's imagine that you eat a piece of fruit or a candy bar, or drink a glass of milk. Simple sugars (like the ones found in these foods) are immediately released into your bloodstream and trigger the pancreas to pump a rush of insulin into the blood. The insulin transports sugar to the cells, but this hormone also pushes fat into them, especially in that dangerous area around the midsection. Remember, insulin is the primary regulator of fat cells, and only sugar will trigger insulin.

Then why track carbohydrates? Technically, carbohydrates are big sugars that your body needs time to break down. They affect your insulin because they're broken down into sugar, which is then released into your bloodstream. The difference is that these complex sugars are released at a much slower rate than simple sugars and therefore cause a more modest release of insulin. In order to release stored belly fat, though, you must keep your insulin level low and track your carbohydrate intake.

What Do the Numbers 15/6 Mean?

Even though this program is founded on the most recent breakthrough nutritional research, it is very much a return to our roots. Ancient humans had very limited access to sugar because fruit was incredibly rare and seasonal. In fact, the primary sugars we consume today, such as refined sugarcane and corn syrup, didn't even exist. Neither did processed carbohydrates like flour and white bread, which didn't become a part of our diets until after the Industrial Revolution.

Rather than representing the latest "fad diet," this program is doing quite the opposite: we are taking the next step forward by taking a smart step backward; that is, a return to 15 grams of sugar and 6 servings of carbohydrates.

Carbohydrate servings are counted as follows:

- 0 to 4 carbohydrate grams = not counted

- 5 to 20 carbohydrate grams = 1 serving

- 21 to 40 carbohydrate grams = 2 servings

- 41 to 60 carbohydrate grams = 3 servings

Always remember that a total daily S/C Value of 15/6 is the golden rule that you must implement each and every day to remain successful on this program.

I created this S/C Value by studying not only the daily diet of our ancestors, but also by working with my clients . . . modern, busy women and men just like you! I discovered that 15/6 is the perfect goal that allows people to lose belly fat rapidly but still feel satisfied and able to eat the carbs they love. This book was designed to keep you on track to stay at or below 15/6 every day. You'll find out that 15/6 is your guide to creating a perfectly healthful life!

Fiber

Another key element for weight loss is getting adequate fiber—at least 25 grams per day—which is why it's one of the nutrients shown in the product list in this book. Typically, if your 6 servings of carbohydrates come from whole-grain or vegetable sources, then you're going to meet or exceed your daily requirement of fiber.

However, if you're not having at least one good bowel movement per day, try adding additional fiber by selecting foods that are higher in it. You can also check out some solutions to slow movements that I have included on the FAQ section of my Website: **JorgeCruise.com/belly-fat-cure-faqs**.

Cholesterol

A breakthrough study published in 2009 in *Circulation,* a journal of the American Heart Association, has shattered the myth that eating cholesterol and fat leads to high cholesterol and heart disease. The study made it clear that a diet high in refined sugar and processed carbohydrates will have a far greater impact on blood cholesterol. In the same way that a cow eats grass or corn and turns it into meat, your own body consumes nutrients like cholesterol and repackages them for other essential uses.

Portion Size

The portion size is very specific for sugars and carbohydrates, as these two elements will affect your insulin. However, the portion size for fats and proteins is chosen by you and will vary, depending on the amount your body needs to feel physically satisfied . . . no more and no less. I recommend starting with an amount that could easily fit into the palm of one hand, and then adding more if you're still physically hungry. But remember, just because I don't tell you how much cheese to use, this doesn't mean you can eat the whole block and still expect your best results!

Simply knowing the truth about hidden sugars, insulin, and fat storage is not enough to maximize your success. You must have a plan or a map. The most successful people I've coached through my Website and on Facebook began their journey not just with the appropriate vehicle, but also with a simple, clear map for reaching the ultimate destination. So, read on for your map!

Your Simple Map:
The Belly Good Menu™

The next part of this book will totally empower you. You're about to learn how much dangerous hidden sugar is found in so many foods and products you've been told are healthy. Take this guide with you to the supermarket or when you're grabbing a bite, and you'll make the smartest and healthiest decisions for you and your family.

Taken alone, however, this list of more than 7,500 items can be somewhat overwhelming and cannot promise success with respect to continued weight loss and rejuvenation. That's why I have included the final piece of the puzzle, your road map to the destination of your best self: my magical Belly Good Menu.

I'm about to give you two examples of a Belly Good Menu, as well as an outline that will teach you how to make your own fat-melting menu every day. These next few pages are the most powerful and important in the entire book! The Belly Good Menu is the map that absolutely guarantees you will reach your destination. If you use it with the resources provided in the rest of the book, you will lose up to 9 pounds a week and transform your health and your life.

How Should You Use
the Belly Good Menu?

My most important recommendation for you, especially if you want to see fast, assured results this week, is to follow either or both of the completed menus I provide (note that they include items that can be found in the food list in the next chapter). Once you've used my sample menus for at least a week and have begun to see rapid fat-loss results, you'll be ready to create specialized fat-melting menus for your own specific tastes.

Sample Belly Good Menu #1

TIME OF DAY	MEAL
Breakfast	2 or 3 eggs any style with 1 piece of whole-grain toast and butter, ¼ cup blackberries, and tea or coffee with cream
Snack	String cheese
Lunch	*Wrap:* grilled chicken strips, cheddar cheese, lettuce, and 1 Tbsp. mayo in a whole-grain wrap; with 5 baby carrots and ranch dressing
Snack	¼ cup walnuts
Dinner	Mozzarella cheese melted over a grilled chicken breast, on ½ cup spaghetti with ¼ cup pasta sauce; and a spinach salad with low-sugar dressing

Sample Belly Good Menu #2

TIME OF DAY	MEAL
Breakfast	Sausage patty, egg, and cheese on ½ whole-grain English muffin; with ¼ cup raspberries and tea or coffee with cream
Snack	15 almonds
Lunch	*Tuna sandwich:* tuna with 1 Tbsp. mayo, 1 slice tomato, and lettuce on 2 slices of whole-grain bread
Snack	String cheese
Dinner	Grilled steak with ½ cup sautéed mushrooms, ¼ cup sautéed onions, a whole-grain roll with butter, and a spinach salad with low-sugar dressing

Whether following the Belly Good Menus in this chapter or creating your own, you should always check product labels (no matter what!), because so many items contain danger-ous artificial or hidden sweeteners. For example, most ranch dressing is sugar free, but some brands add high-fructose corn syrup. Also, many of the "light," "low fat," or "healthy" options and replacements out there exchange fats for sugars, artificial sweeteners, or hydrogenated oils—all of which will actually have an adverse impact on your weight loss.

So, when making your choice:

1. Select the natural option and let go of the nutrition science of 30 years ago. Yes, that means use butter and eggs!

2. Of the natural choices, pick the one with the least sugar and carbs. Yes, that means cream is better than skim milk, because cream has no sugar!

3. "Sugar free" often means "full of excitotoxins"! Avoid all artificial sweeteners, such as sucralose (Splenda), aspartame (Equal), and saccharin (Sweet'N Low), which can overstimulate the neurons in the brain, causing many to self-destruct. Even if this book gives a particular product a low enough S/C Value, always check the label for those unhealthy sweeteners!

Ready to Create Your Own?

After following the two completed menus I've included here for at least a week, you'll probably want to start coming up with your own.

First, it is very important to create a menu at the beginning of each day so that you remove the danger of making the wrong choices as the day goes on. It is also important because what you can eat for dinner is determined by what you ate earlier in the day. For simplicity, I recommend not having more than 5 grams of sugar or 2 servings of carbs at any one meal to ensure that you never go over 15/6 for the day or spike your insulin level.

Here's how the carb servings work per meal: Let's say that I have three items at lunch. One has 4 grams of carbohydrates, another has 6 grams, and the last item has 21 grams. When I add up the total grams of carbohydrates for the meal, I get 31 grams—or 2 servings—of carbohydrates. This shows that I am staying on track with my 6 carb servings for the day.

Second, the initial building blocks of each meal should be proteins and fat. These two nutrients satisfy hunger best and for longer periods of time, so you don't feel like you're starving yourself and you don't have a craving that causes you to "cheat." These two nutrients also don't affect your insulin, so you can play with the portion size of the protein and fat to make sure that you're satisfied. Once you've checked the protein and fat off your list, you can add your carbohydrate.

Let's start with a sample breakfast:

TIME OF DAY	PROTEIN	FAT	CARB
Breakfast	3 whole eggs, any style	Egg yolks Butter	1 slice of toast

You can then determine the exact S/C Value of the meal (which in this example depends on the type of bread) by either looking at the sugar and carbohydrate values on the packaging or searching for the bread in the reference section of this book.

Snacks on this menu are best used to get you safely from one meal to the next, without a craving that might cause you to break from your plan. The best snacks are those that are almost exclusively protein or fat based, with little to no sugar or carbs. Here is an example:

TIME OF DAY	PROTEIN	FAT	CARBS
Snack	1 hard-boiled egg	1 (1 oz. serving) string cheese	0 (no carbs)

Using those principles, the following Belly Good Menu outline becomes the most powerful and effective way to plan your day. When you combine the Belly Good Menu with the reference material in the rest of the book, you'll be well on your way to losing up to 9 pounds in a week.

Belly Good Menu Outline

TIME OF DAY	PROTEIN	FAT	CARBS (1–2 servings whole-grain or vegetable carbs)
Breakfast			
Snack			
Lunch			
Snack			
Dinner			

The Belly Fat Cure Success Planner

Another thing that may help keep you on track is a daily planner, which you can carry around with you. It's so simple to use: Just cross off one sugar box for every gram of sugar consumed and one carbohydrate box for each serving of carbs consumed. Once you have checked off all your boxes, you've reached your daily limit.

EAT USING THE S/C VALUE

INSTRUCTIONS: Cross off one sugar per gram consumed, and cross off one carbohydrate per serving consumed.

SUGAR (15 Grams) ○○○○○○○○○○○○○○○

CARBS* (6 Servings) ○○○○○○

*NOTE: 1 serving of carbs is 5 to 20 grams.

Be sure to make seven copies to take you through the week, or you can download copies from Hay House for free:

JorgeCruise.com

• •

Now that you know that insulin is the key component driving weight gain and fat loss, and that the Belly Good Menu system is your guarantee of success, you possess the tools to achieve the healthy weight you've always dreamed of. You won't accomplish this by starving yourself or starting a diet or workout regimen that you can't maintain, but by making smart choices that leave you satisfied and happy every day. With this book, today becomes the first day of the rest of your healthy lifestyle.

I offer a range of services and information that can help you further adapt your current lifestyle to the fat-melting one you have just discovered. For the smart and healthy chef in you, check out *The Belly Fat Cure,* which has more than 100 recipes that will show you how to make everything from pizza and burgers to pasta and salads . . . the Belly Fat Cure way!

Finally, if you're interested in more already-completed Belly Good Menus or personal nutrition coaching, please visit JorgeCruise.com to get my newest Belly Good Menu and join my free e-mail club.

• • • •

2

The Belly Fat Cure
Food List

Before we get to the list, here are a few things to note. You'll see that fiber, which is so important for proper digestion, is listed along with sugar and carbs. (Please note that, while serving sizes vary, all of the fiber, sugar, and carbs in the list are in grams.)

The reference material in this book was compiled using a number of sources, and all information was accurate at the time of printing. However, manufacturers often change ingredients and formulations, so please check nutrition labels for the most up-to-date information.

I understand that it may be a little confusing to read these labels, so let's use an example from a bag of Mission Tortilla Triangles (see next page).

The "S" arrow points to the sugar content, which is a 0. The "C" arrow points to the carbohydrate content, which is 17 grams—using the S/C Value, this means it's a 1. So a serving of

Nutrition Facts

Serving Size 1oz (28g/about 10 chips)
Servings Per Package 14

Amount Per Serving

Calories 160   Calories from Fat 80

% Daily Value*

Total Fat 9g	**14%**
Saturated Fat 4g	**20%**
Trans Fat 0g	
Cholesterol 0mg	**0%**
Sodium 150mg	**6%**
Total Carbohydrate 17g	**6%**
Dietary Fiber 1g	**4%**
Sugars 0g	
Protein 2g	

Vitamin A	0%	• Vitamin C	0%
Calcium	2%	• Iron	2%

*Percent Daily Values are based on a 2,000 calorie diet. Your daily values may be higher or lower depending on your calorie needs:

	Calories:	2,000	2,500
Total Fat	Less Than	65g	80g
Saturated Fat	Less Than	20g	25g
Cholesterol	Less Than	300mg	300mg
Sodium	Less Than	2,400mg	2,400mg
Total Carbohydrate		300g	375g
Dietary Fiber		25g	30g

Calories per gram:
Fat 9   •   Carbohydrate 4   •   Protein 4

Mission Tortilla Triangles
(10 chips)
S/C Value 0/1

these tortilla chips has an S/C Value of 0/1.

Note that the sugar and carbohydrate values of meat will not be affected by different cooking methods or removing the skin. But do be aware of added sauces and dressings, especially anything that is honey, maple, brown sugar, or barbecue flavored. Many prepackaged and precooked items (such as deli meat) have added sugars, so again, always check the nutrition label.

For each category, the food list in this chapter gives information on generic items first, followed by any brand-name products. Please keep in mind that nutritional values vary based on serving size, brand, and ingredients. "Average" listed after certain item names means that the nutritional information for that item is based on an average size for that item. I have also included "fridge" or "freezer" after certain meats to indicate where the product might be found.

A Word about Serving Sizes

When scales and measuring cups are impractical, the handy guide below will help you get a rough idea of what portion sizes should look like:

- 3 oz meat = 1 deck of cards or the palm of your hand (w/o fingers)

- 3 oz fish = 1 checkbook

- 1 cup fruits or vegetables = 1 baseball or your fist

- ½ cup pasta or rice = 1 hockey puck

- 1 pancake or waffle = 1 CD

- 1 oz cheese = 4 dice

- 1 oz nuts or candy = 1 small handful

- 2 Tbsp of spread = 1 golf ball

- 1 tsp of spread = 1 dice

- 1 tsp of sauce = 1 poker chip or 4 dimes

Abbreviations and Measurement Conversions

ABBREVIATIONS

- Crust = cst
- Cup = c
- Ounce = oz
- Package = pkg
- Packet = pkt
- Piece = pc
- Scoop = scp
- Slice = slc
- Spray = spr
- Tablespoon = T
- Teaspoon = t

CONVERSIONS

- 1 gallon = 4 quarts
- 1 quart = 2 pints
- 1 pint = 16 oz
- 8 oz = 1 cup
- 1 cup = 16 Tbsp
- 1 Tbsp = 3 tsp
- 4 Tbsp = ¼ cup

• • • •

FOOD	Svg Size	Fbr	Sgr	Cbs	S/C Val
Chicken, most preparations	any	0	0	0	0/0
Chicken, canned, Swanson, chunk breast in water	2 oz	0	0	1	0/0
Chicken, canned, Tyson, premium chunk	2 oz	0	0	0	0/0
Chicken, canned, Tyson, premium chunk breast	2 oz	0	0	0	0/0
Chicken, fridge, Butterball, breast strips, grilled	3 oz	0	0	2	0/0
Chicken, fridge, Butterball, breast strips, oven roasted	3 oz	0	0	1	0/0
Chicken, fridge, Foster Farms, grilled chicken breast strips	3 oz	0	0	2	0/0
Chicken, fridge, Foster Farms, honey roasted chicken breast strips	3 oz	0	0	6	0/1
Chicken, fridge, Hormel, grilled chicken strips	2 oz	0	0	0	0/0
Chicken, fridge, Oscar Mayer, breast cuts, honey roasted	3 oz	0	3	3	3/0
Chicken, fridge, Oscar Mayer, breast cuts, oven roasted	3 oz	0	1	1	1/0
Chicken, fridge, Perdue Short Cuts, grilled Italian style	½ c	0	1	2	1/0
Chicken, fridge, Perdue Short Cuts, honey roasted	½ c	0	2	2	2/0
Chicken, fridge, Tyson, grilled breast strips	3 oz	0	1	3	1/0
Chicken, fridge, Tyson, oven roasted diced breast	3 oz	0	1	2	1/0
Chicken, frozen, Foster Farms, crispy strips	3 oz	0	0	14	0/1
Chicken, frozen, Foster Farms, grilled strips	3 oz	0	0	2	0/0
Chicken, frozen, Foster Farms, honey BBQ wings	4	0	0	5	0/1
Chicken, frozen, Tyson, Any'tizers, barbeque style wings	3	0	7	7	7/1
Chicken, frozen, Tyson, Any'tizers, homestyle chicken fries	7	1	0	19	0/1
Chicken, frozen, Tyson, Any'tizers, honey BBQ wings	3	0	7	9	7/1
Chicken, frozen, Tyson, Any'tizers, hot 'n spicy wings	3	0	0	1	0/0
Chicken, frozen, Tyson, Any'tizers, popcorn chicken	6	1	1	19	1/1
Chicken, frozen, Tyson, breast patties	1	1	1	12	1/1
Chicken, frozen, Tyson, crispy strips	2	1	0	13	0/1
Chicken, frozen, Tyson, honey breast tenders	5	2	3	13	3/1
Chicken, frozen, Tyson, nuggets	5	0	0	15	0/1
Chicken, pâté	1 oz	0	0	2	0/0
Cornish game hen, most preparations	any	0	0	0	0/0
Deli, chicken, Boar's Head, breast, hickory smoked	2 oz	0	0	0	0/0
Deli, chicken, Boar's Head, breast, oven roasted	2 oz	0	0	0	0/0
Deli, chicken, Buddig, extra thin	9 pcs	0	1	2	1/0
Deli, chicken, Butterball, breast, oven roasted, thin sliced	4 pcs	0	1	3	1/0
Deli, chicken, Foster Farms, bologna	1 pc	0	0	0	0/0
Deli, chicken, Foster Farms, breast, oven roasted	1 pc	0	0	0	0/0
Deli, chicken, Hillshire Farm, breast, oven roasted	6 pcs	0	1	2	1/0
Deli, chicken, Hormel, rotisserie style breast	2 oz	0	0	0	0/0
Deli, chicken, Oscar Mayer, breast, oven roasted	2 oz	0	1	2	1/0
Deli, chicken, Oscar Mayer, breast, rotisserie, shaved	6 pcs	0	1	2	1/0
Deli, chicken, Sara Lee, oven roasted breast	4 pcs	0	0	0	0/0
Deli, Lunchables, chicken & American sub sandwich	1 pkg	1	3	25	3/2
Deli, Lunchables, chicken strips	1 pkg	1	6	17	6/1
Deli, Lunchables, turkey & cheddar sub sandwich	1 pkg	1	3	25	3/2
Deli, Lunchables, turkey & cheddar w/ crackers	1 pkg	1	6	23	6/2

FOOD	Svg Size	Fbr	Sgr	Cbs	S/C Val
Deli, Lunchables, turkey, mozzarella & mini Ritz	1 pkg	0	2	9	2/1
Deli, turkey, bologna	1 oz	0	1	1	1/0
Deli, turkey, pastrami	2 oz	0	2	1	2/0
Deli, turkey, salami	1 oz	0	0	0	0/0
Deli, turkey, Boars' Head, breast, cracked pepper, smoked	2 oz	0	1	1	1/0
Deli, turkey, Boars' Head, breast, maple glazed	2 oz	0	2	2	2/0
Deli, turkey, Boars' Head, breast, Ovengold	2 oz	0	0	1	0/0
Deli, turkey, Buddig, extra thin	9 pcs	0	1	2	1/0
Deli, turkey, Buddig, honey, extra thin	9 pcs	0	2	3	2/0
Deli, turkey, Butterball, deep fried, original, extra thin sliced	7 pcs	0	1	3	1/0
Deli, turkey, Butterball, honey roasted, thick sliced	1 pc	0	2	3	2/0
Deli, turkey, Butterball, honey roasted, thin sliced	4 pcs	0	3	5	3/1
Deli, turkey, Butterball, oven roasted, thin sliced	4 pcs	0	1	3	1/0
Deli, turkey, Foster Farms, bologna	1 pc	0	0	0	0/0
Deli, turkey, Foster Farms, honey roasted & smoked, thin sliced	4 pcs	0	0	3	0/0
Deli, turkey, Foster Farms, oven roasted, thin sliced	4 pcs	0	0	1	0/0
Deli, turkey, Hillshire Farm, breast, honey roasted	6 pcs	0	3	5	3/1
Deli, turkey, Hillshire Farm, breast, mesquite smoked	6 pcs	0	2	3	2/0
Deli, turkey, Hillshire Farm, breast, oven roasted	6 pcs	0	1	3	1/0
Deli, turkey, Hormel Natural Choice, breast, oven roasted	3 pcs	0	1	1	1/0
Deli, turkey, Hormel Natural Choice, smoked	3 pcs	0	1	1	1/0
Deli, turkey, Hormel, pepperoni	1 oz	0	0	0	0/0
Deli, turkey, Jennie-O, ham	2 oz	0	1	2	1/0
Deli, turkey, Jennie-O, pastrami	2 oz	0	1	3	1/0
Deli, turkey, Oscar Mayer, bologna	1 pc	0	0	1	0/0
Deli, turkey, Oscar Mayer, breast, honey smoked	1 pc	0	1	3	1/0
Deli, turkey, Oscar Mayer, white, oven roasted	1 pc	0	0	0	0/0
Deli, turkey, Sara Lee, breast, cracked pepper	4 pcs	0	0	1	0/0
Deli, turkey, Sara Lee, breast, hardwood smoked	4 pcs	0	0	1	0/0
Duck, most preparations	any	0	0	0	0/0
Egg, large	1	0	0	0	0/0
Egg, beaten	1 c	0	2	2	2/0
Egg, Egg Beaters, original	¼ c	0	0	1	0/0
Egg, Egg Beaters, whites	3 T	0	0	1	0/0
Egg, Real Egg, Kirkland Signature, 99% pure egg whites	¼ c	0	0	1	0/0
Egg substitute, Egg Replacer, Bob's Red Mill	1 T	1	1	2	1/0
Egg substitute, Egg Replacer, Ener-G	1½ t	0	0	4	0/0
Goose, most preparations	any	0	0	0	0/0
Goose, pâté (foie gras)	1 oz	0	0	1	0/0
Hot dog, chicken, Foster Farms, franks	1	0	0	1	0/0
Hot dog, chicken, Zacky Farms, jumbo franks	1	0	1	4	1/0
Hot dog, turkey, Ball Park, franks	1	0	2	6	2/1
Hot dog, turkey, Ball Park, smoked white franks	1	0	3	5	3/1
Hot dog, turkey, Butterball, franks	1	0	1	2	1/0

FOOD	Svg Size	Fbr	Sgr	Cbs	S/C Val
Hot dog, turkey, Butterball, jumbo franks	1	0	1	3	1/0
Hot dog, turkey, Foster Farms, franks	1	0	0	1	0/0
Hot dog, turkey, Jennie-O, franks	1	0	0	1	0/0
Hot dog, turkey, Oscar Mayer, franks	1	0	1	2	1/0
Jerky, turkey, Jack Link's	1 oz	0	3	3	3/0
Jerky, turkey, Oberto	1 oz	0	6	9	6/1
Jerky, turkey, Pacific Gold	1 oz	0	5	8	5/1
Pheasant, most preparations	any	0	0	0	0/0
Quail, most preparations	any	0	0	0	0/0
Sausage, chicken, Aidells, Cajun style andouille	1	0	2	2	2/0
Sausage, chicken, Aidells, chicken & apple	1	0	2	3	2/0
Sausage, chicken, Al Fresco, breakfast, apple maple	1	0	4	4	4/0
Sausage, chicken, Al Fresco, breakfast, country style	1	0	0	0	0/0
Sausage, chicken, Al Fresco, Buffalo style	1	0	2	4	2/0
Sausage, chicken, Al Fresco, chipotle chorizo	1	0	3	5	3/1
Sausage, chicken, Al Fresco, sweet apple	1	0	9	10	9/1
Sausage, chicken, Armour, Vienna in broth	2 oz	0	0	1	0/0
Sausage, chicken, Hillshire Farm, hardwood smoked	2 oz	0	1	3	1/0
Sausage, chicken, Libby's, Vienna	3 pcs	0	0	1	0/0
Sausage, chicken & turkey, Aidells, artichoke & garlic	1	1	0	1	0/0
Sausage, chicken & turkey, Aidells, Italian style	1	0	0	2	0/0
Sausage, chicken & turkey, Aidells, portobello mushroom	1	1	2	3	2/0
Sausage, chicken & turkey, Aidells, sun-dried tomato	1	2	1	3	1/0
Sausage, turkey, Butterball, bratwurst	1	0	0	1	0/0
Sausage, turkey, Butterball, breakfast links	3	0	0	0	0/0
Sausage, turkey, Butterball, hardwood smoked	1	0	1	7	1/1
Sausage, turkey, Butterball, Polska kielbasa	2 oz	0	1	4	1/0
Sausage, turkey, Hillshire Farm, cocktail, Lit'l Smokies	5	0	2	4	2/0
Sausage, turkey, Hillshire Farm, Polska kielbasa	2 oz	0	1	3	1/0
Sausage, turkey, Hillshire Farm, smoked	2 oz	0	1	3	1/0
Sausage, turkey, Jennie-O, beer bratwurst	1	0	3	4	3/0
Sausage, turkey, Jennie-O, sweet Italian	1	0	0	0	0/0
Sausage, turkey, Jimmy Dean, Fully Cooked, links	3	0	1	1	1/0
Sausage, turkey, Jimmy Dean, Fully Cooked, patties	1	0	1	1	1/0
Sausage, turkey, Johnsonville, smoked	1	0	2	4	2/0
Sausage, turkey, Perdue, breakfast, roll	2 oz	0	0	0	0/0
Sausage, turkey, Perdue, sweet Italian, links	1	0	1	4	1/0
Sausage, turkey, Perdue, sweet Italian, roll	2 oz	0	1	2	1/0
Squab, most preparations	any	0	0	0	0/0
Turkey, most preparations	any	0	0	0	0/0
Turkey, canned	1 c	0	0	0	0/0
Turkey, canned, Spam	2 oz	0	0	2	0/0
Turkey, fridge, Butterball, breast medallions, oven roasted	3 oz	0	0	1	0/0
Turkey, fridge, Butterball, breast strips, oven roasted	3 oz	0	0	2	0/0

POULTRY & EGGS, cont'd.

FOOD	Svg Size	Fbr	Sgr	Cbs	S/C Val
Turkey, fridge, Foster Farms, meatballs, homestyle	3	0	0	8	0/1
Turkey, fridge, Perdue, meatballs, Italian style	4	0	0	5	0/1
Turkey, fridge, Perdue, Oven Ready, whole seasoned roaster	4 oz	0	1	1	1/0
Turkey, frozen, Butterball, breast tenderloins, lemon pepper	4 oz	0	2	3	2/0
Turkey, frozen, Butterball, breast tenderloins, teriyaki	4 oz	0	3	4	3/0
Turkey, frozen, Butterball, burger, seasoned	1	0	0	0	0/0
Turkey, frozen, Butterball, whole breast	4 oz	0	1	1	1/0
Turkey, frozen, Foster Farms, meatballs, homestyle	3	0	0	3	0/0
Turkey, frozen, Foster Farms, meatballs, Italian style	3	0	1	5	1/1
Turkey, frozen, Jennie-O, burger	4 oz	0	0	0	0/0
Turkey, rotisserie, white meat	3 oz	0	4	7	4/1
Turkey bacon	1 oz	0	0	1	0/0

MEATS

FOOD	Svg Size	Fbr	Sgr	Cbs	S/C Val
Bacon, most styles, unflavored	any	0	0	0	0/0
Bacon, Hormel, Black Label, original	2 slcs	0	0	0	0/0
Bacon, Jimmy Dean, maple, thick sliced, precooked	3 slcs	0	1	1	1/0
Bacon, Tyson, hickory	2 slcs	0	0	0	0/0
Beef, most preparations	any	0	0	0	0/0
Beef, canned, corned, Hormel	2 oz	0	0	0	0/0
Beef, canned, corned, Libby's	2 oz	0	0	0	0/0
Bison, most preparations	any	0	0	0	0/0
Canadian bacon	2 oz	0	0	1	0/0
Canadian bacon, Hormel, sandwich style	3 slcs	0	0	0	0/0
Deli, bologna, beef	1 oz	0	0	1	0/0
Deli, bologna, mixed meats	1 oz	0	1	1	1/0
Deli, bologna, pork	1 oz	0	0	0	0/0
Deli, bologna, Boar's Head, beef	2 oz	0	0	0	0/0
Deli, bologna, Boar's Head, pork & beef	2 oz	0	0	0	0/0
Deli, bologna, Hebrew National, beef	1 pc	0	0	0	0/0
Deli, bologna, Hebrew National, beef, lean	4 pcs	0	0	1	0/0
Deli, bologna, Johnsonville, beef ring	2 oz	0	0	1	0/0
Deli, bologna, Johnsonville, original ring	2 oz	0	0	1	0/0
Deli, bologna, Oscar Mayer	1 pc	0	0	0	0/0
Deli, bologna, Oscar Mayer, beef, light	1 pc	0	0	2	0/0
Deli, bologna, Oscar Mayer, beef, thin	3 pcs	0	0	1	0/0
Deli, corned beef	3 oz	0	0	0	0/0
Deli, corned beef, Hillshire Farm	7 pcs	0	0	0	0/0
Deli, corned beef, Sara Lee	2 oz	0	0	1	0/0
Deli, ham, Buddig	2 oz	0	1	1	1/0
Deli, ham, Buddig, honey	2 oz	0	2	2	2/0
Deli, ham, Hillshire Farm, baked	6 pcs	0	1	1	1/0
Deli, ham, Hillshire Farm, baked, brown sugar	6 pcs	0	3	3	3/0

FOOD	Svg Size	Fbr	Sgr	Cbs	S/C Val
Deli, ham, Hillshire Farm, honey	6 pcs	0	3	3	3/0
Deli, ham, Hormel Natural Choice, honey	4 pcs	0	3	3	3/0
Deli, ham, Oscar Mayer, boiled	3 pcs	0	1	1	1/0
Deli, ham, Oscar Mayer, brown sugar	3 pcs	0	4	4	4/0
Deli, ham, Oscar Mayer, honey	3 pcs	0	2	2	2/0
Deli, liverwurst, pork	1 oz	0	0	1	0/0
Deli, Lunchables, ham & American sub sandwich	1 pkg	1	3	25	3/2
Deli, Lunchables, ham & cheddar w/ crackers	1 pkg	1	6	23	6/2
Deli, Lunchables, ham & Swiss w/ crackers	1 pkg	1	6	23	6/2
Deli, Lunchables, ham, cheddar & mini Ritz	1 pkg	0	2	10	2/1
Deli, Lunchables, pepperoni pizza	1 pkg	3	6	30	6/2
Deli, mortadella, beef or pork	1 oz	0	0	1	0/0
Deli, pastrami, beef	1 oz	0	0	0	0/0
Deli, pastrami, Boar's Head	2 oz	0	0	0	0/0
Deli, pastrami, Buddig	2 oz	0	1	1	1/0
Deli, pastrami, Hillshire Farm	7 pcs	0	0	0	0/0
Deli, pepperoni, beef or pork	1 oz	0	0	0	0/0
Deli, pepperoni, Gallo	10 pcs	0	0	0	0/0
Deli, pepperoni, Hormel	14 pcs	0	0	0	0/0
Deli, roast beef, Hillshire Farm	7 pcs	0	0	0	0/0
Deli, roast beef, Hormel Natural Choice	2 oz	0	0	0	0/0
Deli, roast beef, Oscar Mayer, slow roasted, shaved	6 pcs	0	0	0	0/0
Deli, salami, beef	1 oz	0	0	1	0/0
Deli, salami, pork	1 oz	0	0	0	0/0
Deli, salami, Gallo, Italian dry salame	5 pcs	0	0	1	0/0
Deli, salami, Hebrew National, beef	3 pcs	0	0	0	0/0
Deli, salami, Hebrew National, beef, lean	4 pcs	0	0	1	0/0
Deli, salami, Hillshire Farm, hard, ultra thin	1 oz	0	0	0	0/0
Deli, salami, Hormel Natural Choice, hard, uncured	1 oz	0	0	0	0/0
Deli, salami, Oberto, Italian dry	1 oz	0	1	0	1/0
Deli, salami, Oscar Mayer, cotto	1 pc	0	0	0	0/0
Deli, salami, Oscar Mayer, hard	3 pcs	0	0	0	0/0
Escargot (snail)	3 oz	0	0	2	0/0
Hot dog, Ball Park, Angus beef franks	1	0	1	3	1/0
Hot dog, Ball Park, beef franks	1	0	2	4	2/0
Hot dog, Ball Park, beef franks, fat free	1	0	2	6	2/1
Hot dog, Ball Park, franks	1	0	2	5	2/1
Hot dog, Ball Park, franks, fat free	1	0	2	4	2/0
Hot dog, Ball Park, franks, lite	1	0	1	3	1/0
Hot dog, Farmer John, beef franks	1	0	0	2	0/0
Hot dog, Farmer John, wieners	1	0	0	0	0/0
Hot dog, Hebrew National, beef franks	1	0	0	1	0/0
Hot dog, Hebrew National, beef franks, quarter pound	1	0	0	3	0/0
Hot dog, Hebrew National, cocktail beef franks	5	0	0	1	0/0

MEATS, cont'd.

FOOD	Svg Size	Fbr	Sgr	Cbs	S/C Val
Hot dog, Hormel Wranglers, beef	1	0	1	1	1/0
Hot dog, Hormel Wranglers, original	1	0	1	1	1/0
Hot dog, Johnsonville, beef, stadium style	1	0	0	2	0/0
Hot dog, Oscar Mayer, beef franks	1	0	0	1	0/0
Hot dog, Oscar Mayer, beef franks, bun length	1	0	0	1	0/0
Hot dog, Oscar Mayer, beef franks, light	1	0	0	2	0/0
Hot dog, Oscar Mayer, wieners	1	0	0	0	0/0
Jerky, beef	1 oz	1	3	3	3/0
Jerky, Jack Link's, beef, original	1 oz	1	3	3	3/0
Jerky, Jack Link's, beef, peppered	1 oz	0	3	4	3/0
Jerky, Jack Link's, beef, teriyaki	1 oz	0	5	5	5/1
Jerky, Jack Link's, buffalo, original	1 oz	0	3	3	3/0
Jerky, Jack Link's, ham, maple & brown sugar	1 oz	0	6	7	6/1
Jerky, Jack Link's, meat stick, X-Stick original	1 oz	0	1	2	1/0
Jerky, Oberto, beef, original	1 oz	0	4	7	4/1
Jerky, Oberto, beef, peppered	1 oz	0	5	6	5/1
Jerky, Oberto, beef, teriyaki	1 oz	0	5	7	5/1
Jerky, Oberto, meat stick, cocktail pep	2 oz	0	2	4	2/0
Jerky, Oberto, meat stick, pepperoni	2 oz	0	2	6	2/1
Jerky, Oberto, meat stick, teriyaki	2 oz	0	2	6	2/1
Jerky, Pacific Gold, beef, original	1 oz	0	6	9	6/1
Jerky, Pacific Gold, beef, peppered	1 oz	0	6	7	6/1
Jerky, Pacific Gold, beef, teriyaki	1 oz	0	6	7	6/1
Jerky, Slim Jim, beef, original	1 oz	0	0	1	0/0
Jerky, Slim Jim, beef, Tabasco	1 oz	0	4	4	4/0
Jerky, Slim Jim, beef steak, original	1 pkg	0	0	3	0/0
Jerky, Slim Jim, beef steak, peppered	1 pkg	0	11	11	11/1
Jerky, Slim Jim, beef steak, teriyaki	1 pkg	0	11	12	11/1
Jerky, Slim Jim, meat stick, deli, all flavors	1 pkg	0	2	7	2/1
Jerky, Slim Jim, meat stick, giant, most flavors	1 oz	0	0	2	0/0
Jerky, Slim Jim, meat stick, giant, pepperoni	1 oz	0	0	3	0/0
Jerky, Slim Jim, meat stick, original	0.28 oz	0	0	0	0/0
Lamb, most preparations	any	0	0	0	0/0
Mutton, most preparations	any	0	0	0	0/0
Pork, most preparations	any	0	0	0	0/0
Pork, pâté	1 oz	0	1	1	1/0
Pork, pâté, en croute	1 oz	0	0	3	0/0
Rabbit, most preparations	any	0	0	0	0/0
Sausage, Farmer John, chorizo	2.5 oz	0	0	2	0/0
Sausage, Farmer John, links, original	3	0	0	1	0/0
Sausage, Farmer John, links, pork	2	0	0	0	0/0
Sausage, Farmer John, links, pork, maple	2	0	2	2	2/0
Sausage, Farmer John, liverwurst	2 oz	0	0	3	0/0
Sausage, Farmer John, patty, original	1	0	0	1	0/0

MEATS, cont'd.

FOOD	Svg Size	Fbr	Sgr	Cbs	S/C Val
Sausage, Hebrew National, Polish, beef	1	0	1	1	1/0
Sausage, Hebrew National, Polish, knockwurst	1	0	0	2	0/0
Sausage, Hillshire Farm, bratwurst, smoked	1	1	1	4	1/0
Sausage, Hillshire Farm, cocktail, Lit'l Beef Franks	6	0	1	2	1/0
Sausage, Hillshire Farm, cocktail, Lit'l Polskas	5	0	1	2	1/0
Sausage, Hillshire Farm, cocktail, Lit'l Smokies	5	0	1	2	1/0
Sausage, Hillshire Farm, cocktail, Lit'l Smokies, beef	5	0	1	2	1/0
Sausage, Hillshire Farm, cocktail, Lit'l Wieners	6	0	1	3	1/0
Sausage, Hillshire Farm, hot links	1	1	2	4	2/0
Sausage, Hillshire Farm, hot links, beef	1	1	2	3	2/0
Sausage, Hillshire Farm, Polska kielbasa	2 oz	0	1	3	1/0
Sausage, Hillshire Farm, Polska kielbasa, beef	2 oz	0	1	3	1/0
Sausage, Hillshire Farm, Polska kielbasa, lite	2 oz	0	0	0	0/0
Sausage, Hillshire Farm, smoked	2 oz	0	1	3	1/0
Sausage, Hillshire Farm, smoked, beef	2 oz	1	1	3	1/0
Sausage, Hillshire Farm, smoked, lite	2 oz	0	0	0	0/0
Sausage, Hormel, Little Sizzlers, pork, maple	3 pcs	0	2	2	2/0
Sausage, Hormel, Little Sizzlers, pork, original	3 pcs	0	0	0	0/0
Sausage, Jimmy Dean, links, maple	3	0	2	3	2/0
Sausage, Jimmy Dean, links, original	3	0	1	1	1/0
Sausage, Jimmy Dean, patties, maple	2	0	2	2	2/0
Sausage, Jimmy Dean, patties, original	2	0	0	1	0/0
Sausage, Jimmy Dean, roll, pork, hot	2 oz	0	0	1	0/0
Sausage, Jimmy Dean, roll, pork, maple	2 oz	0	1	1	1/0
Sausage, Jimmy Dean, roll, pork, reduced fat	2 oz	0	0	1	0/0
Sausage, Jimmy Dean, Fully Cooked, maple, links	3	0	2	2	2/0
Sausage, Jimmy Dean, Fully Cooked, maple, patties	2	0	3	3	3/0
Sausage, Jimmy Dean, Fully Cooked, original, sandwich size patties	1	0	0	0	0/0
Sausage, Jimmy Dean, Heat 'n Serve, links, maple	3	0	3	4	3/0
Sausage, Jimmy Dean, Heat 'n Serve, links, regular	3	0	1	1	1/0
Sausage, Johnsonville, bratwurst	1	0	1	2	1/0
Sausage, Johnsonville, bratwurst, beef	1	0	0	3	0/0
Sausage, Johnsonville, breakfast links, brown sugar & honey	3	0	4	4	4/0
Sausage, Johnsonville, breakfast links, original	3	0	0	2	0/0
Sausage, Johnsonville, breakfast links, Vermont maple	3	0	0	2	0/0
Sausage, Johnsonville, Italian, sweet	1	0	2	3	2/0
Sausage, Johnsonville, Polish	1	0	1	3	1/0
Sausage, Oberto, beef, summer	2 oz	0	1	2	1/0
Sausage, Oscar Mayer, precooked	0.5 oz	0	0	0	0/0
Sausage, Oscar Mayer, smoked, uncured	0.5 oz	0	1	0	1/0
Sausage, Vienna	1 oz	0	0	1	0/0
Sausage, Vienna, Armour, lite	2 oz	0	1	1	1/0
Sausage, Vienna, Armour, original	2 oz	0	0	2	0/0
Sausage, Vienna, Libby's	3 pcs	0	0	1	0/0

MEATS, cont'd.

FOOD	Svg Size	Fbr	Sgr	Cbs	S/C Val
Spam, lite	2 oz	0	0	1	0/0
Spam, original	2 oz	0	0	1	0/0
Spam, spread	2 oz	0	1	1	1/0
Steak, most preparations	any	0	0	0	0/0
Veal, most preparations	any	0	0	0	0/0
Venison, most preparations	any	0	0	0	0/0

SEAFOOD

FOOD	Svg Size	Fbr	Sgr	Cbs	S/C Val
Abalone	3 oz	0	0	5	0/1
Abalone, fried	3 oz	0	0	9	0/1
Ahi, most preparations	any	0	0	0	0/0
Anchovies, canned, most varieties	any	0	0	0	0/0
Arctic char, most preparations	any	0	0	0	0/0
Barramundi, most preparations	any	0	0	0	0/0
Bass, most preparations	any	0	0	0	0/0
Catfish, most preparations	any	0	0	0	0/0
Caviar, black or red	1 T	0	0	1	0/0
Clams, canned, Bumble Bee, chopped	¼ c	0	0	2	0/0
Clams, canned, Bumble Bee, minced	¼ c	0	0	2	0/0
Clams, canned, Bumble Bee, smoked	¼ c	0	0	1	0/0
Clams, canned, Bumble Bee, whole baby	¼ c	0	0	2	0/0
Clams, canned, Chicken of the Sea, chopped	¼ c	0	0	2	0/0
Clams, canned, Chicken of the Sea, minced	¼ c	0	1	2	1/0
Clams, canned, Chicken of the Sea, whole baby	¼ c	0	0	1	0/0
Clams, cooked, small	10	0	0	5	0/1
Clams, raw	½ c	0	0	3	0/0
Cod, most preparations	any	0	0	0	0/0
Crab, blue, average	1	0	0	0	0/0
Crab, Dungeness, average	1	0	0	1	0/0
Crab, king, average leg	1	0	0	0	0/0
Crab, queen, average	1	0	0	0	0/0
Crab, canned, Bumble Bee	2 oz	0	0	0	0/0
Crab, canned, Chicken of the Sea	2 oz	0	1	1	1/0
Eel, most preparations	any	0	0	0	0/0
Fish, most species, most preparations	any	0	0	0	0/0
Flounder, most preparations	any	0	0	0	0/0
Grouper, most preparations	any	0	0	0	0/0
Halibut, most preparations	any	0	0	0	0/0
Herring, most preparations	any	0	0	0	0/0
Imitation crab (surimi)	3 oz	0	0	6	0/1
Lobster, northern, average	1	0	0	1	0/0
Lobster, spiny, average	1	0	0	5	0/1

FOOD	Svg Size	Fbr	Sgr	Cbs	S/C Val
Mackerel, most preparations	any	0	0	0	0/0
Mackerel, canned, Bumble Bee	¼ c	0	0	0	0/0
Mackerel, canned, Chicken of the Sea, in tomato sauce	¼ c	0	1	2	1/0
Mackerel, canned, Chicken of the Sea, in water	⅓ c	0	0	0	0/0
Mahimahi, most preparations	any	0	0	0	0/0
Mussels	1 c	0	0	6	0/1
Octopus	3 oz	0	0	2	0/0
Orange roughy, most preparations	any	0	0	0	0/0
Oysters, eastern, farmed, medium size	6	0	0	5	0/1
Oysters, eastern, wild, medium size	6	0	0	3	0/0
Oysters, Pacific, medium size	2	0	0	5	0/1
Oysters, canned, Bumble Bee, smoked	¼ c	0	0	6	0/1
Oysters, canned, Bumble Bee, whole	¼ c	0	0	3	0/0
Oysters, canned, Chicken of the Sea	2 oz	0	0	6	0/1
Pollock, most preparations	any	0	0	0	0/0
Roe, fish	4 T	0	0	1	0/0
Salmon, most preparations	any	0	0	0	0/0
Salmon, canned, Bumble Bee, all varieties	1 can	0	0	0	0/0
Salmon, canned, Chicken of the Sea, all varieties	1 can	0	0	0	0/0
Salmon, pâté	2.25 oz	0	1	6	1/1
Salmon, smoked (lox)	any	0	0	0	0/0
Salmon, smoked, Chicken of the Sea, pouch	3 oz	0	1	1	1/0
Sardines, most preparations	any	0	0	0	0/0
Sardines, canned, Bumble Bee, in mustard	3.75 oz	1	1	2	1/0
Sardines, canned, Bumble Bee, in oil or water	3.75 oz	0	0	0	0/0
Sardines, canned, Chicken of the Sea, in oil, smoked	3.75 oz	0	0	2	0/0
Sardines, canned, Chicken of the Sea, in tomato sauce	3.75 oz	2	2	2	2/0
Sardines, canned, Chicken of the Sea, in water	3.75 oz	0	0	2	0/0
Scallops, bay & sea	3 oz	0	0	0	0/0
Scallops, mixed species	3 oz	0	0	2	0/0
Sea bass, most preparations	any	0	0	0	0/0
Sea urchin (uni)	1 oz	0	0	3	0/0
Shark, most preparations	any	0	0	0	0/0
Shrimp	3 oz	0	0	1	0/0
Shrimp, canned, Bumble Bee	2 oz	0	1	0	1/0
Shrimp, canned, Chicken of the Sea	2 oz	0	1	1	1/0
Shrimp, pâté	2.25 oz	0	1	7	1/1
Snapper, most preparations	any	0	0	0	0/0
Sole, most preparations	any	0	0	0	0/0
Squid, fried (calamari)	3 oz	0	0	7	0/1
Squid, raw	3 oz	0	0	3	0/0
Swordfish, most preparations	any	0	0	0	0/0
Tilapia, most preparations	any	0	0	0	0/0
Trout, most preparations	any	0	0	0	0/0

FOOD	Svg Size	Fbr	Sgr	Cbs	S/C Val
Tuna, most preparations	any	0	0	0	0/0
Tuna, canned in oil or water	1 can	0	0	0	0/0
Tuna, canned, Bumble Bee, all varieties	1 can	0	0	0	0/0
Tuna, canned, Chicken of the Sea, all varieties	1 can	0	0	0	0/0
Yellowtail, most preparations	any	0	0	0	0/0

FROZEN SEAFOOD

FOOD	Svg Size	Fbr	Sgr	Cbs	S/C Val
Crab, Fisher Boy, cake	1	1	3	16	3/1
Crab, Mrs. Paul's, deviled cake	1	3	0	12	0/1
Crab, Phillips, crab & spinach dip	2 T	0	1	1	1/0
Crab, Phillips, Maryland style cake	1	0	0	6	0/1
Crab, Phillips, Maryland style cakes, minis	4	0	0	6	0/1
Crab, SeaPack, Maryland style cake, w/ 1 oz sauce	1	1	3	19	3/1
Fish, Fisher Boy, fillet, battered	1	0	1	16	1/1
Fish, Fisher Boy, sticks	6	2	2	24	2/2
Fish, Gorton's, fillet, classic grilled salmon	1	0	1	2	1/0
Fish, Gorton's, fillet, crispy battered	2	3	3	22	3/2
Fish, Gorton's, fillet, crunchy breaded	2	0	3	23	3/2
Fish, Gorton's, fillet, grilled, most flavors	1	0	0	1	0/0
Fish, Gorton's, fillet, potato crunch	2	2	3	20	3/1
Fish, Gorton's, fillet, tilapia	1	1	1	23	1/2
Fish, Gorton's, sticks, crunchy breaded	6	1	3	20	3/1
Fish, Gorton's, tenders, beer batter	3	2	4	18	4/1
Fish, Gorton's, tenders, original batter	3	2	3	23	3/2
Fish, Mrs. Paul's, fillet, beer battered	2	1	4	23	4/2
Fish, Mrs. Paul's, fillet, crunchy fish	2	0	3	23	3/2
Fish, Mrs. Paul's, fillet, lightly breaded haddock	1	1	4	17	4/1
Fish, Mrs. Paul's, fillet, lightly breaded tilapia	1	0	0	17	0/1
Fish, Mrs. Paul's, popcorn, golden breading	4 oz	2	5	18	5/1
Fish, Mrs. Paul's, sticks, crunchy fish	6	0	2	22	2/2
Fish, Phillips, coconut mahi mahi	3	1	11	31	11/2
Fish, Phillips, salmon cake	1	3	1	3	1/0
Fish, SeaPack, salmon burger	1	0	0	1	0/0
Fish, SeaPack, salmon nuggets	4	1	1	19	1/1
Fish, Van de Kamp's, fillet, beer battered	2	0	0	18	0/1
Fish, Van de Kamp's, fillet, breaded fish, Healthy Selects	2	0	0	24	0/2
Fish, Van de Kamp's, fillet, crispy fish	2	0	2	23	2/2
Fish, Van de Kamp's, fillet, crispy haddock	2	0	1	22	1/2
Fish, Van de Kamp's, fillet, crispy halibut	3	0	2	24	2/2
Fish, Van de Kamp's, fillet, crunchy fish	2	0	0	20	0/1
Fish, Van de Kamp's, popcorn, crunchy	8	0	1	25	1/2
Fish, Van de Kamp's, sticks, crunchy	6	0	0	20	0/1
Fish, Van de Kamp's, sticks, crunchy, Healthy Selects	6	0	4	26	4/2
Fish, Van de Kamp's, sticks, crunchy, xtra large	4	0	0	18	0/1
Fish, Van de Kamp's, tenders, crispy	3	0	1	21	1/2

SEAFOOD, cont'd.

FOOD	Svg Size	Fbr	Sgr	Cbs	S/C Val
Scallops, Mrs. Paul's, fried	13	0	3	28	3/2
Shrimp, Fisher Boy, Crunchers, coconut	16	1	4	21	4/2
Shrimp, Fisher Boy, Poppers	3 oz	2	1	25	1/2
Shrimp, Gorton's, beer batter	5	0	2	25	2/2
Shrimp, Gorton's, butterfly	5	4	4	27	4/2
Shrimp, Gorton's, grilled, classic	8	0	1	5	1/1
Shrimp, Gorton's, grilled, scampi	8	0	1	3	1/0
Shrimp, Gorton's, popcorn, crunchy golden breaded	22	0	3	26	3/2
Shrimp, Gorton's, scampi	4 oz	0	0	8	0/1
Shrimp, Phillips, breaded	5	2	3	20	3/1
Shrimp, Phillips, Buffalo	5	2	7	26	7/2
Shrimp, Phillips, coconut	5	1	8	27	8/2
Shrimp, Phillips, honey chipotle	8	0	3	5	3/1
Shrimp, Phillips, steamed spiced	8	0	0	2	0/0
Shrimp, SeaPack, butterfly	7	0	2	20	2/1
Shrimp, SeaPack, coconut, w/ sauce	4	1	19	36	19/2
Shrimp, SeaPack, popcorn	15	1	2	20	2/1
Shrimp, SeaPack, scampi	6	0	1	4	1/0
Shrimp, SeaPack, tempura, w/ sauce	4	7	13	35	13/2
Shrimp, Van de Kamp's, butterfly	7	1	2	31	2/2

MEAT ALTERNATIVES

FOOD	Svg Size	Fbr	Sgr	Cbs	S/C Val
"Beef," Boca, ground crumbles	2 oz	3	0	6	0/1
"Beef," Boca, ground crumbles, w/ all natural ingredients	2 oz	3	0	6	0/1
"Beef," El Burrito, NeatLoaf	2 oz	3	1	8	1/1
"Beef," El Burrito, SoyLoaf	2 oz	3	1	8	1/1
"Beef," El Burrito, SoySteak	1	5	3	49	3/3
"Beef," El Burrito, SoyTaco	1 oz	2	0	3	0/0
"Beef," Lightlife, Gimme Lean, ground beef style	2 oz	2	1	10	1/1
"Beef," Lightlife, Smart Ground, veggie protein crumbles, Mexican style	⅓ c	3	1	7	1/1
"Beef," Lightlife, Smart Ground, veggie protein crumbles, original	⅓ c	3	0	6	0/1
"Beef," Lightlife, Smart Strips, steak style strips	3 oz	5	0	6	0/1
"Beef," Morningstar Farms, Meal Starters, Grillers Recipe Crumbles	⅔ c	3	0	5	0/1
"Beef," Yves, classic veggie meatballs	4	2	0	8	0/1
"Beef," Yves, meatless beef strips, Heart's Desire	3 oz	1	0	4	0/0
"Beef," Yves, meatless ground	⅓ c	2	1	5	1/1
"Beef," Yves, meatless ground, lettuce wraps	⅓ c	2	4	8	4/1
"Beef," Yves, meatless taco stuffers	⅓ c	2	1	5	1/1
Burger patty, Amy's, all American burger	1	4	2	12	2/1
Burger patty, Amy's, bistro burger	1	2	1	16	1/1
Burger patty, Amy's, California veggie burger	1	4	2	21	2/2
Burger patty, Amy's, California veggie burger, light in sodium	1	3	1	16	1/1
Burger patty, Amy's, cheddar veggie burger	1	3	2	16	2/1

MEAT ALTERNATIVES, cont'd.

FOOD	Svg Size	Fbr	Sgr	Cbs	S/C Val
Burger patty, Amy's, quarter pound veggie burger	1	6	5	23	5/2
Burger patty, Amy's, Texas veggie burger	1	3	2	14	2/1
Burger patty, Boca, all American flame grilled	1	5	0	6	0/1
Burger patty, Boca, all American w/ organic soy	1	4	1	9	1/1
Burger patty, Boca, bruschetta	1	5	0	9	0/1
Burger patty, Boca, cheeseburger	1	4	1	6	1/1
Burger patty, Boca, grilled vegetable	1	4	1	7	1/1
Burger patty, Boca, original vegan	1	4	0	6	0/1
Burger patty, Boca, original vegan, big burgers, family pack	1	6	1	8	1/1
Burger patty, Boca, savory mushroom mozzarella	1	4	0	8	0/1
Burger patty, Boca, vegan w/ organic soy	1	4	1	9	1/1
Burger patty, Follow Your Heart, Heart Smart Burger	1	16	1	3	1/0
Burger patty, Gardenburger, black bean chipotle	1	5	1	16	1/1
Burger patty, Gardenburger, California burger	1	3	1	15	1/1
Burger patty, Gardenburger, garden vegan	1	4	0	12	0/1
Burger patty, Gardenburger, original	1	5	0	18	0/1
Burger patty, Gardenburger, portabella	1	5	0	17	0/1
Burger patty, Gardenburger, sun-dried tomato basil	1	4	2	17	2/1
Burger patty, Gardenburger, veggie medley	1	5	1	17	1/1
Burger patty, Lightlife, Light Burgers, mushroom	1	3	1	13	1/1
Burger patty, Lightlife, Light Burgers, original	1	3	0	12	0/1
Burger patty, Lightlife, Light Burgers, veggie	1	4	2	16	2/1
Burger patty, Morningstar Farms, Asian veggie patties	1	2	3	10	3/1
Burger patty, Morningstar Farms, chipotle black bean burger	1	7	2	24	2/2
Burger patty, Morningstar Farms, garden veggie patties	1	3	1	9	1/1
Burger patty, Morningstar Farms, Grillers California turk'y	1	5	0	7	0/1
Burger patty, Morningstar Farms, Grillers original	1	2	0	5	0/1
Burger patty, Morningstar Farms, Grillers Prime	1	2	0	4	0/0
Burger patty, Morningstar Farms, Grillers ¼ pound burger	1	3	0	10	0/1
Burger patty, Morningstar Farms, Grillers vegan	1	4	0	7	0/1
Burger patty, Morningstar Farms, mushroom lover's burger	1	0	1	8	1/1
Burger patty, Morningstar Farms, spicy black bean burger	1	4	2	13	2/1
Burger patty, Morningstar Farms, tomato & basil pizza burger	1	3	2	7	2/1
Burger patty, Yves, meatless beef burger	1	2	0	8	0/1
Burger patty, Yves, meatless chicken burger	1	2	0	5	0/1
"Chicken," Boca, original Chik'n nuggets	¼ pkg	3	2	17	2/1
"Chicken," Boca, original Chik'n nuggets, w/ all natural ingredients	¼ pkg	3	2	17	2/1
"Chicken," Boca, original Chik'n patty	1	2	1	15	1/1
"Chicken," Boca, original Chik'n patty, w/ all natural ingredients	1	2	1	15	1/1
"Chicken," Follow Your Heart, Chicken-Free Chicken	2 oz	0	1	5	1/1
"Chicken," Lightlife, Smart Strips, Chick'n style strips	3 oz	4	0	6	0/1
"Chicken," Lightlife, Smart Tenders, lemon pepper	3 pcs	4	0	8	0/1
"Chicken," Lightlife, Smart Tenders, savory Chick'n	3 pcs	0	3	7	3/1
"Chicken," Lightlife, Smart Wings, Buffalo	4 pcs	4	0	6	0/1

FOOD	Svg Size	Fbr	Sgr	Cbs	S/C Val
"Chicken," Lightlife, Smart Wings, honey BBQ	4 pcs	4	9	16	9/1
"Chicken," Morningstar Farms, Buffalo wings	5 pcs	3	2	20	2/1
"Chicken," Morningstar Farms, Chik Patties, Italian herb	1	2	1	22	1/2
"Chicken," Morningstar Farms, Chik Patties, original	1	2	1	16	1/1
"Chicken," Morningstar Farms, Chik'n nuggets	4 pcs	4	2	19	2/1
"Chicken," Morningstar Farms, Chik'n tenders, original	2 pcs	3	1	20	1/1
"Chicken," Morningstar Farms, Grillers Chik'n	1	5	0	7	0/1
"Chicken," Morningstar Farms, Meal Starters, Chik'n strips	12 pcs	1	1	6	1/1
"Chicken," Morningstar Farms, Meal Starters, Chik'n strips, vegan	12 pcs	1	1	6	1/1
"Chicken," Yves, curry flavor vindaloo sauce veggie breast	½ pkg	3	4	13	4/1
"Chicken," Yves, lemon herb chicken skewers	1	4	2	7	2/1
"Chicken," Yves, meatless chicken strips, Heart's Desire	3 oz	0	1	3	1/0
Deli "meat," Lightlife, Smart Deli, baked ham style	4 pcs	0	2	3	2/0
Deli "meat," Lightlife, Smart Deli, bologna style	4 pcs	0	1	4	1/0
Deli "meat," Lightlife, Smart Deli, pepperoni style	13 pcs	1	0	2	0/0
Deli "meat," Lightlife, Smart Deli, roast turkey style	4 pcs	2	0	5	0/1
Deli "meat," Tofurky, cranberry & stuffing	5 pcs	3	2	8	2/1
Deli "meat," Tofurky, hickory smoked	5 pcs	3	1	6	1/1
Deli "meat," Tofurky, Italian deli	5 pcs	4	2	7	2/1
Deli "meat," Tofurky, oven roasted	5 pcs	3	1	6	1/1
Deli "meat," Tofurky, peppered	5 pcs	3	1	6	1/1
Deli "meat," Tofurky, "Philly style" steak	5 pcs	3	0	7	0/1
Deli "meat," Yves, meatless deli bologna	4 pcs	0	0	2	0/0
Deli "meat," Yves, meatless deli salami	4 pcs	0	0	4	0/0
Deli "meat," Yves, meatless deli turkey	4 pcs	0	0	5	0/1
Deli "meat," Yves, meatless ham	4 pcs	0	0	5	0/1
Deli "meat," Yves, meatless pepperoni	6 pcs	0	0	4	0/0
Deli "meat," Yves, Meatless Roast Without the Beef	4 pcs	1	1	4	1/0
Deli "meat," Yves, meatless smoked chicken	4 pcs	0	1	5	1/1
Hot dog, Lightlife, Smart Dogs, veggie protein link	1	1	1	2	1/0
Hot dog, Lightlife, Smart Dogs, veggie protein link, jumbo	1	2	1	3	1/0
Hot dog, Lightlife, Tofu Pups	1	1	0	2	0/0
Hot dog, Tofurky, chipotle franks	1	1	1	3	1/0
Hot dog, Tofurky, franks	1	3	1	5	1/1
Hot dog, Yves, the good dog	1	0	0	1	0/0
Hot dog, Yves, meatless hot dog	1	0	0	2	0/0
Hot dog, Yves, meatless jumbo dog	1	0	2	5	2/1
Hot dog, Yves, tofu dog	1	0	0	2	0/0
Hot dog, Yves, Veggie Brats, classic	1	1	2	9	2/1
Hot dog, Yves, Veggie Brats, zesty Italian	1	2	2	9	2/1
Jerky, Primal Strips, hickory smoked	1 pkg	1	3	8	3/1
Jerky, Primal Strips, hot & spicy	1 pkg	6	3	12	3/1
Jerky, Primal Strips, mesquite lime	1 pkg	0	4	7	4/1
Jerky, Primal Strips, teriyaki	1 pkg	1	3	7	3/1

FOOD	Svg Size	Fbr	Sgr	Cbs	S/C Val
Jerky, Primal Strips, Texas BBQ	1 pkg	1	5	11	5/1
Jerky, Primal Strips, Thai peanut	1 pkg	1	4	8	4/1
Jerky, Tofurky, original jurky	4 pcs	1	3	9	3/1
Jerky, Tofurky, peppered jurky	4 pcs	1	3	9	3/1
"Pork," Lightlife, Smart Bacon, bacon style strips	1 pc	0	0	0	0/0
"Pork," Morningstar Farms, bacon strips	2 pcs	1	0	2	0/0
"Pork," Morningstar Farms, hickory BBQ riblets	1	5	24	35	24/2
"Pork," Yves, meatless Canadian bacon	3 pcs	0	0	2	0/0
Sausage, Boca, breakfast links	2 pcs	2	2	5	2/1
Sausage, El Burrito, Soy Breakfast Sausage roll	1 oz	2	0	3	0/0
Sausage, El Burrito, SoyKnox	1 pc	0	4	0	4/0
Sausage, El Burrito, SoyRizo	1.75 oz	0	2	0	2/0
Sausage, El Burrito, Soy Sausage, Santa Fe	1 pc	1	0	2	0/0
Sausage, El Burrito, Soy Sausage, soy chicken	1 pc	0	4	4	4/0
Sausage, El Burrito, Soy Sausage, soy kielbasa	1 pc	0	1	2	1/0
Sausage, El Burrito, Soy Sausage, sundried tomato & basil	1 pc	0	1	3	1/0
Sausage, Lightlife, Gimme Lean, ground sausage style	2 oz	3	0	7	0/1
Sausage, Lightlife, Smart Links, breakfast sausage style	2 pcs	3	0	8	0/1
Sausage, Lightlife, Smart Sausages, chorizo style	1 pc	0	0	5	0/1
Sausage, Lightlife, Smart Sausages, Italian style	1 pc	1	0	7	0/1
Sausage, Lightlife, Smart Sausages, smoked style	1 pc	2	3	9	3/1
Sausage, Morningstar Farms, breakfast patty	1	1	0	4	0/0
Sausage, Morningstar Farms, hot & spicy sausage patty	1	1	0	3	0/0
Sausage, Morningstar Farms, Italian sausage link	1	1	0	7	0/1
Sausage, Morningstar Farms, maple flavored sausage patty	1	0	2	5	2/1
Sausage, Morningstar Farms, sausage-style recipe crumbles	2/3 c	3	0	5	0/1
Sausage, Morningstar Farms, veggie sausage link	1	2	0	3	0/0
Sausage, Morningstar Farms, veggie sausage patty	1	1	0	3	0/0
Sausage, Tofurky, beer brat	1	5	2	8	2/1
Sausage, Tofurky, breakfast link	1	2	1	6	1/1
Sausage, Tofurky, Italian sausage	1	8	2	12	2/1
Sausage, Tofurky, kielbasa	1	8	2	12	2/1
Sausage, Yves, meatless breakfast patties	2	2	1	4	1/0
Sausage, Yves, veggie chorizo	1/3 pc	2	0	6	0/1
Seitan, White Wave, chicken style	1 pc	2	1	4	1/0
Seitan, White Wave, traditional	3 oz	1	0	3	0/0
Seitan, White Wave, vegetarian stir-fry strips	3 oz	1	0	2	0/0
Tempeh, Lightlife, fakin' bacon, organic	3 slcs	4	2	10	2/1
Tempeh, Lightlife, flax, organic	½ pkg	11	0	16	0/1
Tempeh, Lightlife, garden veggie, organic	½ pkg	10	1	17	1/1
Tempeh, Lightlife, soy, organic	½ pkg	12	0	16	0/1
Tempeh, Lightlife, three grain, organic	½ pkg	9	0	16	0/1
Tempeh, Lightlife, wild rice, organic	½ pkg	11	1	12	1/1
Tempeh, Tofurky, five grain, organic	3 oz	6	0	20	0/1

MEAT ALTERNATIVES, cont'd.

FOOD	Svg Size	Fbr	Sgr	Cbs	S/C Val
Tempeh, Tofurky, soy, organic	3 oz	7	0	20	0/1
Tempeh, Tofurky, spicy veggie	3 oz	7	0	20	0/1
Tempeh, marinated, Lightlife Tempehtations, classic BBQ	3 oz	5	10	17	10/1
Tempeh, marinated, Lightlife Tempehtations, ginger teriyaki	3 oz	5	9	18	9/1
Tempeh, marinated, Lightlife Tempehtations, zesty lemon	3 oz	6	1	10	1/1
Tempeh, marinated, Tofurky, coconut curry	6 pcs	5	8	13	8/1
Tempeh, marinated, Tofurky, lemon pepper	6 pcs	7	2	15	2/1
Tempeh, marinated, Tofurky, sesame garlic	6 pcs	3	2	5	2/1
Tempeh, marinated, Tofurky, smoky maple bacon	7 pcs	5	3	17	3/1
Tofu, House Foods, extra firm	3 oz	0	0	1	0/0
Tofu, House Foods, extra firm, organic	3 oz	0	0	0	0/0
Tofu, House Foods, extra soft	3 oz	0	1	2	1/0
Tofu, House Foods, firm	3 oz	0	0	2	0/0
Tofu, House Foods, firm, organic	3 oz	0	0	0	0/0
Tofu, House Foods, medium firm	3 oz	0	0	1	0/0
Tofu, House Foods, medium firm, organic	3 oz	0	0	1	0/0
Tofu, House Foods, soft	3 oz	0	0	2	0/0
Tofu, House Foods, soft, organic	3 oz	0	0	0	0/0
Tofu, Nasoya, extra firm	⅕ pkg	0	1	2	1/0
Tofu, Nasoya, firm	⅕ pkg	0	0	2	0/0
Tofu, Nasoya, firm, lite	⅕ pkg	0	0	1	0/0
Tofu, Nasoya, silken	⅕ pkg	0	0	1	0/0
Tofu, Nasoya, silken, lite	⅕ pkg	0	0	0	0/0
Tofu, Nasoya, soft	⅕ pkg	0	0	1	0/0
Tofu, Woodstock Farms, extra firm, organic	3 oz	0	0	0	0/0
Tofu, Woodstock Farms, firm, organic	3 oz	0	0	1	0/0
"Turkey," Tofurky, roast & gravy	⅕ pkg	3	1	13	1/1
"Turkey," Yves, meatless ground turkey	⅓ c	2	0	4	0/0

DAIRY & DAIRY ALTERNATIVES

FOOD	Svg Size	Fbr	Sgr	Cbs	S/C Val
Almond milk, refrigerated, chocolate, Almond Breeze	1 c	1	20	22	20/2
Almond milk, refrigerated, original, Almond Breeze	1 c	1	7	8	7/1
Almond milk, refrigerated, original, Silk Pure Almond	1 c	1	7	8	7/1
Almond milk, refrigerated, vanilla, Almond Breeze	1 c	1	15	16	15/1
Almond milk, refrigerated, vanilla, Silk Pure Almond	1 c	1	15	16	15/1
Almond milk, refrigerated, vanilla, unsweetened, Almond Breeze	1 c	1	0	2	0/0
Almond milk, shelf stable, chocolate, Almond Breeze	1 c	1	20	22	20/2
Almond milk, shelf stable, chocolate, unsweetened, Almond Breeze	1 c	1	0	3	0/0
Almond milk, shelf stable, original, Almond Breeze	1 c	1	7	8	7/1
Almond milk, shelf stable, original, Almond Dream	1 c	0	5	6	5/1
Almond milk, shelf stable, original, Pacific Natural Foods	1 c	0	6	8	6/1
Almond milk, shelf stable, original, unsweetened, Almond Breeze	1 c	1	0	2	0/0
Almond milk, shelf stable, original, unsweetened, Almond Dream	1 c	0	0	1	0/0

FOOD	Svg Size	Fbr	Sgr	Cbs	S/C Val
Almond milk, shelf stable, original, unsweetened, Pacific Natural Foods	1 c	0	0	2	0/0
Almond milk, shelf stable, vanilla, Almond Breeze	1 c	1	15	16	15/1
Almond milk, shelf stable, vanilla, Pacific Natural Foods	1 c	0	9	11	9/1
Almond milk, shelf stable, vanilla, unsweetened, Almond Breeze	1 c	1	0	2	0/0
Almond milk, shelf stable, vanilla, unsweetened, Pacific Natural Foods	1 c	0	0	3	0/0
Butter	1 c	0	0	0	0/0
Buttermilk	1 c	0	13	13	13/1
Buttermilk, Alta Dena	1 c	0	14	14	14/1
Buttermilk, light, Friendship	1 c	0	12	12	12/1
Cheese, American	1 oz	0	0	1	0/0
Cheese, blue	1 oz	0	0	1	0/0
Cheese, Brie	1 oz	0	0	0	0/0
Cheese, Camembert	1 oz	0	0	0	0/0
Cheese, cheddar	1 oz	0	0	0	0/0
Cheese, Colby	1 oz	0	0	1	0/0
Cheese, Edam	1 oz	0	0	0	0/0
Cheese, feta	1 oz	0	1	1	1/0
Cheese, fontina	1 oz	0	0	0	0/0
Cheese, goat, hard	1 oz	0	1	1	1/0
Cheese, goat, soft	1 oz	0	0	0	0/0
Cheese, Gouda	1 oz	0	1	1	1/0
Cheese, Gruyère	1 oz	0	0	0	0/0
Cheese, Limburger	1 oz	0	0	0	0/0
Cheese, Monterey Jack	1 oz	0	0	0	0/0
Cheese, mozzarella	1 oz	0	0	1	0/0
Cheese, mozzarella, string	1 oz	0	0	1	0/0
Cheese, Muenster	1 oz	0	0	0	0/0
Cheese, Neufchâtel	1 oz	0	1	1	1/0
Cheese, Parmesan	1 oz	0	0	1	0/0
Cheese, provolone	1 oz	0	0	1	0/0
Cheese, queso añejo	1 oz	0	1	1	1/0
Cheese, queso asadero	1 oz	0	1	1	1/0
Cheese, queso fresco	1 oz	0	0	0	0/0
Cheese, ricotta	1 oz	0	0	1	0/0
Cheese, Romano	1 oz	0	0	1	0/0
Cheese, Swiss	1 oz	0	0	2	0/0
Cheese, Frigo Cheese Heads, string, mozzarella	1 pc	0	0	1	0/0
Cheese, Kraft Singles, American	1 slc	0	1	2	1/0
Cheese, Kraft Singles, American, fat free	1 slc	0	1	2	1/0
Cheese, Kraft Singles, pepperjack, 2% milk	1 slc	0	0	2	0/0
Cheese, Kraft Singles, sharp cheddar	1 slc	0	1	2	1/0
Cheese, Kraft Singles, sharp cheddar, fat free	1 slc	0	1	2	1/0
Cheese, Kraft Singles, sharp cheddar, 2% milk	1 slc	0	1	1	1/0
Cheese, Kraft Singles, Swiss, fat free	1 slc	0	1	2	1/0

FOOD	Svg Size	Fbr	Sgr	Cbs	S/C Val
Cheese, Kraft Singles, Swiss, 2% milk	1 slc	0	1	2	1/0
Cheese, Kraft Singles, white American	1 slc	0	2	2	2/0
Cheese, Kraft Singles, white American, fat free	1 slc	0	1	2	1/0
Cheese, Kraft Singles, white American, 2% milk	1 slc	0	1	2	1/0
Cheese, Kraft, string, mozzarella	1 pc	0	0	1	0/0
Cheese, Sargento, string, mozzarella	1 pc	0	0	1	0/0
Cheese, Sargento, string, mozzarella, light	1 pc	0	0	1	0/0
Cheese, The Laughing Cow, Light Gourmet Cheese Bites	5 pcs	0	1	1	1/0
Cheese, The Laughing Cow, Mini Babybel, all varieties	1 pc	0	0	0	0/0
Cheese, Velveeta, most flavors	1 oz	0	2	3	2/0
Cheese, Velveeta, 2% milk	1 oz	0	2	4	2/0
Cheese, Velveeta slices	1 slc	0	2	2	2/0
Cheese, Velveeta slices, extra thick	1 slc	0	3	3	3/0
Cheese alternative, American, Toffuti	1 slc	0	0	2	0/0
Cheese alternative, cheddar, Daiya, shredded	¼ c	1	0	7	0/1
Cheese alternative, cheddar, Follow Your Heart, Vegan Gourmet	1 oz	2	0	2	0/0
Cheese alternative, cheddar, Teese	1 oz	0	0	5	0/1
Cheese alternative, Monterey Jack, Follow Your Heart, Vegan Gourmet	1 oz	2	0	2	0/0
Cheese alternative, mozzarella, Daiya, shredded	¼ c	1	0	7	0/1
Cheese alternative, mozzarella, Follow Your Heart, Vegan Gourmet	1 oz	1	0	1	0/0
Cheese alternative, mozzarella, Teese	1 oz	0	0	5	0/1
Cheese alternative, mozzarella, Toffuti	1 slc	0	0	2	0/0
Cheese alternative, nacho cheese, Follow Your Heart, Vegan Gourmet	1 oz	2	0	2	0/0
Cheese alternative, nacho cheese, Teese	1 oz	0	0	5	0/1
Cheese curds, Heluva Good!, cheddar	1 oz	0	0	0	0/0
Cheese spread, Alouette, creamy onion & shallot	2 T	0	0	1	0/0
Cheese spread, Alouette, cucumber dill, light	2 T	0	2	2	2/0
Cheese spread, Alouette, garlic & herbs	2 T	0	0	1	0/0
Cheese spread, Alouette, garlic & herbs, light	2 T	0	2	2	2/0
Cheese spread, Alouette, peppercorn parmesan	2 T	0	0	1	0/0
Cheese spread, Alouette, pepper medley	2 T	0	1	3	1/0
Cheese spread, Alouette, savory vegetable	2 T	0	0	1	0/0
Cheese spread, Alouette, spinach artichoke	2 T	0	0	1	0/0
Cheese spread, Alouette, sundried tomato & basil	2 T	0	0	1	0/0
Cheese spread, Alouette, Crème de Brie	2 T	0	0	0	0/0
Cheese spread, Alouette, Crème de Brie, garlic & herbs	2 T	0	0	0	0/0
Cheese spread, Alouette, Elégante, all flavors	2 T	0	1	2	1/0
Cheese spread, Heluva Good!, cheddar & horseradish	2 T	3	3	3	3/0
Cheese spread, Heluva Good!, port wine	2 T	3	3	3	3/0
Cheese spread, Heluva Good!, sharp cheddar	2 T	3	3	3	3/0
Cheese spread, Kaukauna, port wine	2 T	0	3	4	3/0
Cheese spread, Kaukauna, port wine, lite	2 T	0	3	4	3/0
Cheese spread, Kaukauna, sharp cheddar	2 T	0	3	3	3/0
Cheese spread, Kaukauna, sharp cheddar, lite	2 T	0	5	4	5/0

FOOD	Svg Size	Fbr	Sgr	Cbs	S/C Val
Cheese spread, Kraft Bacon	2 T	0	0	1	0/0
Cheese spread, Kraft Cheez Whiz	2 T	0	2	4	2/0
Cheese spread, Kraft Cheez Whiz, light	2 T	0	4	6	4/1
Cheese spread, Kraft Easy Cheese, American	2 T	0	1	2	1/0
Cheese spread, Kraft Easy Cheese, cheddar	2 T	0	1	2	1/0
Cheese spread, Kraft Easy Cheese, cheddar 'n bacon	2 T	0	1	2	1/0
Cheese spread, Kraft Easy Cheese, sharp cheddar	2 T	0	2	2	2/0
Cheese spread, Kraft Old English	2 T	0	0	1	0/0
Cheese spread, Kraft Olive & Pimento	2 T	0	2	3	2/0
Cheese spread, Kraft Pimento	2 T	0	2	3	2/0
Cheese spread, Kraft Pineapple	2 T	0	4	4	4/0
Cheese spread, Kraft Roka Blue	2 T	0	1	2	1/0
Cheese spread, Président, Rondelé, garlic & herbs, light	2 T	0	1	2	1/0
Cheese spread, Président, Rondelé, most flavors	2 T	0	1	1	1/0
Cheese spread, The Laughing Cow, wedges, all flavors	1 pc	0	1	1	1/0
Coconut milk, refrigerated, original, So Delicious	1 c	0	6	7	6/1
Coconut milk, refrigerated, unsweetened, So Delicious	1 c	0	0	1	0/0
Coconut milk, refrigerated, vanilla, So Delicious	1 c	0	7	9	7/1
Cottage cheese	½ c	0	3	3	3/0
Cottage cheese, fat free, Alta Dena	½ c	0	5	5	5/1
Cottage cheese, fat free, Breakstone's	½ c	0	6	8	6/1
Cottage cheese, fat free, Friendship	½ c	0	5	6	5/1
Cottage cheese, 1% fat, Friendship	½ c	0	3	3	3/0
Cottage cheese, 2% fat, Alta Dena	½ c	0	4	4	4/0
Cottage cheese, 2% fat, Breakstone's	½ c	0	4	6	4/1
Cottage cheese, 2% fat, Friendship	½ c	0	2	3	2/0
Cottage cheese, 2% fat, Friendship, digestive health	½ c	3	2	5	2/1
Cottage cheese, 2% fat, Knudsen	½ c	0	4	6	4/1
Cottage cheese, 2% fat, Lactaid	½ c	0	3	7	3/1
Cottage cheese, 4% fat, Alta Dena	½ c	0	3	3	3/0
Cottage cheese, 4% fat, Breakstone's	½ c	0	5	6	5/1
Cottage cheese, 4% fat, Friendship	½ c	0	3	3	3/0
Cream, heavy whipping	½ c	0	0	3	0/0
Cream, light whipping	½ c	0	0	4	0/0
Cream cheese	2 T	0	1	1	1/0
Cream cheese, Philadelphia	2 T	0	1	2	1/0
Cream cheese, Philadelphia, fat free	2 T	0	1	2	1/0
Cream cheese, Philadelphia, garden vegetable	2 T	0	1	2	1/0
Cream cheese, Philadelphia, honey nut	2 T	0	4	4	4/0
Cream cheese, Philadelphia, light	2 T	0	2	2	2/0
Cream cheese, nondairy, Follow Your Heart, Vegan Gourmet	2 T	2	0	3	0/0
Cream cheese, nondairy, Toffuti, Better Than Cream Cheese, all flavors	2 T	0	2	9	2/1
Cream cheese, nondairy, Toffuti, Better Than Cream Cheese, non-hydrogenated	2 T	0	2	13	2/1
Creamer, Coffee-mate, liquid, amaretto	1 T	0	5	1	5/0

FOOD	Svg Size	Fbr	Sgr	Cbs	S/C Val
Creamer, Coffee-mate, liquid, cinnamon bun	1 T	0	5	5	5/1
Creamer, Coffee-mate, liquid, French vanilla	1 T	0	5	5	5/1
Creamer, Coffee-mate, liquid, French vanilla, fat free	4 t	0	6	11	6/1
Creamer, Coffee-mate, liquid, French vanilla, sugar free	1 T	0	0	1	0/0
Creamer, Coffee-mate, liquid, hazelnut	1 T	0	5	5	5/1
Creamer, Coffee-mate, liquid, hazelnut, fat free	1 T	0	4	5	4/1
Creamer, Coffee-mate, liquid, hazelnut, sugar free	1 T	0	0	1	0/0
Creamer, Coffee-mate, liquid, original	1 T	0	1	2	1/0
Creamer, Coffee-mate, liquid, original, fat free	1 T	0	0	2	0/0
Creamer, Coffee-mate, liquid, original, low fat	1 T	0	0	1	0/0
Creamer, Coffee-mate, liquid, vanilla caramel	1 T	0	5	5	5/1
Creamer, Coffee-mate, liquid, vanilla caramel, fat free	1 T	0	5	5	5/1
Creamer, Coffee-mate, liquid, vanilla caramel, sugar free	1 T	0	0	1	0/0
Creamer, Coffee-mate, powder, creamy chocolate	4 t	0	7	9	7/1
Creamer, Coffee-mate, powder, French vanilla	4 t	0	7	9	7/1
Creamer, Coffee-mate, powder, French vanilla, fat free	4 t	0	6	11	6/1
Creamer, Coffee-mate, powder, French vanilla, sugar free	1 T	0	0	2	0/0
Creamer, Coffee-mate, powder, hazelnut	4 t	0	7	9	7/1
Creamer, Coffee-mate, powder, hazelnut, sugar free	1 T	0	0	2	0/0
Creamer, Coffee-mate, powder, original	1 t	0	0	1	0/0
Creamer, Coffee-mate, powder, original, fat free	1 t	0	0	2	0/0
Creamer, Coffee-mate, powder, original, lite	1 t	0	0	2	0/0
Creamer, Coffee-mate, powder, vanilla caramel	4 t	0	7	9	7/1
Creamer, Coffee-mate, powder, vanilla caramel, sugar free	1 T	0	0	2	0/0
Creamer, International Delight, amaretto	1 T	0	6	7	6/1
Creamer, International Delight, French vanilla	1 T	0	6	6	6/1
Creamer, International Delight, French vanilla, fat free	1 T	0	5	7	5/1
Creamer, International Delight, French vanilla, sugar free	1 T	0	0	1	0/0
Creamer, International Delight, hazelnut	1 T	0	5	6	5/1
Creamer, International Delight, hazelnut, sugar free	1 T	0	0	1	0/0
Creamer, International Delight, Irish crème	1 T	0	6	7	6/1
Crème frâiche	2 T	0	0	1	0/0
Crème frâiche, Alouette Cuisine	2 T	0	0	0	0/0
Crème frâiche, Alta Dena	2 T	0	1	1	1/0
Eggnog	½ c	0	20	21	20/2
Eggnog, Alta Dena, holiday	½ c	0	29	29	29/2
Eggnog, Hood, golden	½ c	0	21	22	21/2
Eggnog, Hood, light	½ c	0	21	22	21/2
Eggnog, Lactaid, lactose free	½ c	0	19	20	19/1
Eggnog, Silk, soymilk nog	½ c	0	12	15	12/1
Goat milk	1 c	0	11	11	11/1
Half & half	2 T	0	0	1	0/0
Half & half, Alta Dena	2 T	0	1	1	1/0
Half & half, Horizon Organic	2 T	0	1	1	1/0

FOOD	Svg Size	Fbr	Sgr	Cbs	S/C Val
Half & half, Land O' Lakes, Mini Moo's	1 pkg	0	0	0	0/0
Hazelnut milk, shelf stable, chocolate, Pacific Natural Foods	1 c	1	15	19	15/1
Hazelnut milk, shelf stable, original, Pacific Natural Foods	1 c	1	14	18	14/1
Hemp milk, shelf stable, original, Hemp Dream	1 c	0	6	8	6/1
Hemp milk, shelf stable, original, Living Harvest	1 c	0	6	10	6/1
Hemp milk, shelf stable, original, Pacific Natural Foods	1 c	1	14	20	14/1
Hemp milk, shelf stable, original unsweetened, Living Harvest	1 c	0	0	1	0/0
Hemp milk, shelf stable, vanilla, Hemp Dream	1 c	0	9	11	9/1
Hemp milk, shelf stable, vanilla, Living Harvest	1 c	0	9	12	9/1
Hemp milk, shelf stable, vanilla, Pacific Natural Foods	1 c	1	16	24	16/2
Hemp milk, shelf stable, vanilla unsweetened, Living Harvest	1 c	0	0	1	0/0
Kefir, Alta Dena	2 T	0	2	2	2/0
Kefir, Helios, plain, organic	1 c	2	10	12	10/1
Kefir, Lifeway, Greek style	1 c	0	11	12	11/1
Kefir, Lifeway, original	1 c	3	12	15	12/1
Kefir, Lifeway, plain, lowfat, unsweetened, organic	1 c	3	8	12	8/1
Kefir, Lifeway, plain, nonfat, unsweetened	1 c	3	12	15	12/1
Kefir, Lifeway, plain, whole milk, organic	1 c	3	8	12	8/1
Kefir, Lifeway, Slim6, plain, lowfat	1 c	2	6	8	6/1
Margarine, most varieties	1 T	0	0	0	0/0
Milk	1 c	0	13	12	13/1
Milk, banana, Nesquik, reduced fat	1 c	0	31	32	31/2
Milk, chocolate, Alta Dena, 1% low fat	1 c	0	32	32	32/2
Milk, chocolate, Alta Dena, whole	1 c	1	37	37	37/2
Milk, chocolate, Hood Organic, 1% low fat	1 c	0	27	27	27/2
Milk, chocolate, Hood Simply Smart, fat free	1 c	0	26	28	26/2
Milk, chocolate, Lactaid, 1% low fat	1 c	0	23	24	23/2
Milk, chocolate, Nesquik, fat free	1 c	0	28	29	28/2
Milk, chocolate, Nesquik, low fat	1 c	0	28	29	28/2
Milk, chocolate, Nesquik, low fat, 100 calories, no sugar added	1 c	0	12	13	12/1
Milk, chocolate, Nesquik, reduced fat	1 c	0	28	29	28/2
Milk, condensed, sweetened	2 T	0	21	21	21/2
Milk, condensed, sweetened, Eagle Brand	2 T	0	22	23	22/2
Milk, condensed, sweetened, Eagle Brand, fat free	2 T	0	25	25	25/2
Milk, condensed, sweetened, Eagle Brand, low fat	2 T	0	23	23	23/2
Milk, evaporated	2 T	0	4	4	4/0
Milk, evaporated, Nestlé, Carnation	2 T	0	3	3	3/0
Milk, evaporated, Nestlé, Carnation, fat free	2 T	0	3	3	3/0
Milk, evaporated, Nestlé, Carnation, low fat	2 T	0	4	4	4/0
Milk, strawberry, Nesquik, 1% low fat	1 c	0	30	31	30/2
Milk, strawberry, Nesquik, 2% reduced fat	1 c	0	30	31	30/2
Milk, vanilla, Nesquik, 1% low fat	1 c	0	29	30	29/2
Milk, vanilla, Nesquik, 2% reduced fat	1 c	0	29	30	29/2
Oat milk, shelf stable, original, Pacific Natural Foods	1 c	1	19	24	19/2

FOOD	Svg Size	Fbr	Sgr	Cbs	S/C Val
Oat milk, shelf stable, vanilla, Pacific Natural Foods	1 c	2	20	25	20/2
Rice milk, refrigerated, original, Rice Dream	1 c	0	10	23	10/2
Rice milk, refrigerated, vanilla, Rice Dream	1 c	0	12	26	12/2
Rice milk, shelf stable, carob, Rice Dream	1 c	0	26	30	26/2
Rice milk, shelf stable, chocolate, enriched, Rice Dream	1 c	0	28	34	28/2
Rice milk, shelf stable, original, Rice Dream	1 c	0	11	24	11/2
Rice milk, shelf stable, original, enriched, Rice Dream	1 c	0	10	23	10/2
Rice milk, shelf stable, plain, Pacific Natural Foods	1 c	0	14	27	14/2
Rice milk, shelf stable, vanilla, Pacific Natural Foods	1 c	0	14	27	14/2
Rice milk, shelf stable, vanilla, Rice Dream	1 c	0	12	27	12/2
Rice milk, shelf stable, vanilla, enriched, Rice Dream	1 c	0	12	26	12/2
Sour cream, cultured	2 T	0	1	1	1/0
Sour cream, Daisy	2 T	0	1	1	1/0
Sour cream, Friendship	2 T	0	1	2	1/0
Sour cream, Hood	2 T	0	1	2	1/0
Sour cream, Horizon Organic	2 T	0	1	1	1/0
Sour cream, fat free, Hood	2 T	0	2	4	2/0
Sour cream, fat free, Knudsen	2 T	0	2	5	2/1
Sour cream, light, Alta Dena	2 T	0	1	1	1/0
Sour cream, light, Friendship	2 T	0	2	2	2/0
Sour cream, light, Knudsen	2 T	0	2	2	2/0
Sour cream, low fat, Hood	2 T	0	2	3	2/0
Sour cream, low fat, Horizon Organic	2 T	0	2	3	2/0
Sour cream, nondairy, Sour Supreme Better Than Sour Cream, Toffuti	2 T	0	2	9	2/1
Sour cream, nondairy, Vegan Gourmet, Follow Your Heart	2 T	2	0	3	0/0
Soy milk, refrigerated, chocolate, Silk	1 c	2	19	23	19/2
Soy milk, refrigerated, chocolate, light, 8th Continent	1 c	0	12	12	12/1
Soy milk, refrigerated, chocolate, light, Silk	1 c	2	14	15	14/1
Soy milk, refrigerated, original, Silk	1 c	1	6	8	6/1
Soy milk, refrigerated, original, Soy Dream	1 c	2	9	16	9/1
Soy milk, refrigerated, original, light, 8th Continent	1 c	0	2	2	2/0
Soy milk, refrigerated, original, light, Silk	1 c	1	6	8	6/1
Soy milk, refrigerated, unsweetened, Silk	1 c	1	1	4	1/0
Soy milk, refrigerated, vanilla, Silk	1 c	1	8	11	8/1
Soy milk, refrigerated, vanilla, Soy Dream	1 c	2	10	14	10/1
Soy milk, refrigerated, vanilla, light, 8th Continent	1 c	0	5	5	5/1
Soy milk, refrigerated, vanilla, light, Silk	1 c	1	7	10	7/1
Soy milk, refrigerated, very vanilla, Silk	1 c	1	16	19	16/1
Soy milk, shelf stable, chocolate, Silk	1 c	2	21	25	21/2
Soy milk, shelf stable, chocolate, Soy Dream	1 c	3	15	21	15/2
Soy milk, shelf stable, original, Silk	1 c	1	6	8	6/1
Soy milk, shelf stable, original, Soy Dream	1 c	2	4	8	4/1
Soy milk, shelf stable, unsweetened, Silk	1 c	1	1	4	1/0
Soy milk, shelf stable, vanilla, Silk	1 c	1	7	10	7/1

FOOD	Svg Size	Fbr	Sgr	Cbs	S/C Val
Soy milk, shelf stable, vanilla, Soy Dream	1 c	2	10	18	10/1
Whipped cream, Alta Dena	2 T	0	1	1	0/0
Whipped cream, Hood	2 T	0	0	0	0/0
Whipped cream, Land O' Lakes	2 T	0	0	0	0/0
Whipped cream, Reddi-Wip	2 T	0	1	0	1/0
Whipped cream, Reddi-Wip, chocolate	2 T	0	1	1	1/0
Whipped cream, Reddi-Wip, fat free	2 T	0	1	1	1/0
Whipped topping, Cool Whip, Kraft	2 T	0	1	2	1/0
Whipped topping, Cool Whip, Kraft, lite	2 T	0	1	3	1/0
Whipped topping, Cool Whip, Kraft, sugar free	2 T	0	0	3	0/0
Whipped topping, 365 Everyday Value, nonfat, real dairy	2 T	0	1	0	1/0
Yogurt, Breyers, Fruit on the Bottom, black cherry	6 oz	0	29	33	29/2
Yogurt, Breyers, Fruit on the Bottom, blueberry	6 oz	1	27	32	27/2
Yogurt, Breyers, Fruit on the Bottom, mixed berry	6 oz	0	27	32	27/2
Yogurt, Breyers, Fruit on the Bottom, peach	6 oz	0	28	32	28/2
Yogurt, Breyers, Fruit on the Bottom, strawberry	6 oz	0	28	33	28/2
Yogurt, Breyers, Fruit on the Bottom, strawberry banana	6 oz	0	27	32	27/2
Yogurt, Breyers, Light, black cherry jubilee	6 oz	0	8	12	8/1
Yogurt, Breyers, Light, blueberries 'n cream	6 oz	0	8	12	8/1
Yogurt, Breyers, Light, key lime pie	6 oz	0	7	11	7/1
Yogurt, Breyers, Light, lemon chiffon	6 oz	0	7	11	7/1
Yogurt, Breyers, Light, peaches 'n cream	6 oz	0	7	12	7/1
Yogurt, Breyers, Light, raspberries 'n cream	6 oz	0	7	12	7/1
Yogurt, Breyers, Light, strawberry	6 oz	0	7	12	7/1
Yogurt, Breyers, Light, strawberry cheesecake	6 oz	0	7	12	7/1
Yogurt, Breyers, Light, vanilla bean	6 oz	0	7	11	7/1
Yogurt, Breyers, Smooth & Creamy, peaches 'n cream	6 oz	0	29	34	29/2
Yogurt, Breyers, Smooth & Creamy, strawberry	6 oz	0	29	34	29/2
Yogurt, Breyers, Smooth & Creamy, strawberry cheesecake	6 oz	0	28	33	28/2
Yogurt, Dannon, coffee	6 oz	0	25	25	25/2
Yogurt, Dannon, lemon	6 oz	0	25	25	25/2
Yogurt, Dannon, plain	6 oz	0	12	12	12/1
Yogurt, Dannon, vanilla	6 oz	0	25	25	25/2
Yogurt, Dannon, Activia, blueberry	4 oz	0	17	19	17/1
Yogurt, Dannon, Activia, cherry	4 oz	0	18	19	18/1
Yogurt, Dannon, Activia, mixed berry	4 oz	0	17	19	17/1
Yogurt, Dannon, Activia, peach	4 oz	0	17	19	17/1
Yogurt, Dannon, Activia, plain	4 oz	0	9	10	9/1
Yogurt, Dannon, Activia, prune	4 oz	0	17	19	17/1
Yogurt, Dannon, Activia, strawberry	4 oz	0	17	19	17/1
Yogurt, Dannon, Activia, vanilla	4 oz	0	17	19	17/1
Yogurt, Dannon, Activia, Fiber, peach	4 oz	3	17	19	17/1
Yogurt, Dannon, Activia, Fiber, strawberry	4 oz	3	17	19	17/1
Yogurt, Dannon, Activia, Fiber, vanilla	4 oz	3	17	19	17/1

FOOD	Svg Size	Fbr	Sgr	Cbs	S/C Val
Yogurt, Dannon, Activia, Light, blueberry	4 oz	2	9	13	9/1
Yogurt, Dannon, Activia, Light, peach	4 oz	2	8	12	8/1
Yogurt, Dannon, Activia, Light, raspberry	4 oz	2	8	13	8/1
Yogurt, Dannon, Activia, Light, strawberry	4 oz	2	8	13	8/1
Yogurt, Dannon, Activia, Light, vanilla	4 oz	3	7	14	7/1
Yogurt, Dannon, Fruit on the Bottom, blueberry	6 oz	0	25	26	25/2
Yogurt, Dannon, Fruit on the Bottom, cherry	6 oz	0	24	26	24/2
Yogurt, Dannon, Fruit on the Bottom, mixed berry	6 oz	0	27	27	27/2
Yogurt, Dannon, Fruit on the Bottom, peach	6 oz	0	27	28	27/2
Yogurt, Dannon, Fruit on the Bottom, raspberry	6 oz	0	26	28	26/2
Yogurt, Dannon, Fruit on the Bottom, strawberry	6 oz	0	26	28	26/2
Yogurt, Dannon, Greek, blueberry	5.3 oz	0	16	17	16/1
Yogurt, Dannon, Greek, honey	5.3 oz	0	21	23	21/2
Yogurt, Dannon, Greek, plain	5.3 oz	0	6	6	6/1
Yogurt, Dannon, Greek, strawberry	5.3 oz	0	16	17	16/1
Yogurt, Dannon, Greek, vanilla	5.3 oz	0	16	17	16/1
Yogurt, Dannon, Light & Fit, blackberry	6 oz	0	11	16	11/1
Yogurt, Dannon, Light & Fit, blueberry	6 oz	0	11	16	11/1
Yogurt, Dannon, Light & Fit, cherry	6 oz	0	11	16	11/1
Yogurt, Dannon, Light & Fit, lemon chiffon	6 oz	0	11	15	11/1
Yogurt, Dannon, Light & Fit, mixed berry	6 oz	0	10	15	10/1
Yogurt, Dannon, Light & Fit, peach	6 oz	0	11	16	11/1
Yogurt, Dannon, Light & Fit, raspberry	6 oz	0	11	16	11/1
Yogurt, Dannon, Light & Fit, strawberry kiwi	6 oz	0	11	16	11/1
Yogurt, Dannon, Light & Fit, vanilla	6 oz	0	11	16	11/1
Yogurt, Dannon, Light & Fit, Carb & Sugar Control, all flavors	4 oz	0	2	3	2/0
Yogurt, Fage Total, cherry	5.3 oz	0	16	17	16/1
Yogurt, Fage Total, cherry, 2%	5.3 oz	0	17	18	17/1
Yogurt, Fage Total, classic	8 oz	0	7	7	7/1
Yogurt, Fage Total, classic, 0%	8 oz	0	9	9	9/1
Yogurt, Fage Total, classic, 2%	8 oz	0	9	9	9/1
Yogurt, Fage Total, classic w/ honey	5.3 oz	0	28	28	28/2
Yogurt, Fage Total, classic w/ honey, 2%	5.3 oz	0	29	29	29/2
Yogurt, Fage Total, peach	5.3 oz	0	16	17	16/1
Yogurt, Fage Total, peach, 2%	5.3 oz	0	17	18	17/1
Yogurt, Fage Total, strawberry	5.3 oz	0	16	17	16/1
Yogurt, Fage Total, strawberry, 2%	5.3 oz	0	17	18	17/1
Yogurt, Stonyfield, fruit on the bottom, blueberry, fat free	6 oz	0	20	22	20/2
Yogurt, Stonyfield, fruit on the bottom, strawberries & cream, cream top	6 oz	0	19	20	19/1
Yogurt, Stonyfield, fruit on the bottom, strawberry, fat free	6 oz	0	21	22	21/2
Yogurt, Stonyfield, fruit on the bottom, Super Fruits, fat free	6 oz	0	22	22	22/2
Yogurt, Stonyfield, Oikos, blueberry	5.3 oz	0	15	16	15/1
Yogurt, Stonyfield, Oikos, honey	5.3 oz	0	17	18	17/1
Yogurt, Stonyfield, Oikos, plain	5.3 oz	0	6	6	6/1

DAIRY & DAIRY ALTERNATIVES, cont'd.

FOOD	Svg Size	Fbr	Sgr	Cbs	S/C Val
Yogurt, Stonyfield, O'Soy, fruit on the bottom, blueberry	6 oz	2	26	29	26/2
Yogurt, Stonyfield, O'Soy, fruit on the bottom, peach	6 oz	2	28	30	28/2
Yogurt, Stonyfield, O'Soy, fruit on the bottom, strawberry	6 oz	2	26	29	26/2
Yogurt, Stonyfield, O'Soy, smooth & creamy, chocolate	6 oz	2	22	25	22/2
Yogurt, Stonyfield, O'Soy, smooth & creamy, vanilla	6 oz	1	21	24	21/2
Yogurt, Stonyfield, probiotic, French vanilla, fat free	4 oz	0	16	16	16/1
Yogurt, Stonyfield, probiotic, strawberry, fat free	4 oz	0	16	17	16/1
Yogurt, Stonyfield, smooth & creamy, French vanilla, cream top	6 oz	0	22	23	22/2
Yogurt, Stonyfield, smooth & creamy, French vanilla, fat free	6 oz	0	24	25	24/2
Yogurt, Stonyfield, smooth & creamy, French vanilla, low fat	6 oz	0	21	22	21/2
Yogurt, Stonyfield, smooth & creamy, peach, fat free	6 oz	0	25	25	25/2
Yogurt, Stonyfield, smooth & creamy, plain, fat free	6 oz	0	11	11	11/1
Yogurt, Stonyfield, smooth & creamy, plain, low fat	6 oz	0	11	11	11/1
Yogurt, Stonyfield, smooth & creamy, pomegranate berry, fat free	6 oz	0	24	25	24/2
Yogurt, Stonyfield, smooth & creamy, strawberry, fat free	6 oz	0	25	26	25/2
Yogurt, Stonyfield, smooth & creamy, white chocolate raspberry, cream top	6 oz	0	23	23	23/2
Yogurt, Yoplait, Fiber One, all flavors	4 oz	5	4	13	4/1
Yogurt, Yoplait, Greek, plain	6 oz	0	9	10	9/1
Yogurt, Yoplait, Greek, strawberry	6 oz	0	18	19	18/1
Yogurt, Yoplait, Light, fruit flavors	6 oz	0	14	19	14/1
Yogurt, Yoplait, Light, indulgent flavors	6 oz	0	15	20	15/1
Yogurt, Yoplait, Original, most flavors	6 oz	0	27	33	27/2
Yogurt, Yoplait, Original, coconut cream pie	6 oz	0	27	34	27/2
Yogurt, Yoplait, Original, lemon burst	6 oz	0	31	36	31/2
Yogurt, Yoplait, Original, piña colada	6 oz	0	28	33	28/2
Yogurt, Yoplait, Thick & Creamy, fruit flavors	6 oz	0	28	32	28/2
Yogurt, Yoplait, Thick & Creamy, Light, fruit flavors	6 oz	0	14	20	14/1
Yogurt, Yoplait, Whips!, chocolate flavors	4 oz	0	23	26	23/2
Yogurt, Yoplait, Whips!, fruit flavors	4 oz	0	21	25	21/2

NUTS, SEEDS & LEGUMES

FOOD	Svg Size	Fbr	Sgr	Cbs	S/C Val
Almond butter	2 T	1	2	7	2/1
Almond butter, Earth Balance	2 T	4	2	6	2/1
Almond butter, MaraNatha, most varieties	2 T	4	2	6	2/1
Almond butter, MaraNatha, honey	2 T	3	5	9	5/1
Almond butter, Woodstock Farms, all varieties	2 T	4	2	7	2/1
Almonds, raw	¼ c	4	0	6	0/1
Almonds, roasted	¼ c	4	2	7	2/1
Baked beans, plain	½ c	5	10	27	10/2
Baked beans, Amy's, vegetarian	½ c	6	9	28	9/2
Baked beans, Bush's, original	½ c	5	12	29	12/2
Baked beans, Bush's, vegetarian	½ c	5	12	29	12/2
Baked beans, Campbell's	½ c	5	12	29	12/2

NUTS, SEEDS & LEGUMES, cont'd.

FOOD	Svg Size	Fbr	Sgr	Cbs	S/C Val
Baked beans, Van Camp's, original	1 can	8	8	29	8/2
Baked beans, Van Camp's, pork & beans	½ c	6	7	23	7/2
Black beans	¼ c	7	1	30	1/2
Black-eyed peas, cooked	¼ c	2	1	8	1/1
Brazil nuts	1 oz	2	1	3	1/0
Broad beans (fava beans)	¼ c	9	2	22	2/2
Cashew butter, roasted, MaraNatha	2 T	2	2	10	2/1
Cashew butter, Woodstock Farms	2 T	0	2	9	2/1
Cashews, dry roasted	1 oz	1	1	9	1/1
Cashews, oil roasted	1 oz	1	1	9	1/1
Cashews, raw	1 oz	1	2	9	2/1
Chickpeas (garbanzo beans)	¼ c	9	5	30	5/2
Cowpeas	¼ c	4	3	25	3/2
Edamame (soybeans), cooked	½ c	4	2	8	2/1
Fava beans (broad beans)	¼ c	9	2	22	2/2
Garbanzo beans (chickpeas)	¼ c	9	5	30	5/2
Great northern beans	¼ c	9	1	29	1/2
Great northern beans, HamBeens, w/ ham flavor, cooked	½ c	11	1	22	1/2
Kidney beans, most varieties	¼ c	12	1	28	1/2
Kidney beans, red	¼ c	7	1	28	1/2
Lentils, boiled	½ c	8	2	19	2/1
Lentils, raw	½ c	29	2	58	2/3
Lentils, Hurst's, garlic & herb, cooked	½ c	5	2	22	2/2
Lentils, Hurst's, red curry, cooked	½ c	5	2	23	2/2
Lima beans	¼ c	9	4	28	4/2
Lima beans, baby, HamBeens, w/ ham flavor, cooked	½ c	9	1	22	1/2
Macadamia nut butter, MaraNatha, roasted	2 T	2	2	10	2/1
Macadamia nuts, dry roasted	1 oz	2	1	4	1/0
Macadamia nuts, raw	1 oz	2	1	4	1/0
Miso	1 T	1	1	5	1/1
Mixed nuts, Emerald Nuts	1 oz	2	1	6	1/1
Mixed nuts, Emerald Nuts, deluxe	1 oz	2	1	6	1/1
Mixed nuts, Planters	1 oz	2	1	5	1/1
Mixed nuts, Planters, deluxe	1 oz	2	1	6	1/1
Mixed nuts, Planters, honey roasted	1 oz	2	5	9	5/1
Mung beans	¼ c	8	3	32	3/2
Navy beans	¼ c	12	2	32	2/2
Navy beans, HamBeens, w/ ham flavor, cooked	½ c	11	1	20	1/1
Peanut butter, chunky	2 T	2	4	6	4/1
Peanut butter, smooth	2 T	2	3	6	3/1
Peanut butter, Better'n Peanut Butter, original	2 T	0	2	13	2/1
Peanut butter, Earth Balance	2 T	3	2	7	2/1
Peanut butter, Jif, creamy, natural	2 T	2	3	7	3/1
Peanut butter, Jif, creamy, regular	2 T	2	3	7	3/1

FOOD	Svg Size	Fbr	Sgr	Cbs	S/C Val
Peanut butter, Jif, creamy, simply	2 T	2	2	6	2/1
Peanut butter, Jif, creamy, w/ honey	2 T	2	6	10	6/1
Peanut butter, Jif, crunchy, reduced fat	2 T	2	4	15	4/1
Peanut butter, Joseph's, sugar-free creamy Valencia	2 T	1	0	6	0/1
Peanut butter, Joseph's, sugar-free crunchy Valencia	2 T	1	0	6	0/1
Peanut butter, Kirkland Signature, organic creamy	2 T	2	2	7	2/1
Peanut butter, Laura Scudder's, most flavors	2 T	2	1	6	1/1
Peanut butter, Laura Scudder's, reduced fat	2 T	2	2	12	2/1
Peanut butter, MaraNatha, natural	2 T	3	1	7	1/1
Peanut butter, MaraNatha, natural, no stir	2 T	2	3	8	3/1
Peanut butter, MaraNatha, organic	2 T	3	1	7	1/1
Peanut butter, MaraNatha, organic, no stir	2 T	2	3	7	3/1
Peanut butter, Peter Pan, creamy	2 T	2	3	6	3/1
Peanut butter, Peter Pan, creamy, honey roast	2 T	2	8	10	8/1
Peanut butter, Peter Pan, creamy, reduced fat	2 T	2	4	14	4/1
Peanut butter, Peter Pan, creamy, whipped	2 T	2	2	5	2/1
Peanut butter, Peter Pan, crunchy, honey roast	2 T	2	7	11	7/1
Peanut butter, Peter Pan, crunchy, reduced fat	2 T	2	4	14	4/1
Peanut butter, Skippy, creamy	2 T	2	3	7	3/1
Peanut butter, Skippy, creamy, natural	2 T	2	3	6	3/1
Peanut butter, Skippy, creamy, reduced fat	2 T	2	4	15	4/1
Peanut butter, Skippy, creamy, roasted honey nut	2 T	2	3	7	3/1
Peanut butter, Skippy, super chunk	2 T	2	3	7	3/1
Peanut butter, Smart Balance	2 T	2	3	8	3/1
Peanut butter, Smucker's, chunky	2 T	2	1	6	1/1
Peanut butter, Smucker's, creamy	2 T	2	1	6	1/1
Peanut butter, Smucker's, creamy, honey	2 T	2	4	9	4/1
Peanut butter, Smucker's, creamy, reduced fat	2 T	2	2	12	2/1
Peanut butter, Woodstock Farms, most varieties	2 T	2	2	7	2/1
Peanut butter, Woodstock Farms, organic, crunchy	2 T	2	1	6	1/1
Peanut butter, Woodstock Farms, organic, smooth, unsalted	2 T	2	1	6	1/1
Peanuts, all varieties, dry roasted	1 oz	2	1	6	1/1
Peanuts, all varieties, oil roasted	1 oz	2	1	5	1/1
Peanuts, all varieties, raw	1 oz	2	1	5	1/1
Peas, edible pod	10	1	1	3	1/0
Peas, green	½ c	4	4	10	4/1
Pecans	1 oz	3	1	4	1/0
Pecans, candied	1 oz	5	4	10	4/1
Pine nuts	¼ c	1	1	4	1/0
Pink beans	¼ c	7	1	34	1/2
Pinto beans, cooked	¼ c	8	1	30	1/2
Pinto beans, HamBeens, w/ ham flavor, cooked	½ c	6	1	20	1/1
Pistachios	1 oz	3	2	8	2/1
Pumpkin seeds	¼ c	2	0	3	0/0

FOOD	Svg Size	Fbr	Sgr	Cbs	S/C Val
Refried beans, traditional	¼ c	3	0	9	0/1
Refried beans, vegetarian	¼ c	3	0	8	0/1
Refried beans, Amy's, black beans	½ c	6	1	21	1/2
Refried beans, Amy's, traditional	½ c	6	1	22	1/2
Refried beans, Old El Paso	½ c	6	1	18	1/1
Refried beans, Rosarita	½ c	6	0	18	0/1
Refried beans, Rosarita, black	½ c	8	0	19	0/1
Refried beans, Rosarita, vegetarian	½ c	7	0	19	0/1
Sesame butter	1 T	1	0	4	0/0
Sesame seeds	¼ c	4	0	9	0/1
Soybeans (edamame)	½ c	4	2	8	2/1
Split peas	¼ c	13	4	30	4/2
Split peas, HamPeas, w/ ham flavor	½ c	4	1	21	1/2
Sunflower seeds, dry roasted	¼ c	4	1	8	1/1
Sunflower seeds, in shells	¼ c	1	0	2	0/0
Sunflower seed butter, Sunbutter, most varieties	2 T	4	3	7	3/1
Sunflower seed butter, Sunbutter, unsweetened organic	2 T	2	1	5	1/1
Tahini	1 T	1	0	4	0/0
Tahini, MaraNatha, raw or roasted	2 T	1	0	7	0/1
Tahini, Woodstock Farms	2 T	4	0	4	0/0
Walnuts, black	¼ c	2	0	3	0/0
Walnuts, English	¼ c	2	1	4	1/0
White beans	¼ c	8	1	30	1/2

BREADS, WRAPS & GRAINS

FOOD	Svg Size	Fbr	Sgr	Cbs	S/C Val
Bagel, cinnamon raisin, 4" diameter	1	2	6	58	6/3
Bagel, oat bran, 4" diameter	1	4	2	56	2/3
Bagel, onion, 4" diameter	1	3	6	57	6/3
Bagel, plain, 4" diameter	1	3	6	57	6/3
Bagel, poppy seed, 4" diameter	1	3	6	57	6/3
Bagel, Alvarado Street Bakery, sprouted spelt	1	12	4	52	4/3
Bagel, Alvarado Street Bakery, sprouted wheat	1	3	2	51	2/3
Bagel, Alvarado Street Bakery, sprouted wheat, cinnamon raisin	1	3	28	59	28/3
Bagel, Alvarado Street Bakery, sprouted wheat, onion & poppyseed	1	2	8	66	8/4
Bagel, Alvarado Street Bakery, sprouted wheat, sesame seed	1	2	7	64	7/4
Bagel, Fiber One, cinnamon raisin	1	10	13	58	13/3
Bagel, Fiber One, multigrain	1	10	7	55	7/3
Bagel, Lender's, blueberry	1	1	5	32	5/2
Bagel, Lender's, cinnamon raisin, mini	1	2	6	32	6/2
Bagel, Lender's, cinnamon raisin swirl	1	3	11	51	11/3
Bagel, Lender's, egg	1	2	5	49	5/3
Bagel, Lender's, everything	1	2	5	49	5/3
Bagel, Lender's, multigrain, whole grain	1	2	5	49	5/3

BREADS, WRAPS & GRAINS, cont'd.

FOOD	Svg Size	Fbr	Sgr	Cbs	S/C Val
Bagel, Lender's, 100% whole wheat	1	6	6	41	6/3
Bagel, Lender's, onion	1	2	4	49	4/3
Bagel, Lender's, plain	1	2	6	46	6/3
Bagel, Lender's, plain, frozen	1	1	2	29	2/2
Bagel, Lender's, plain, frozen, New York style	1	2	3	48	3/3
Bagel, Lender's, plain, mini	1	1	2	29	2/2
Bagel, Lender's, plain, refrigerated	1	2	3	43	3/3
Bagel, Lender's, plain, refrigerated, Little Lender's	1	0	0	13	0/1
Bagel, Lender's, plain, refrigerated, 100 Calories	1	0	1	18	1/1
Bagel, Lender's, plain, whole grain	1	2	5	49	5/3
Bagel, Oroweat, honey wheat	1	2	5	34	5/2
Bagel, Oroweat, 100% whole wheat	1	5	3	24	3/2
Bagel, Oroweat, plain	1	4	3	25	3/2
Bagel, Pepperidge Farm, brown sugar cinnamon, mini	1	2	6	24	6/2
Bagel, Pepperidge Farm, cinnamon raisin, mini	1	1	6	23	6/2
Bagel, Pepperidge Farm, everything	1	2	9	53	9/3
Bagel, Pepperidge Farm, 100% whole wheat	1	6	6	49	6/3
Bagel, Pepperidge Farm, 100% whole wheat, mini	1	3	3	20	3/1
Bagel, Pepperidge Farm, plain	1	3	3	54	3/3
Bagel, Pepperidge Farm, plain, mini	1	1	4	22	4/2
Bagel, Sara Lee, blueberry	1	2	9	61	9/4
Bagel, Sara Lee, cinnamon raisin	1	2	11	60	11/3
Bagel, Sara Lee, everything	1	1	7	55	7/3
Bagel, Sara Lee, honey wheat	1	4	10	61	10/4
Bagel, Sara Lee, onion	1	3	5	58	5/3
Bagel, Sara Lee, plain	1	2	3	57	3/3
Bagel, Thomas', everything	1	3	6	50	6/3
Bagel, Thomas', everything, Bagel Thins	1	5	3	24	3/2
Bagel, Thomas', 100% whole wheat, Bagel Thins	1	5	3	24	3/2
Bagel, Thomas', 100% whole wheat, Hearty Grains	1	7	7	49	7/3
Bagel, Thomas', 100% whole wheat, mini	1	3	4	25	4/2
Bagel, Thomas', onion	1	3	6	51	6/3
Bagel, Thomas', plain	1	2	6	51	6/3
Bagel, Thomas', plain, Bagel Thins	1	4	3	25	3/2
Bagel, Thomas', plain, mini	1	0	3	24	3/2
Bagel, Thomas', plain, mini, 100 calories	1	4	0	22	0/2
Biscuit, Pillsbury, buttermilk	3	1	4	29	4/2
Biscuit, Pillsbury, Grands!, frozen, buttermilk	1	0	2	22	2/2
Biscuit, Pillsbury, Grands!, frozen, sandwich style	1	1	3	34	3/2
Biscuit, Pillsbury, Grands!, homestyle, buttermilk	1	0	4	25	4/2
Biscuit, Pillsbury, Grands!, homestyle, buttermilk, reduced fat	1	0	4	25	4/2
Biscuit, Pillsbury, Grands!, homestyle, golden wheat, reduced fat	1	2	5	29	5/2
Biscuit, Pillsbury, Grands!, homestyle, original	1	0	4	25	4/2
Bread, egg	1 slc	1	1	14	1/1

FOOD	Svg Size	Fbr	Sgr	Cbs	S/C Val
Bread, French	1 slc	1	1	16	1/1
Bread, Italian	1 slc	1	0	14	0/1
Bread, multigrain	1 slc	2	2	12	2/1
Bread, oat bran	1 slc	1	2	11	2/1
Bread, oatmeal	1 slc	1	2	14	2/1
Bread, pumpernickel	1 slc	2	0	13	0/1
Bread, rye	1 slc	2	1	14	1/1
Bread, wheat	1 slc	1	2	13	2/1
Bread, white	1 slc	1	1	14	1/1
Bread, whole wheat	1 slc	2	2	12	2/1
Bread, Alvarado Street Bakery, California style, complete protein	1 slc	2	2	15	2/1
Bread, Alvarado Street Bakery, Diabetic Lifestyles, low glycemic	1 slc	2	2	15	2/1
Bread, Alvarado Street Bakery, essential flax seed	2 slcs	3	2	15	2/1
Bread, Alvarado Street Bakery, sprouted barley	1 slc	2	3	15	3/1
Bread, Alvarado Street Bakery, sprouted rye seed	1 slc	2	2	15	2/1
Bread, Alvarado Street Bakery, sprouted sourdough	1 slc	2	2	15	2/1
Bread, Alvarado Street Bakery, sprouted sourdough, French	1 slc	2	2	15	2/1
Bread, Alvarado Street Bakery, sprouted soy crunch	1 slc	2	1	15	1/1
Bread, Alvarado Street Bakery, sprouted wheat, cinnamon raisin	1 slc	2	6	16	6/1
Bread, Alvarado Street Bakery, sprouted wheat, multi-grain	1 slc	2	2	15	2/1
Bread, Alvarado Street Bakery, sprouted whole wheat	1 slc	3	3	19	3/1
Bread, Alvarado Street Bakery, Ultimate Kids	1 slc	2	3	16	3/1
Bread, Arnold, active health, Grains & More	1 slc	5	3	22	3/2
Bread, Arnold, ancient grains, Grains & More	1 slc	3	4	21	4/2
Bread, Arnold, butter split top, Dutch Country	1 slc	1	2	18	2/1
Bread, Arnold, country oat bran	1 slc	1	3	21	3/2
Bread, Arnold, country wheat	1 slc	2	4	22	4/2
Bread, Arnold, country white	1 slc	1	3	22	3/2
Bread, Arnold, country white, whole grain	1 slc	2	3	21	3/2
Bread, Arnold, double fiber, Grains & More	1 slc	6	2	21	2/2
Bread, Arnold, double protein, Grains & More	1 slc	3	2	18	2/1
Bread, Arnold, extra fiber, Dutch Country	1 slc	4	3	18	3/1
Bread, Arnold, flax & fiber, Grains & More	1 slc	5	3	21	3/2
Bread, Arnold, German dark wheat, whole grains	1 slc	2	3	21	3/2
Bread, Arnold, grain lover's, Grains & More	1 slc	3	4	21	4/2
Bread, Arnold, health nut, whole grains	1 slc	2	3	21	3/2
Bread, Arnold, honey wheat, Sandwich Thins	1	5	2	22	2/2
Bread, Arnold, honey wheat, Soft Family	2 slcs	2	4	25	4/2
Bread, Arnold, honey whole wheat, whole grains	1 slc	3	4	20	4/1
Bread, Arnold, Italian, premium	1 slc	1	3	16	3/1
Bread, Arnold, multi-grain, Sandwich Thins	1	5	2	22	2/2
Bread, Arnold, multi-grain, sugar free, Carb Counting	1 slc	3	0	9	0/1
Bread, Arnold, multi-grain, whole grains	1 slc	4	4	20	4/1
Bread, Arnold, oatnut, whole grains	1 slc	2	4	22	4/2

FOOD	Svg Size	Fbr	Sgr	Cbs	S/C Val
Bread, Arnold, 100% whole wheat, Dutch Country	1 slc	3	3	18	3/1
Bread, Arnold, 100% whole wheat, light	2 slcs	5	2	18	2/1
Bread, Arnold, 100% whole wheat, Sandwich Thins	1 slc	5	2	21	2/2
Bread, Arnold, 100% whole wheat, Soft Family	2 slcs	3	4	23	4/2
Bread, Arnold, 100% whole wheat, stone ground	1 slc	3	4	22	4/2
Bread, Arnold, 100% whole wheat, Triple Health, Grains & More	1 slc	6	3	20	3/1
Bread, Arnold, 100% whole wheat, whole grains	1 slc	3	4	20	4/1
Bread, Arnold, potato, premium, Dutch Country	1 slc	1	3	18	3/1
Bread, Arnold, rye, dark	1 slc	0	1	15	1/1
Bread, Arnold, rye, everything	1 slc	0	1	16	1/1
Bread, Arnold, rye, melba thin	2 slcs	0	2	20	2/1
Bread, Arnold, rye, seedless	2 slcs	0	2	20	2/1
Bread, Arnold, rye, seedless, Sandwich Thins	1	5	2	23	2/2
Bread, Arnold, rye, w/ seeds	1 slc	0	1	14	1/1
Bread, Arnold, rye & pump	1 slc	0	1	14	1/1
Bread, Arnold, 7 grain, whole grains	1 slc	3	3	21	3/2
Bread, Arnold, 12 grain, whole grains	1 slc	3	3	21	3/2
Bread, Arnold, white, classic, Soft Family	2 slcs	1	5	26	5/2
Bread, Arnold, white, premium, Brick Oven	1 slc	0	3	17	3/1
Bread, Arnold, white, premium, Dutch Country	1 slc	0	2	17	2/1
Bread, Arnold, white, whole grain, Sandwich Thins	1	5	2	22	2/2
Bread, Arnold, white, whole grain, Soft Family	2 slcs	2	4	25	4/2
Bread, Ener-G Foods, light brown rice loaf	1 slc	1	1	7	1/1
Bread, Fiber One, country white	1 slc	6	4	24	4/2
Bread, Fiber One, multigrain	1 slc	6	4	25	4/2
Bread, Fiber One, oatmeal	1 slc	6	4	25	4/2
Bread, Fiber One, 100% whole wheat	1 slc	7	4	23	4/2
Bread, Food for Life, 7 sprouted grains	1 slc	3	1	15	1/1
Bread, Food for Life, Ezekiel 4:9, sprouted grain, low sodium	1 slc	3	0	14	0/1
Bread, Food for Life, Ezekiel 4:9, sprouted grain, sesame	1 slc	3	0	14	0/1
Bread, Food for Life, Ezekiel 4:9, sprouted 100% whole grain	1 slc	3	0	15	0/1
Bread, Healthy Choice, hearty 7-grain	1 slc	3	3	18	3/1
Bread, Healthy Choice, 100% whole grain	1 slc	3	3	18	3/1
Bread, King's Hawaiian, Hawaiian sweet	½" slc	2	12	32	12/2
Bread, King's Hawaiian, Hawaiian sweet, sandwich rolls	1	2	16	42	16/3
Bread, King's Hawaiian, Hawaiian sweet, snacker rolls	1	2	14	36	14/2
Bread, King's Hawaiian, honey wheat	½" slc	2	8	28	8/2
Bread, Kirkland Signature, split top wheat	1 slc	3	2	17	2/1
Bread, Milton's, multi-grain	1 slc	3	5	22	5/2
Bread, Milton's, multi-grain plus	1 slc	4	7	25	7/2
Bread, Milton's, 100% whole wheat, whole grains	1 slc	5	4	22	4/2
Bread, Milton's, whole grain	1 slc	5	3	16	3/1
Bread, Oroweat, country buttermilk	1 slc	0	3	19	3/1
Bread, Oroweat, country potato	1 slc	0	2	19	2/1

FOOD	Svg Size	Fbr	Sgr	Cbs	S/C Val
Bread, Oroweat, country white	1 slc	0	3	19	3/1
Bread, Oroweat, country white, whole grain	1 slc	1	4	19	4/1
Bread, Oroweat, double fiber, whole grain	1 slc	6	2	16	2/1
Bread, Oroweat, extra fiber, Dutch Country	1 slc	4	3	18	3/1
Bread, Oroweat, Hawaiian, sweet	1 slc	0	4	19	4/1
Bread, Oroweat, Health Nut	1 slc	2	2	18	2/1
Bread, Oroweat, honey wheat, Sandwich Thins	1 slc	5	2	22	2/2
Bread, Oroweat, honey wheat, Soft Family	2 slcs	2	4	25	4/2
Bread, Oroweat, honey wheat berry	1 slc	2	3	17	3/1
Bread, Oroweat, honey whole wheat, whole grain	1 slc	2	4	18	4/1
Bread, Oroweat, Italian, premium	1 slc	0	0	15	0/1
Bread, Oroweat, multi-grain, healthy	1 slc	2	4	17	4/1
Bread, Oroweat, multi-grain, Sandwich Thins	1	5	2	22	2/2
Bread, Oroweat, natural ancient grains	1 slc	2	3	18	3/1
Bread, Oroweat, 9 grain, whole grain	1 slc	3	3	17	3/1
Bread, Oroweat, oatnut, original	1 slc	1	3	19	3/1
Bread, Oroweat, oatnut, 3-seed	1 slc	2	4	18	4/1
Bread, Oroweat, 100% whole wheat, Country	1 slc	3	3	18	3/1
Bread, Oroweat, 100% whole wheat, Dutch Country	1 slc	3	3	18	3/1
Bread, Oroweat, 100% whole wheat, light	2 slcs	7	3	18	3/1
Bread, Oroweat, 100% whole wheat, Sandwich Thins	1	5	2	21	2/2
Bread, Oroweat, 100% whole wheat, Triple Health	1 slc	5	3	18	3/1
Bread, Oroweat, 100% whole wheat, whole grain	1 slc	3	3	17	3/1
Bread, Oroweat, potato, premium, Dutch Country	1 slc	0	3	18	3/1
Bread, Oroweat, raisin cinnamon	1 slc	1	7	20	7/1
Bread, Oroweat, raisin cinnamon swirl	1 slc	1	6	17	6/1
Bread, Oroweat, rye, dark	1 slc	1	0	13	0/1
Bread, Oroweat, rye, dill	1 slc	1	0	14	0/1
Bread, Oroweat, rye, extra sour New York style	1 slc	1	0	14	0/1
Bread, Oroweat, rye, Jewish	1 slc	1	1	13	1/1
Bread, Oroweat, rye, Russian	1 slc	1	0	13	0/1
Bread, Oroweat, 7 grain	1 slc	2	3	19	3/1
Bread, Oroweat, 12 grain	1 slc	2	3	18	3/1
Bread, Oroweat, white, classic, Soft Family	2 slcs	1	5	26	5/2
Bread, Oroweat, white, whole grain, Sandwich Thins	1	5	2	22	2/2
Bread, Oroweat, white, whole grain, Soft Family	2 slcs	2	4	25	4/2
Bread, Oroweat, whole grain & flax	1 slc	4	3	17	3/1
Bread, Oroweat, winter wheat, Master's Best	1 slc	2	3	14	3/1
Bread, Pepperidge Farm, brown sugar cinnamon swirl	1 slc	1	6	17	6/1
Bread, Pepperidge Farm, buttermilk, Farmhouse	1 slc	1	4	23	4/2
Bread, Pepperidge Farm, cinnamon swirl	1 slc	0	4	15	4/1
Bread, Pepperidge Farm, double fiber, whole grain	1 slc	6	2	21	2/2
Bread, Pepperidge Farm, extra fiber wheat, Light Style	3 slcs	6	3	26	3/2
Bread, Pepperidge Farm, 15 grain, Small Slice	1 slc	3	2	13	2/1

FOOD	Svg Size	Fbr	Sgr	Cbs	S/C Val
Bread, Pepperidge Farm, 15 grain, whole grain	1 slc	4	3	20	3/1
Bread, Pepperidge Farm, German dark wheat, 100% Natural	1 slc	3	2	17	2/1
Bread, Pepperidge Farm, Italian sesame	1 slc	0	1	15	1/1
Bread, Pepperidge Farm, Italian wheat	1 slc	3	1	16	1/1
Bread, Pepperidge Farm, Italian white	1 slc	1	1	15	1/1
Bread, Pepperidge Farm, 9 grain, 100% Natural	1 slc	3	3	18	3/1
Bread, Pepperidge Farm, oatmeal	1 slc	4	3	20	3/1
Bread, Pepperidge Farm, oatmeal, Farmhouse	1 slc	1	3	21	3/2
Bread, Pepperidge Farm, oatmeal, Light Style	3 slcs	2	2	27	2/2
Bread, Pepperidge Farm, oatmeal, whole grain	1 slc	4	4	21	4/2
Bread, Pepperidge Farm, 100% whole wheat, cinnamon w/ raisins swirl	1 slc	2	4	13	4/1
Bread, Pepperidge Farm, 100% whole wheat, Deli Flats	1	5	3	19	3/1
Bread, Pepperidge Farm, 100% whole wheat, Farmhouse	1 slc	3	3	19	3/1
Bread, Pepperidge Farm, 100% whole wheat, 100% Natural	1 slc	3	3	18	3/1
Bread, Pepperidge Farm, 100% whole wheat, Small Slice	1 slc	3	2	13	2/1
Bread, Pepperidge Farm, 100% whole wheat, stone ground	1 slc	2	1	12	1/1
Bread, Pepperidge Farm, 100% whole wheat, Very Thin	3 slcs	3	3	20	3/1
Bread, Pepperidge Farm, 100% whole wheat, whole grain	1 slc	4	4	21	4/2
Bread, Pepperidge Farm, pumpernickel, dark pump	1 slc	1	1	15	1/1
Bread, Pepperidge Farm, raisin cinnamon swirl	1 slc	0	5	15	5/1
Bread, Pepperidge Farm, rye, seeded	1 slc	2	1	15	1/1
Bread, Pepperidge Farm, rye, seeded, whole grain	1 slc	2	0	14	0/1
Bread, Pepperidge Farm, rye, seedless	1 slc	1	0	14	0/1
Bread, Pepperidge Farm, 7 grain, Deli Flats	1	5	3	19	3/1
Bread, Pepperidge Farm, 7 grain, Light Style	3 slcs	4	3	26	3/2
Bread, Pepperidge Farm, soft honey oat, whole grain	1 slc	4	3	19	3/1
Bread, Pepperidge Farm, soft honey whole wheat, whole grain	1 slc	4	4	21	4/2
Bread, Pepperidge Farm, soft wheat, Light Style	3 slcs	4	3	25	3/2
Bread, Pepperidge Farm, sourdough, Farmhouse	1 slc	1	2	22	2/2
Bread, Pepperidge Farm, 12 grain, Farmhouse	1 slc	3	3	21	3/2
Bread, Pepperidge Farm, white, original	1 slc	1	2	13	2/1
Bread, Pepperidge Farm, white, sandwich	2 slcs	0	3	23	3/2
Bread, Pepperidge Farm, white, Very Thin	3 slcs	1	2	24	2/2
Bread, Pillsbury, French	⅛ pkg	0	2	24	2/2
Bread, Pillsbury, Italian	⅛ pkg	0	2	22	2/2
Bread, Sara Lee, buttermilk, whole grain, Hearty & Delicious	1 slc	1	5	22	5/2
Bread, Sara Lee, country white, whole grain, Hearty & Delicious	1 slc	1	5	24	5/2
Bread, Sara Lee, honey wheat	1 slc	1	3	14	3/1
Bread, Sara Lee, 100% multi-grain, 45 Calories & Delightful	2 slcs	4	3	18	3/1
Bread, Sara Lee, 100% multi-grain, Hearty & Delicious	1 slc	3	4	20	4/1
Bread, Sara Lee, 100% whole wheat	1 slc	2	2	13	2/1
Bread, Sara Lee, 100% whole wheat, Hearty & Delicious	1 slc	3	5	21	5/2
Bread, Sara Lee, 100% whole wheat, Soft & Smooth	1 slc	2	3	12	3/1
Bread, Sara Lee, 100% whole wheat, w/ honey, 45 Calories & Delightful	2 slcs	5	3	18	3/1

FOOD	Svg Size	Fbr	Sgr	Cbs	S/C Val
Bread, Sara Lee, 100% whole wheat, w/ honey, Hearty & Delicious	1 slc	4	3	21	3/2
Bread, Sara Lee, potato, whole grain, Hearty & Delicious	1 slc	1	4	23	4/2
Bread, Sara Lee, wheat, 45 Calories & Delightful	2 slcs	5	2	18	2/1
Bread, Sara Lee, white, 45 Calories & Delightful	2 slcs	4	2	18	2/1
Bread, Sara Lee, white, classic, Soft & Smooth	2 slcs	1	4	30	4/2
Bread, Sara Lee, white, whole grain, Soft & Smooth	2 slcs	1	5	28	5/2
Bread, Wonder, buttermilk	1 slc	0	2	13	2/1
Bread, Wonder, classic white	1 slc	0	2	14	2/1
Bread, Wonder, classic white, sandwich	1 slc	0	2	13	2/1
Bread, Wonder, kids	1 slc	2	2	12	2/1
Bread, Wonder, potato	1 slc	0	3	14	3/1
Bread, Wonder, Smartwhite	2 slcs	5	4	23	4/2
Bread, Wonder, Texas toast	1 slc	1	2	19	2/1
Bread, Wonder, wheat, light	2 slcs	5	3	18	3/1
Bread, Wonder, wheat, 100% whole, soft	2 slcs	3	3	20	3/1
Bread, Wonder, wheat, 100% whole, stoneground	2 slcs	4	5	32	5/2
Bread, Wonder, wheat, whole grain	2 slcs	4	4	26	4/2
Bread, Wonder, white, light	2 slcs	5	3	18	3/1
Bread, Wonder, white, whole grain	2 slcs	4	4	25	4/2
English muffin, Fiber One, multigrain, light	1	8	2	24	2/2
English muffin, Fiber One, 100% whole wheat	1	6	3	22	3/2
English muffin, Fiber One, original	1	6	2	23	2/2
English muffin, Fiber One, wheat multigrain, light	1	8	2	24	2/2
English muffin, Food for Life, Ezekiel 4:9, sprouted whole grain	1	3	0	15	0/1
English muffin, Oroweat, cinnamon raisin	1	4	11	36	11/2
English muffin, Oroweat, double fiber	1	8	5	29	5/2
English muffin, Oroweat, extra crisp	1	1	1	27	1/2
English muffin, Oroweat, 100% whole wheat, whole grain	1	4	6	27	6/2
English muffin, Oroweat, sourdough	1	1	1	28	1/2
English muffin, Oroweat, whole grain & flax	1	5	5	28	5/2
English muffin, Pepperidge Farm, 100% whole wheat, whole grain	1	3	4	26	4/2
English muffin, Pepperidge Farm, original	1	1	1	25	1/2
English muffin, Thomas', honey wheat	1	1	3	26	3/2
English muffin, Thomas', original	1	1	1	25	1/2
English muffin, Thomas', original, sandwich size	1	2	2	38	2/2
English muffin, Thomas', original, whole grain	1	2	1	26	1/2
English muffin, Thomas', sourdough	1	1	2	26	2/2
English muffin, Thomas', Better Start, high fiber, 100 calories	1	5	0	24	0/2
English muffin, Thomas', Better Start, light, multi-grain	1	8	0	24	0/2
English muffin, Thomas', Hearty Grains, double fiber honey wheat	1	5	2	27	2/2
English muffin, Thomas', Hearty Grains, multi-grain	1	2	3	27	3/2
English muffin, Thomas', Hearty Grains, 100% whole wheat	1	3	2	23	2/2
English muffin, Thomas', Hearty Grains, 12 grain	1	2	1	25	1/2
Fillo, Athens, 9" x 14" sheet	5 pcs	1	0	37	0/2

BREADS, WRAPS & GRAINS, cont'd.

FOOD	Svg Size	Fbr	Sgr	Cbs	S/C Val
Fillo, Athens, 14" x 18" sheet	5 pcs	1	1	37	1/2
Fillo, Athens, shredded dough (kataifi)	2 oz	0	0	22	0/2
Hamburger bun, Alvarado Street Bakery, sprouted wheat	1	3	4	27	4/2
Hamburger bun, Arnold, white	1	1	4	30	4/2
Hamburger bun, Fiber One	1	5	4	25	4/2
Hamburger bun, Food for Life, Ezekiel 4:9, sprouted grain	1	6	0	32	0/2
Hamburger bun, Food for Life, Ezekiel 4:9, sprouted grain, sesame	1	6	0	32	0/2
Hamburger bun, Oroweat, country potato	1	2	5	36	5/2
Hamburger bun, Oroweat, golden seeded	1	2	5	34	5/2
Hamburger bun, Oroweat, 100% whole wheat, whole grain	1	7	3	32	3/2
Hamburger bun, Oroweat, onion	1	2	6	35	6/2
Hamburger bun, Pepperidge Farm, classic	1	1	3	22	3/2
Hamburger bun, Pepperidge Farm, classic 100% whole grain white	1	2	2	18	2/1
Hamburger bun, Pepperidge Farm, classic 100% whole wheat	1	2	3	18	3/1
Hamburger bun, Sara Lee, wheat	1	1	3	22	3/2
Hamburger bun, Sara Lee, white	1	1	4	23	4/2
Hamburger bun, Wonder, wheat	1	2	4	21	4/2
Hamburger bun, Wonder, white	1	1	3	21	3/2
Hot dog bun, Alvarado Street Bakery, sprouted wheat	1	3	4	27	4/2
Hot dog bun, Arnold, Chicago	1	1	3	25	3/2
Hot dog bun, Arnold, New England	1	1	3	23	3/2
Hot dog bun, Arnold, potato	1	1	4	28	4/2
Hot dog bun, Arnold, wheat	1	2	5	25	5/2
Hot dog bun, Arnold, white	1	1	4	26	4/2
Hot dog bun, Fiber One	1	5	4	25	4/2
Hot dog bun, Food for Life, Ezekiel 4:9, sprouted grain	1	6	0	34	0/2
Hot dog bun, Oroweat, country potato	1	0	2	19	2/1
Hot dog bun, Oroweat, 100% whole wheat, whole grain	1	6	2	28	2/2
Hot dog bun, Pepperidge Farm, classic	1	0	4	26	4/2
Hot dog bun, Pepperidge Farm, classic whole grain white	1	2	2	21	2/2
Hot dog bun, Sara Lee, wheat	1	1	3	22	3/2
Hot dog bun, Sara Lee, white	1	1	4	22	4/2
Hot dog bun, Sara Lee, white, whole grain	1	1	4	22	4/2
Hot dog bun, Wonder, wheat	1	2	4	21	4/2
Hot dog bun, Wonder, white	1	1	3	21	3/2
Matzo, plain	1 pc	1	0	23	0/2
Matzo, Manischewitz, egg	1 pc	1	2	28	2/2
Matzo, Manischewitz, thin unsalted	1 pc	0	1	20	1/1
Matzo, Manischewitz, whole wheat	1 pc	3	1	21	1/2
Pie crust, Arrowhead Mills, graham cracker, 9"	⅛ cst	0	6	14	6/1
Pie crust, Nilla	⅙ cst	0	10	18	10/1
Pie crust, Oreo	⅙ cst	1	9	19	9/1
Pie crust, Pillsbury, 9"	⅛ cst	0	1	9	1/1
Pie crust, Pillsbury, deep dish, 9"	⅛ cst	0	1	11	1/1

BREADS, WRAPS & GRAINS, cont'd.

FOOD	Svg Size	Fbr	Sgr	Cbs	S/C Val
Pita, white, 6.5" diameter	1	1	1	33	1/2
Pita, whole wheat, 6.5" diameter	1	5	1	35	1/2
Pita, Food for Life, Ezekiel 4:9, prophets pocket	1	6	1	24	1/2
Pizza crust, Alvarado Street Bakery, California style pizza bread	⅛ cst	1	1	35	1/2
Pizza crust, Boboli, 100% whole wheat 8"	½ cst	6	3	34	3/2
Pizza crust, Boboli, 100% whole wheat 12"	⅙ cst	4	2	22	2/2
Pizza crust, Boboli, original 8"	½ cst	1	1	35	1/2
Pizza crust, Boboli, original 12"	⅙ cst	1	1	32	1/2
Pizza crust, Boboli, thin 12"	⅙ cst	0	0	23	0/2
Pizza crust, Pillsbury, classic	⅙ cst	0	4	31	4/2
Puff pastry, Pepperidge Farm, sheet	⅙ pc	0	1	14	1/1
Puff pastry, Pepperidge Farm, shell	1 pc	0	1	16	1/1
Roll, dinner, egg	1	1	2	18	2/1
Roll, dinner, plain	1	1	2	15	2/1
Roll, dinner, rye	1	2	0	19	0/1
Roll, dinner, wheat	1	1	0	13	0/1
Roll, dinner, whole wheat	1	2	2	14	2/1
Roll, French	1	1	0	19	0/1
Roll, pumpernickel	1	2	0	15	0/1
Roll, Alvarado Street Bakery, sprouted wheat	1	2	2	15	2/1
Roll, Arnold, dinner	1	0	3	21	3/2
Roll, Arnold, French	1	2	2	43	2/3
Roll, Arnold, steak	1	1	2	37	2/2
Roll, King's Hawaiian, Hawaiian sweet	1	1	7	18	7/1
Roll, King's Hawaiian, honey wheat	1	1	4	15	4/1
Roll, King's Hawaiian, savory butter	1	1	3	15	3/1
Roll, Oroweat, country potato	1	1	3	23	3/2
Roll, Oroweat, Hawaiian	1	1	7	25	7/2
Roll, Oroweat, 100% whole wheat	1	3	3	17	3/1
Roll, Pepperidge Farm, dinner rolls, soft country style	1	1	3	17	3/1
Roll, Pillsbury, cinnamon	1	0	9	23	9/2
Roll, Pillsbury, cinnamon, Grands!	1	1	23	54	23/3
Roll, Pillsbury, cinnamon, mini-bites	3	0	11	26	11/2
Roll, Pillsbury, crescent, big & buttery	1	0	4	20	4/1
Roll, Pillsbury, crescent, big & flaky	1	0	4	20	4/1
Roll, Pillsbury, crescent, original	1	0	2	11	2/1
Roll, Pillsbury, crescent, reduced fat	1	0	2	12	2/1
Roll, Pillsbury, dinner	1	0	3	20	3/1
Roll, Sara Lee, dinner rolls, classic	1	1	4	21	4/2
Roll, Sara Lee, dinner rolls, wheat & honey	1	1	3	20	3/1
Taco shells, Mission	3	2	0	20	0/1
Taco shells, Old El Paso	3	1	0	19	0/1
Tortilla, corn	1	2	0	11	0/1
Tortilla, flour, 10"	1	2	1	36	1/2

FOOD	Svg Size	Fbr	Sgr	Cbs	S/C Val
Tortilla, Alvarado Street Bakery, sprouted wheat, burrito size	1	6	0	30	0/2
Tortilla, Alvarado Street Bakery, sprouted wheat, fajita size	1	1	0	23	0/2
Tortilla, Food for Life, brown rice	1	2	0	24	0/2
Tortilla, Food for Life, sprouted corn	2	6	0	25	0/2
Tortilla, La Tortilla Factory, white corn	1	1	0	14	0/1
Tortilla, La Tortilla Factory, yellow corn	1	1	0	14	0/1
Tortilla, La Tortilla Factory, Smart & Delicious, low carb, large whole wheat	1	12	1	18	1/1
Tortilla, La Tortilla Factory, Smart & Delicious, low carb, original whole wheat	1	7	0	10	0/1
Tortilla, La Tortilla Factory, Smart & Delicious, 100 calorie, traditional	1	8	3	24	3/2
Tortilla, La Tortilla Factory, Smart & Delicious, 100 calorie, whole wheat	1	8	3	24	3/2
Tortilla, Mission, flour, 8"	1	1	1	25	1/2
Tortilla, Mission, flour, 8", fat free, heart healthy	1	3	2	26	2/2
Tortilla, Mission, flour, 10"	1	1	2	36	2/2
Tortilla, Mission, flour, 10", fat free, heart healthy	1	5	2	35	2/2
Tortilla, Mission, flour, Carb Balance, fajita size	1	7	1	12	1/1
Tortilla, Mission, white corn	2	3	2	22	2/2
Tortilla, Mission, whole wheat, Carb Balance, fajita size	1	8	0	12	0/1
Tortilla, Mission, yellow corn, extra thin	2	2	2	16	2/1
Tortilla, Tumaro's, garden spinach & vegetables, 8"	1	1	0	23	0/2
Tortilla, Tumaro's, honey wheat, 8"	1	2	0	23	0/2
Tortilla, Tumaro's, premium white, 8"	1	0	0	23	0/2
Tortilla, Tumaro's, sun-dried tomato & basil, 8"	1	1	0	23	0/2
Tostada shells, Old El Paso	3	1	0	19	0/1
Wrap, La Tortilla Factory, Smart & Delicious, gluten free, dark teff	1	3	0	31	0/2
Wrap, La Tortilla Factory, Smart & Delicious, gluten free, ivory teff	1	3	0	30	0/2
Wrap, La Tortilla Factory, SoftWraps, multigrain	1	12	1	18	1/1
Wrap, La Tortilla Factory, SoftWraps, traditional	1	13	0	20	0/1
Wrap, La Tortilla Factory, SoftWraps, whole grain	1	5	1	28	1/2
Wrap, Mission, multigrain	1	7	2	32	2/2
Wrap, Mission, original	1	4	3	35	3/2
Wrap, Tumaro's, honey wheat, 10"	1	2	0	34	0/2
Wrap, Tumaro's, sun-dried tomato & basil, 10"	1	1	1	34	1/2
Waffles, Eggo, blueberry	2	0	6	29	6/2
Waffles, Eggo, blueberry, Nutri-Grain	2	3	7	31	7/2
Waffles, Eggo, buttermilk	2	1	2	26	2/2
Waffles, Eggo, homestyle	2	0	2	27	2/2
Waffles, Eggo, low fat, Nutri-Grain	2	3	3	27	3/2
Waffles, Eggo, whole wheat, Nutri-Grain	2	3	3	26	3/2
Waffles, Kashi, Golean, blueberry	2	6	4	33	4/2
Waffles, Kashi, Golean, original	2	6	4	33	4/2
Waffles, Kashi, Golean, strawberry flax	2	6	5	31	5/2
Waffles, Kashi, Heart to Heart, original	2	3	6	31	6/2

FOOD	Svg Size	Fbr	Sgr	Cbs	S/C Val
BREAD CRUMBS, COATINGS & STUFFING					
Bread coating, Don's Chuck Wagon, all purpose batter	¼ c	1	0	20	0/1
Bread coating, Kraft, Shake 'n Bake, barbecue glaze	⅛ pkt	0	5	9	5/1
Bread coating, Kraft, Shake 'n Bake, garlic & herb	⅛ pkt	0	1	7	1/1
Bread coating, Kraft, Shake 'n Bake, hot & spicy	⅛ pkt	0	0	7	0/1
Bread coating, Kraft, Shake 'n Bake, Italian	⅛ pkt	0	0	7	0/1
Bread coating, Kraft, Shake 'n Bake, original chicken	⅛ pkt	0	1	7	1/1
Bread coating, Kraft, Shake 'n Bake, Parmesan crusted	⅛ pkt	0	1	7	1/1
Bread coating, Oven Fry, extra crispy chicken	2 T	0	2	10	2/1
Bread coating, Oven Fry, extra crispy pork	2 T	0	1	11	1/1
Bread coating, Oven Fry, fish fry	1½ T	0	0	9	0/1
Bread coating, Oven Fry, home style flour	1½ T	0	0	7	0/1
Bread coating, Zatarain's, Bake & Crisp, chicken	2 T	0	0	9	0/1
Bread coating, Zatarain's, Bake & Crisp, pork	2 T	0	0	10	0/1
Bread coating, Zatarain's, Bake & Crisp, seafood	2 T	0	0	9	0/1
Bread coating, Zatarain's, chicken frying mix	4 T	0	0	16	0/1
Crumbs, bread, dry, grated, plain	¼ c	1	2	19	2/1
Crumbs, bread, Progresso, garlic & herb	¼ c	1	2	20	2/1
Crumbs, bread, Progresso, Italian style	¼ c	1	2	20	2/1
Crumbs, bread, Progresso, Parmesan	¼ c	1	2	19	2/1
Crumbs, bread, Progresso, plain	¼ c	1	2	20	2/1
Crumbs, corn flake, Kellogg's	6 T	0	3	29	3/2
Crumbs, graham cracker, Honey-Maid	2½ T	0	4	13	4/1
Crumbs, graham cracker, Keebler	3 T	1	3	13	3/1
Crumbs, matzo, Manischewitz, Italian herb	¼ c	0	1	22	1/2
Crumbs, panko, Kikkoman	¼ c	0	1	12	1/1
Crumbs, panko, Progresso, Italian	¼ c	0	0	16	0/1
Crumbs, panko, Progresso, plain	¼ c	0	1	19	1/1
Crumbs, saltine crackers, crushed	½ c	1	1	26	1/2
Stuffing, Arnold, cornbread	¾ c	0	2	19	2/1
Stuffing, Arnold, seasoned	¾ c	0	1	20	1/1
Stuffing, Arnold, unspiced	¾ c	0	2	20	2/1
Stuffing, Arrowhead Mills, savory herb	½ c	1	0	20	0/1
Stuffing, Arrowhead Mills, Stuffing Express, garlic herb	½ c	0	0	20	0/1
Stuffing, Kraft, Stove Top, chicken, as prepared	½ c	1	2	20	2/1
Stuffing, Kraft, Stove Top, cornbread, as prepared	½ c	1	2	22	2/2
Stuffing, Kraft, Stove Top, savory herbs, as prepared	½ c	1	2	21	2/2
Stuffing, Kraft, Stove Top, traditional sage, as prepared	½ c	1	2	21	2/2
Stuffing, Kraft, Stove Top, turkey, as prepared	½ c	1	2	21	2/2
Stuffing, Zatarain's, cornbread, as prepared	½ c	0	2	21	2/2
Stuffing, Zatarain's, Creole chicken, as prepared	½ c	1	2	20	2/1
Stuffing, Zatarain's, French bread, as prepared	½ c	1	2	20	2/1

FOOD	Svg Size	Fbr	Sgr	Cbs	S/C Val
FLOURS & GRAINS					
Amaranth, uncooked	½ c	7	2	63	2/4
Arrowroot flour	¼ c	1	0	28	0/2
Barley, hulled	½ c	16	1	68	1/4
Barley, pearled, uncooked	½ c	16	1	78	1/4
Barley flour	½ c	8	1	55	1/3
Buckwheat	¼ c	4	1	30	1/2
Buckwheat flour	½ c	6	2	42	2/3
Bulgur, uncooked	¼ c	6	0	27	0/2
Carob flour	¼ c	10	13	23	13/2
Chickpea flour	½ c	5	5	27	5/2
Corn flour, white, masa	½ c	6	0	43	0/3
Corn flour, white, whole grain	½ c	4	0	45	0/3
Corn flour, yellow, whole grain	½ c	4	0	45	0/3
Cornmeal, white, whole grain	½ c	5	0	47	0/3
Cornmeal, yellow, whole grain	½ c	5	0	47	0/3
Flaxseed, ground	1 T	2	0	2	0/0
Flaxseed, whole	1 t	1	0	1	0/0
Kamut, uncooked	½ c	9	8	65	8/4
Millet, uncooked	½ c	9	0	73	0/4
Oat bran, uncooked	½ c	7	1	31	1/2
Oats, uncooked	½ c	8	0	52	0/3
Peanut flour	½ c	5	2	10	2/1
Potato flour	½ c	5	3	66	3/4
Quinoa, whole grain, uncooked	¼ c	3	1	28	1/2
Rice bran, crude	1 c	25	1	59	1/3
Rice flour, brown	½ c	4	1	60	1/3
Rice flour, white	½ c	2	0	63	0/4
Rye	½ c	13	1	64	1/4
Rye flour, dark	½ c	15	1	44	1/3
Rye flour, light	½ c	4	0	39	0/2
Rye flour, medium	½ c	6	1	38	1/2
Soy flour, defatted	½ c	9	10	29	10/2
Soy flour, full fat, raw	½ c	4	3	15	3/1
Soy flour, full fat, roasted	½ c	4	3	15	3/1
Soy flour, low fat	½ c	7	5	15	5/1
Soy flour, Arrowhead Mills, organic	¼ c	4	0	9	0/1
Spelt, uncooked	¼ c	5	3	31	3/2
Tapioca flour	¼ c	0	0	26	0/2
Teff, uncooked	¼ c	4	1	35	1/2
Wheat bran, crude	¼ c	6	0	9	0/1
Wheat flour, white, all purpose	½ c	2	0	48	0/3
Wheat flour, white, bread	½ c	2	0	50	0/3
Wheat flour, white, cake	½ c	1	0	53	0/3

FOOD	Svg Size	Fbr	Sgr	Cbs	S/C Val
Wheat flour, whole grain	½ c	7	0	44	0/3
Wheat germ, raw	2 T	2	0	10	0/1
BAKING MIXES					
All purpose, Arrowhead Mills	⅓ c	2	2	28	2/2
All purpose, Arrowhead Mills, gluten free	¼ c	0	0	32	0/2
All purpose, Bisquick	⅓ c	1	1	26	1/2
All purpose, Bisquick, Heart Smart	⅓ c	1	3	27	3/2
All purpose, Bob's Red Mill, gluten free	⅓ c	2	2	25	2/2
All purpose, Bob's Red Mill, low carb	¼ c	5	0	11	0/1
All purpose, Hodgson Mill	¼ c	3	0	22	0/2
All purpose, "Jiffy"	¼ c	0	0	21	0/2
Biscuit, Bisquick Complete, buttermilk	⅓ c	0	1	21	1/2
Biscuit, Bisquick Complete, honey butter	⅓ c	0	5	24	5/2
Biscuit, "Jiffy," buttermilk	⅓ c	0	2	27	2/2
Bread, Betty Crocker, banana	1/12 pkg	0	13	25	13/2
Bread, Bob's Red Mill, low carb	1/21 pkg	4	0	9	0/1
Bread, Bob's Red Mill, whole wheat	1/13 pkg	2	3	27	3/2
Bread, Hodgson Mill, gluten free	¼ c	3	3	26	3/2
Bread, Hodgson Mill, honey whole wheat	¼ c	2	2	22	2/2
Bread, Hodgson Mill, white	¼ c	1	2	22	2/2
Corn bread, Aunt Jemima, easy mix	⅓ c	1	5	24	5/2
Corn bread & muffin, Arrowhead Mills	¼ c	2	3	25	3/2
Corn bread & muffin, Betty Crocker	3 T	0	5	24	5/2
Corn bread & muffin, Hodgson Mill	¼ c	3	5	27	5/2
Corn muffin, "Jiffy"	¼ c	0	7	27	7/2
Latkes, Manischewitz	3 T	2	1	18	1/1
Latkes, Streit's	3 T	1	0	20	0/1
Latkes, Streit's, vegetable potato pancake mix	3 T	2	1	19	1/1
Matzo ball, Manischewitz	2 T	1	0	11	0/1
Matzo ball, Streit's	2 T	0	0	12	0/1
Muffin, Betty Crocker, apple streusel, box	¼ c	0	20	37	20/2
Muffin, Betty Crocker, banana nut, box	3 T	0	14	27	14/2
Muffin, Betty Crocker, blueberry, pouch	⅙ pkg	0	11	23	11/2
Muffin, Betty Crocker, lemon poppy seed, pouch	⅙ pkg	0	10	22	10/2
Muffin, Duncan Hines, apple cinnamon, whole grain	1/12 pkg	3	17	33	17/2
Muffin, Duncan Hines, blueberry streusel, whole grain	1/12 pkg	3	19	32	19/2
Muffin, Fiber One, apple cinnamon	¼ c	5	14	29	14/2
Muffin, Fiber One, banana nut	¼ c	5	12	27	12/2
Muffin, Fiber One, blueberry	¼ c	5	13	28	13/2
Pancake, Aunt Jemima, buttermilk	¼ c	1	4	23	4/2
Pancake, Aunt Jemima, original	¼ c	1	7	33	7/2
Pancake, Aunt Jemima, whole wheat	¼ c	3	4	26	4/2
Pancake, Bisquick, Shake 'n Pour	⅓ pkg	1	7	42	7/3
Pancake, Fiber One, buttermilk	½ c	5	4	36	4/2

BREADS, WRAPS & GRAINS, cont'd.

FOOD	Svg Size	Fbr	Sgr	Cbs	S/C Val
Pancake, Fiber One, original	½ c	5	4	36	4/2
Pancake, Krusteaz, buttermilk	½ c	2	6	40	6/2
Pancake, Krusteaz, buttermilk, fat free	½ c	6	8	46	8/3
Pancake, Krusteaz, oat bran, low fat	½ c	4	10	45	10/3
Pancake, Krusteaz, original	½ c	1	5	32	5/2
Pancake, Krusteaz, wheat & honey	½ c	4	6	42	6/3
Pancake & waffle, Arrowhead Mills, buttermilk	¼ c	2	4	27	4/2
Pancake & waffle, Arrowhead Mills, gluten free	¼ c	0	1	36	1/2
Pancake & waffle, Arrowhead Mills, multigrain	¼ c	3	2	27	2/2
Pancake & waffle, Bob's Red Mill, buttermilk	⅓ c	4	3	27	3/2
Pancake & waffle, Bob's Red Mill, high fiber	⅓ c	5	1	26	1/2
Pancake & waffle, Hodgson Mill, gluten free	¼ c	3	0	30	0/2
Pancake & waffle, "Jiffy," buttermilk	⅓ c	0	8	30	8/2
Pie crust, Betty Crocker	¹⁄₁₆ pkg	0	0	19	0/1
Pie crust, "Jiffy"	¹⁄₁₆ pkg	0	0	8	0/1
Pie crust, Krusteaz	2 T	0	0	10	0/1
Pizza crust, Arrowhead Mills	¹⁄₁₂ pkg	1	2	30	2/2
Pizza crust, Arrowhead Mills, gluten free	¹⁄₁₂ pkg	0	2	33	2/2
Pizza crust, Betty Crocker	¼ pkg	1	2	33	2/2
Pizza crust, Hodgson Mill, gluten free	⅛ pkg	2	1	45	1/3
Pizza crust, "Jiffy"	⅕ pkg	0	1	26	1/2
Waffle, Krusteaz, Belgian	½ c	3	12	40	12/2

PASTA & RICE

FOOD	Svg Size	Fbr	Sgr	Cbs	S/C Val
PASTA					
Agnolotti, Buitoni, quattro formaggi	1 c	2	2	35	2/2
Agnolotti, Buitoni, wild mushroom	1 c	3	4	39	4/2
Angel hair, fresh, Buitoni	1¼ c	2	1	43	1/3
Chow mein, cooked	1 c	2	0	26	0/2
Corn pasta, dry, De Boles, gluten free, all varieties	2 oz	5	0	43	0/3
Couscous, cooked	1 c	2	0	37	0/2
Couscous, dry	1 oz	1	0	20	0/1
Egg noodles, cooked	1 c	2	1	40	1/2
Egg noodles, dry	1 oz	1	1	20	1/1
Egg noodles, spinach, cooked	1 c	4	1	39	1/2
Egg noodles, Manischewitz, wide	2 c	2	2	39	2/2
Fettuccine, dry, Food for Life, Ezekiel 4:9, sprouted whole grain	2 oz	7	0	39	0/2
Fettuccine, fresh, Buitoni	1¼ c	2	1	46	1/3
Jerusalem artichoke pasta, dry, De Boles, most varieties	2 oz	1	2	41	2/3
Jerusalem artichoke pasta, dry, De Boles, garlic & parsley	2 oz	2	2	41	2/3
Jerusalem artichoke pasta, dry, De Boles, tomato & basil	2 oz	2	2	41	2/3
Jerusalem artichoke pasta, dry, De Boles, organic, most varieties	2 oz	1	2	43	2/3

FOOD	Svg Size	Fbr	Sgr	Cbs	S/C Val
Jerusalem artichoke pasta, dry, De Boles, organic, w/ spinach	2 oz	3	1	43	1/3
Linguine, fresh, Buitoni	1¼ c	2	1	45	1/3
Linguine, fresh, Buitoni, 100% whole wheat	1¼ c	6	1	41	1/3
Macaroni, cooked	1 c	2	1	41	1/3
Macaroni, dry	1 oz	1	1	21	1/2
Macaroni, whole wheat, cooked	1 c	4	1	37	1/2
Multigrain pasta, dry, De Boles, gluten free, all varieties	2 oz	3	0	46	0/3
Penne, dry, Food for Life, Ezekiel 4:9, sprouted whole grain	2 oz	7	0	39	0/2
Ravioli, Buitoni, chicken & prosciutto, 100% whole wheat	1¼ c	4	3	37	3/2
Ravioli, Buitoni, four cheese	1¼ c	3	3	45	3/3
Ravioli, Buitoni, four cheese, light	1¼ c	2	3	41	3/3
Ravioli, Buitoni, four cheese, 100% whole wheat	1¼ c	5	3	40	3/2
Ravioli, Buitoni, spicy beef & sausage	1 c	3	3	40	3/2
Ravioli, Pasta Prima, spinach & mozzarella	1 c	4	0	29	0/2
Rice noodles, dry	1 oz	1	0	24	0/2
Rice pasta, dry, De Boles, gluten free, most varieties	2 oz	0	0	46	0/3
Rice pasta, dry, De Boles, gluten free, w/ golden flax	2 oz	1	0	44	0/3
Soba noodles, dry	1 oz	1	0	21	0/2
Spaghetti, cooked	1 c	3	1	43	1/3
Spaghetti, dry	1 oz	1	1	21	1/2
Spaghetti, dry, Food for Life, Ezekiel 4:9, sprouted whole grain	2 oz	7	0	33	0/2
Spaghetti, whole wheat, cooked	1 c	6	1	37	1/2
Spinach pasta, dry	2 oz	6	2	43	2/3
Tofu shirataki, House Foods, angel hair	4 oz	2	0	3	0/0
Tofu shirataki, House Foods, fettuccine	4 oz	2	0	3	0/0
Tofu shirataki, House Foods, spaghetti	4 oz	2	0	3	0/0
Tortellini, Buitoni, herb chicken	1 c	3	3	49	3/3
Tortellini, Buitoni, spinach cheese	1 c	3	4	49	4/3
Tortellini, Buitoni, three cheese	1 c	3	4	50	4/3
Tortellini, Buitoni, three cheese, 100% whole wheat	1 c	8	3	44	3/3
Tortelloni, Buitoni, cheese & roasted garlic	1 c	2	3	37	3/2
Tortelloni, Buitoni, chicken & prosciutto	1 c	2	3	46	3/3
Tortelloni, Buitoni, sweet Italian sausage	1 c	3	6	48	6/3
Udon noodles, dry	2 oz	1	0	40	0/2
Whole wheat pasta, dry, De Boles, most varieties	2 oz	5	2	42	2/3
Whole wheat pasta, dry, De Boles, w/ golden flax	2 oz	6	0	38	0/2

PASTA MIXES & SIDE DISHES

FOOD	Svg Size	Fbr	Sgr	Cbs	S/C Val
Back to Nature, macaroni & cheese	½ pkg	1	6	48	6/3
Back to Nature, 100% whole wheat macaroni & white cheddar	½ pkg	7	6	47	6/3
Back to Nature, organic macaroni & cheese	½ pkg	2	8	49	8/3
Back to Nature, organic shells & cheddar	½ pkg	2	10	58	10/3
Back to Nature, organic shells & white cheddar	½ pkg	2	8	49	8/3
Bowl Appétit!, cheddar broccoli pasta	1 pkg	2	8	52	8/3
Bowl Appétit!, homestyle chicken flavored pasta	1 pkg	2	2	44	2/3

PASTA & RICE, cont'd.

FOOD	Svg Size	Fbr	Sgr	Cbs	S/C Val
Bowl Appétit!, pasta Alfredo	1 pkg	2	9	55	9/3
Chicken Helper, creamy chicken & noodles, as prepared	1 c	0	1	20	1/1
Chicken Helper, fettuccine Alfredo, as prepared	1 c	1	1	26	1/2
Hamburger Helper, beef pasta, as prepared	1 c	1	1	21	1/2
Hamburger Helper, cheeseburger macaroni, as prepared	1 c	0	2	23	2/2
Hamburger Helper, cheesy jambalaya, as prepared	1 c	1	2	25	2/2
Hamburger Helper, lasagna, as prepared	1 c	0	4	25	4/2
Hamburger Helper, Salisbury, as prepared	1 c	0	1	24	1/2
Hamburger Helper, spaghetti, as prepared	1 c	1	5	27	5/2
Hamburger Helper, tomato basil penne, as prepared	1 c	1	6	31	6/2
Healthy Choice, Fresh Mixers, chicken cacciatore	1 pkg	6	3	49	3/3
Healthy Choice, Fresh Mixers, rotini & zesty marinara sauce	1 pkg	7	11	56	11/3
Healthy Choice, Fresh Mixers, steak portobello	1 pkg	5	4	42	4/3
Healthy Choice, Fresh Mixers, Szechwan beef w/ Asian style noodles	1 pkg	4	18	65	18/4
Healthy Choice, Fresh Mixers, Tuscan style chicken	1 pkg	6	4	50	4/3
Healthy Choice, Fresh Mixers, ziti & meat sauce	1 pkg	8	10	56	10/3
Knorr, Italian Sides, scampi	½ pkg	12	2	13	2/1
Knorr, Italian Sides, tomato Parmesan	½ pkg	8	4	14	4/1
Knorr, Pasta Sides, Alfredo	½ pkg	4	3	13	3/1
Knorr, Pasta Sides, butter	½ pkg	4	4	14	4/1
Knorr, Pasta Sides, cheddar broccoli	½ pkg	8	4	16	4/1
Knorr, Pasta Sides, stroganoff	½ pkg	4	2	13	2/1
Kraft Easy Mac, cup, Alfredo	2 oz	1	6	39	6/2
Kraft Easy Mac, cup, original	2 oz	1	6	39	6/2
Kraft Easy Mac, packet, original	1 pkt	1	5	42	5/3
Kraft Easy Mac, packet, original, Big Packs	1 pkt	2	8	63	8/4
Kraft Macaroni & Cheese, cheesy Alfredo	2.5 oz	2	7	50	7/3
Kraft Macaroni & Cheese, The Cheesiest	2.5 oz	1	6	48	6/3
Kraft Macaroni & Cheese, thick 'n creamy	2.5 oz	2	8	50	8/3
Kraft Macaroni & Cheese, three cheese	2.5 oz	1	7	50	7/3
Kraft Macaroni & Cheese, white cheddar	2.5 oz	2	7	48	7/3
Kraft Macaroni & Cheese Deluxe, four cheese	3.5 oz	2	3	46	3/3
Kraft Macaroni & Cheese Deluxe, original cheddar, family size	3.5 oz	2	4	44	4/3
Kraft Macaroni & Cheese Deluxe, 2% milk cheese, ½ the fat	3.5 oz	2	6	50	6/3
Kraft Velveeta, rotini & cheese, box, broccoli	4.4 oz	2	6	49	6/3
Kraft Velveeta, rotini & cheese, cup, broccoli	2 oz	1	3	30	3/2
Kraft Velveeta, shells & cheese, box, original	4 oz	2	4	49	4/3
Kraft Velveeta, shells & cheese, box, 2% milk	4 oz	2	7	58	7/3
Kraft Velveeta, shells & cheese, cup, original	2 oz	1	3	29	3/2
Kraft Velveeta, shells & cheese, cup, 2% milk	2 oz	1	4	31	4/2
Pasta Roni, angel hair pasta w/ herbs, as prepared	1 c	2	6	41	6/3
Pasta Roni, butter & garlic, as prepared	1 c	2	4	39	4/2
Pasta Roni, cheddar macaroni, as prepared	1 c	1	4	37	4/2
Pasta Roni, fettuccine Alfredo, as prepared	1 c	2	5	44	5/3

FOOD	Svg Size	Fbr	Sgr	Cbs	S/C Val
Pasta Roni, stroganoff, as prepared	1 c	2	7	48	7/3
Pasta Roni, tomato Parmesan, as prepared	1 c	2	8	40	8/2
Suddenly Salad, Caesar, as prepared	1 c	1	3	38	3/2
Suddenly Salad, classic, as prepared	¾ c	1	4	38	4/2
Suddenly Salad, creamy Italian, as prepared	¾ c	2	4	36	4/2
Suddenly Salad, ranch & bacon, as prepared	¾ c	1	4	34	4/2
Tuna Helper, creamy broccoli, as prepared	1 c	1	2	25	2/2
Tuna Helper, creamy pasta, as prepared	1 c	1	1	21	1/2
Tuna Helper, fettuccine Alfredo, as prepared	1 c	1	1	22	1/2
Tuna Helper, tuna melt, as prepared	1 c	0	2	26	2/2
Zatarain's, gumbo pasta dinner, as prepared	1 c	2	0	23	0/2
Zatarain's, jambalaya pasta dinner, as prepared	1 c	2	1	28	1/2

RICE & RICE DISHES

FOOD	Svg Size	Fbr	Sgr	Cbs	S/C Val
Bowl Appétit!, cheddar broccoli rice	1 pkg	2	6	52	6/3
Bowl Appétit!, herb chicken vegetable flavored rice	1 pkg	2	2	51	2/3
Bowl Appétit!, teriyaki rice	1 pkg	2	6	57	6/3
Healthy Choice, Fresh Mixers, sesame teriyaki chicken	1 pkg	3	16	69	16/4
Healthy Choice, Fresh Mixers, Southwestern style chicken	1 pkg	5	3	60	3/3
Healthy Choice, Fresh Mixers, sweet & sour chicken	1 pkg	5	22	78	22/4
Healthy Choice, Fresh Mixers, sweet hickory BBQ chicken	1 pkg	5	6	70	6/4
Knorr, Asian Sides, chicken fried rice, as prepared	1 c	4	2	16	2/1
Knorr, Asian Sides, teriyaki rice, as prepared	1 c	4	4	17	4/1
Knorr, Rice Sides, chicken broccoli, as prepared	1 c	4	1	17	1/1
Knorr, Rice Sides, mushroom, as prepared	1 c	4	1	17	1/1
Knorr, Rice Sides, rice medley, as prepared	1 c	4	0	15	0/1
Knorr, Rice Sides, rice pilaf, as prepared	1 c	4	0	15	0/1
Rice, brown, long grain, cooked	1 c	4	1	45	1/3
Rice, white, glutinous, cooked	1 c	2	0	37	0/2
Rice, white, long grain, cooked	1 c	1	0	45	0/3
Rice, wild, cooked	1 c	3	1	35	1/2
Rice-A-Roni, broccoli au gratin, as prepared	1 c	2	3	46	3/3
Rice-A-Roni, chicken & broccoli, as prepared	1 c	2	2	40	2/2
Rice-A-Roni, chicken & mushroom, as prepared	1 c	2	3	51	3/3
Rice-A-Roni, chicken teriyaki, as prepared	1 c	2	2	40	2/2
Rice-A-Roni, fried rice, as prepared	1 c	2	4	50	4/3
Rice-A-Roni, red beans & rice, as prepared	1 c	5	3	52	3/3
Uncle Ben's, Country Inn, chicken & broccoli	⅓ pkg	1	1	42	1/3
Uncle Ben's, Country Inn, rice pilaf	⅓ pkg	1	1	43	1/3
Uncle Ben's, Ready Rice, Spanish style	½ pkg	3	3	41	3/3
Uncle Ben's, Ready Rice, teriyaki style	½ pkg	3	2	42	2/3
Uncle Ben's, Ready Whole Grain Medley, Santa Fe	½ pkg	5	1	42	1/3
Uncle Ben's, Ready Whole Grain Medley, vegetable harvest	½ pkg	5	2	44	2/3
Uncle Ben's, whole grain & wild rice, mushroom recipe	⅓ pkg	3	3	42	3/3
Zatarain's, black beans & rice, as prepared	1 c	6	0	47	0/3

PASTA & RICE, cont'd.

FOOD	Svg Size	Fbr	Sgr	Cbs	S/C Val
Zatarain's, black-eyed peas & rice, as prepared	1 c	4	0	46	0/3
Zatarain's, gumbo mix w/ rice, as prepared	1 c	0	0	16	0/1
Zatarain's, jambalaya mix, as prepared	1 c	1	0	30	0/2
Zatarain's, red beans & rice, as prepared	1 c	5	0	40	0/2

CEREALS

FOOD	Svg Size	Fbr	Sgr	Cbs	S/C Val
COLD CEREALS					
All-Bran, Kellogg's, Bran Buds	⅓ c	13	8	24	8/2
All-Bran, Kellogg's, Complete wheat flakes	¾ c	5	5	23	5/2
All-Bran, Kellogg's, original	½ c	10	6	23	6/2
All-Bran, Kellogg's, strawberry medley	1 c	10	10	44	10/3
Alpha-Bits, Post	1 c	2	10	23	10/2
Apple Caramel Pecan Crunch, Post	1 c	5	10	41	10/3
Apple Jacks, Kellogg's	1 c	3	12	25	12/2
Autumn Wheat, Kashi	29 pcs	6	7	43	7/3
Aztec Crunchy Corn & Amaranth, Erewhon, organic	1 c	1	1	26	1/2
Banana Nut Crunch, Post	1 c	4	12	44	12/3
Basic 4, General Mills	1 c	3	14	43	14/3
Berry Basic, Sunbelt	½ c	5	12	41	12/3
Blueberry Morning, Post	¼ c	2	16	45	16/3
Boo Berry, General Mills	1 c	1	12	28	12/2
Bran Flakes, Post	¾ c	5	5	24	5/2
Breakfast O's, Barbara's, organic	1 c	2	1	22	1/2
Brown Rice Crisps, Barbara's, organic	1 c	0	2	25	2/2
Cap'n Crunch, Quaker	¾ c	1	12	23	12/2
Cheerios, General Mills, apple cinnamon	¾ c	1	12	25	12/2
Cheerios, General Mills, banana nut	¾ c	1	9	23	9/2
Cheerios, General Mills, chocolate	¾ c	1	9	23	9/2
Cheerios, General Mills, frosted	¾ c	2	10	23	10/2
Cheerios, General Mills, fruity	¾ c	2	9	23	9/2
Cheerios, General Mills, honey nut	¾ c	2	9	22	9/2
Cheerios, General Mills, multigrain	1 c	3	6	23	6/2
Cheerios, General Mills, oat cluster crunch	¾ c	2	8	22	8/2
Cheerios, General Mills, original	1 c	3	1	20	1/1
Chex, General Mills, chocolate	¾ c	0	8	26	8/2
Chex, General Mills, cinnamon	¾ c	0	8	25	8/2
Chex, General Mills, corn	1 c	1	3	26	3/2
Chex, General Mills, honey nut	¾ c	1	9	28	9/2
Chex, General Mills, multi-bran	¾ c	6	10	39	10/2
Chex, General Mills, rice	1 c	0	2	23	2/2
Chex, General Mills, wheat	¾ c	5	5	38	5/2
Cinnamon Harvest, Kashi	28 pcs	5	9	43	9/3

FOOD	Svg Size	Fbr	Sgr	Cbs	S/C Val
Cinnamon Toast Crunch, General Mills	¾ c	1	10	25	10/2
Cocoa Crispy Brown Rice, Erewhon organic	1 c	1	11	44	11/3
Cocoa Krispies, Kellogg's	¾ c	0	12	27	12/2
Cocoa Pebbles, Post	¾ c	0	11	26	11/2
Cocoa Puffs, General Mills	¾ c	2	11	23	11/2
Cocoa Puffs Combos, General Mills, chocolate & vanilla	¾ c	1	11	23	11/2
Cookie Crisp, General Mills	¾ c	1	10	22	10/2
Corn Flakes, Barbara's, organic	1 c	0	3	25	3/2
Corn Flakes, Erewhon, organic, gluten free	1 c	1	0	30	0/2
Corn Flakes, Kellogg's	1 c	1	2	24	2/2
Corn Flakes, Kellogg's, touch of honey	1 c	1	6	27	6/2
Corn Pops, Kellogg's	1 c	3	10	29	10/2
Count Chocula, General Mills	¾ c	1	12	23	12/2
Cracklin' Oat Bran, Kellogg's	¾ c	6	15	35	15/2
Cranberry Almond Crunch, Post	¾ c	3	14	40	14/2
Crispix, Kellogg's	1 c	0	4	25	4/2
Crispy Brown Rice, Erewhon, gluten free, organic	1 c	0	0	25	0/2
Crispy Brown Rice, Erewhon, no salt added, organic	1 c	1	1	25	1/2
Crispy Brown Rice, Erewhon, original, organic	1 c	1	1	25	1/2
Crispy Brown Rice, Erewhon, w/ mixed berries, gluten free	1 c	1	6	27	6/2
Crunchy Corn Bran, Quaker	¾ c	5	6	23	6/2
Cupcake Pebbles, Post	¾ c	0	11	26	11/2
Dora the Explorer, General Mills	¾ c	3	6	23	6/2
Eggo cereal, Kellogg's, maple syrup	1 c	2	12	25	12/2
Ezekiel 4:9, Food for Life, almond	2 oz	6	0	38	0/2
Ezekiel 4:9, Food for Life, golden flax	2 oz	6	0	37	0/2
Ezekiel 4:9, Food for Life, original	2 oz	6	0	40	0/2
Fiber One, General Mills, caramel delight	1 c	9	11	41	11/3
Fiber One, General Mills, frosted shredded wheat	1 c	9	12	50	12/3
Fiber One, General Mills, honey clusters	1 c	13	6	42	6/3
Fiber One, General Mills, original	½ c	14	0	25	0/2
Fiber One, General Mills, raisin bran clusters	1 c	11	13	45	13/3
Franken Berry, General Mills	1 c	1	12	29	12/2
Froot Loops, Kellogg's	1 c	3	12	25	12/2
Froot Loops, Kellogg's, marshmallow	1 c	2	14	25	14/2
Frosted Flakes, Kellogg's	¾ c	1	11	27	11/2
Frosted Flakes, Kellogg's, reduced sugar	1 c	1	8	28	8/2
Frosted Krispies, Kellogg's	¾ c	0	12	27	12/2
Frosted Mini-Wheats, Kellogg's, cinnamon streusel, bite size	24 pcs	5	12	44	12/3
Frosted Mini-Wheats, Kellogg's, honey nut, little bites	46 pcs	6	12	47	12/3
Frosted Mini-Wheats, Kellogg's, maple & brown sugar, bite size	24 pcs	5	13	44	13/3
Frosted Mini-Wheats, Kellogg's, original, big bite	5 pcs	5	10	41	10/3
Frosted Mini-Wheats, Kellogg's, original, bite size	24 pcs	6	12	48	12/3
Frosted Mini-Wheats, Kellogg's, original, little bites	51 pcs	6	12	46	12/3

CEREALS, cont'd.

FOOD	Svg Size	Fbr	Sgr	Cbs	S/C Val
Fruity Pebbles, Post	¾ c	0	11	26	11/2
Golden Crisp, Post	¾ c	0	14	24	14/2
Golden Grahams, General Mills	¾ c	1	11	26	11/2
Golean, Kashi	1 c	10	6	30	6/2
Golean, Kashi, Crisp!, toasted berry crumble	¾ c	8	10	35	10/2
Golean, Kashi, Crunch!	1 c	8	13	37	13/2
Golean, Kashi, Crunch!, honey almond flax	1 c	8	12	36	12/2
Good Friends, Kashi	1 c	12	10	42	10/3
Good Friends, Kashi, cinna-raisin crunch	1 c	8	13	41	13/3
Granola, Bear Naked, fruit & nut	¼ c	2	6	17	6/1
Granola, Bear Naked, mango agave almond	¼ c	2	6	19	6/1
Granola, Bear Naked, maple pecan	¼ c	2	7	22	7/2
Granola, Bear Naked Fit, triple berry crunch	¼ c	3	4	23	4/2
Granola, Bear Naked Fit, vanilla almond crunch	¼ c	2	4	22	4/2
Granola, Kashi, Apple Orchard	½ c	7	11	38	11/2
Granola, Kashi, Cocoa Beach	½ c	7	11	36	11/2
Granola, Kashi, Mountain Medley	½ c	7	12	38	12/2
Granola, Kashi, Summer Berry	½ c	7	9	39	9/2
Granola, Kellogg's, low fat w/o raisins	½ c	3	14	40	14/2
Granola, Kellogg's, low fat w/ raisins	⅔ c	4	17	48	17/3
Granola, Quaker, low fat	⅔ c	3	18	45	18/3
Granola, Quaker, oats & honey	½ c	3	12	35	12/2
Granola, Quaker, oats, honey & raisins	½ c	3	15	38	15/2
Granola, Sunbelt, bananas & almonds	½ c	3	13	39	13/2
Granola, Sunbelt, cinnamon & raisins	⅔ c	4	16	44	16/3
Granola, Sunbelt, raisins, dates & almonds	½ c	3	18	39	18/2
Grape-Nuts, Post	½ c	7	4	48	4/3
Grape-Nuts Flakes, Post	¾ c	3	4	23	4/2
Great Grains, Post, crunchy pecans	¾ c	5	8	37	8/2
Great Grains, Post, raisins, dates & pecans	¾ c	5	14	40	14/2
Heart to Heart, Kashi, honey toasted	¾ c	5	5	25	5/2
Heart to Heart, Kashi, oat flakes & wild blueberry clusters	1 c	4	12	44	12/3
Heart to Heart, Kashi, warm cinnamon	¾ c	5	5	25	5/2
Honey Bunches of Oats, Post, honey roasted	¾ c	2	6	25	6/2
Honey Bunches of Oats, Post, w/ almonds	¾ c	2	6	25	6/2
Honey Bunches of Oats, Post, w/ chocolate bunches	¾ c	2	7	25	7/2
Honey Bunches of Oats, Post, w/ cinnamon clusters	¾ c	2	6	25	6/2
Honey Bunches of Oats, Post, w/ pecan bunches	¾ c	2	5	24	5/2
Honey Bunches of Oats, Post, w/ real peaches	¾ c	2	8	25	8/2
Honey Bunches of Oats, Post, w/ real strawberries	¾ c	2	8	26	8/2
Honey Bunches of Oats, Post, w/ vanilla bunches	1 c	4	12	46	12/3
Honeycomb, Post, cinna-graham	¾ c	2	10	27	10/2
Honeycomb, Post, original	½ c	1	10	28	10/2
Honey Nut Clusters, General Mills	1 c	3	16	49	16/3

FOOD	Svg Size	Fbr	Sgr	Cbs	S/C Val
Honey Nut O's, Barbara's, organic	1 c	1	11	24	11/2
Honey Smacks, Kellogg's	¾ c	1	15	24	15/2
Honey Sunshine, Kashi	¾ c	6	6	25	6/2
Island Vanilla, Kashi	27 pcs	6	9	44	9/3
Just Bunches!, Post, cinnamon	⅔ c	4	14	43	14/3
Just Bunches!, Post, honey roasted	⅔ c	4	14	43	14/3
Kamut Flakes, Erewhon, organic	⅔ c	4	1	25	1/2
Kix, General Mills, berry berry	¾ c	1	8	22	8/2
Kix, General Mills, honey	1¼ c	3	6	28	6/2
Kix, General Mills, original	1¼ c	3	3	25	3/2
Life, Quaker, cinnamon	¾ c	2	8	25	8/2
Life, Quaker, maple & brown sugar	¾ c	2	8	25	8/2
Life, Quaker, original	¾ c	2	6	25	6/2
Lucky Charms, General Mills	¾ c	1	11	22	11/2
Lucky Charms, General Mills, chocolate	¾ c	1	12	24	12/2
Maple Pecan Crunch, Post	¾ c	3	12	40	12/2
Mighty Bites Honey Crunch, Kashi	1 c	3	5	23	5/2
Mini-Wheats, Kellogg's, unfrosted, bite size	30 pcs	6	1	46	1/3
Müeslix, Kellogg's	⅔ c	4	17	40	17/2
Oatmeal Crisp, General Mills, crunchy almond	1 c	4	16	47	16/3
Oatmeal Crisp, General Mills, hearty raisin	1 c	4	20	51	20/3
Oatmeal Squares, Quaker, brown sugar	1 c	5	10	44	10/3
Oatmeal Squares, Quaker, cinnamon	1 c	5	13	47	13/3
Oatmeal Squares, Quaker, golden maple	1 c	4	12	44	12/3
Oh!s, Quaker, honey graham	¾ c	1	12	23	12/2
Organic Wild Puffs, Barbara's, crunchy cocoa	¾ c	2	7	25	7/2
Organic Wild Puffs, Barbara's, fruit medley	¾ c	2	7	26	7/2
Product 19, Kellogg's	1 c	1	4	25	4/2
Puffed Rice, Quaker	1 c	0	0	9	0/1
Puffed Wheat, Quaker	1 c	1	0	11	0/1
Puffins, Barbara's, honey rice	¾ c	1	6	25	6/2
Puffins, Barbara's, multigrain	¾ c	1	6	25	6/2
Puffins, Barbara's, original	¾ c	4	5	23	5/2
Puffins, Barbara's, peanut butter	¾ c	1	6	23	6/2
Raisin Bran, Erewhon, organic	1 c	6	10	40	10/2
Raisin Bran, Kellogg's	1 c	4	20	45	20/3
Raisin Bran, Post	1 c	8	19	46	19/3
Raisin Bran Crunch, Kellogg's	1 c	4	20	45	20/3
Raisin Bran Extra, Kellogg's	1 c	4	20	45	20/3
Raisin Nut Bran, General Mills	¾ c	5	14	38	14/2
Reese's Puffs, General Mills	¾ c	1	11	22	11/2
Rice Krispies, Kellogg's	1¼ c	0	4	29	4/2
Rice Krispies Treats, Kellogg's	¾ c	0	9	26	9/2
Rice Twice, Erewhon, gluten free	¾ c	0	8	26	8/2

FOOD	Svg Size	Fbr	Sgr	Cbs	S/C Val
7 Whole Grain Flakes, Kashi	1 c	6	4	41	4/3
7 Whole Grain Honey Puffs, Kashi	1 c	2	6	25	6/2
7 Whole Grain Nuggets, Kashi	½ c	7	3	47	3/3
7 Whole Grain Puffs, Kashi	1 c	1	0	15	0/1
Shredded Minis, Barbara's, blueberry burst	1 c	3	14	43	14/3
Shredded Oats, Barbara's, cinnamon crunch	1 c	3	15	43	15/3
Shredded Oats, Barbara's, multigrain	¾ c	3	5	24	5/2
Shredded Oats, Barbara's, original	1¼ c	5	12	46	12/3
Shredded Oats, Barbara's, vanilla almond	1 c	4	15	42	15/3
Shredded Wheat, Barbara's	2 pcs	5	0	31	0/2
Shredded Wheat, Post, honey nut, spoon size	1 c	5	12	44	12/3
Shredded Wheat, Post, lightly frosted, spoon size	1 c	5	12	44	12/3
Shredded Wheat, Post, original	1 c	6	0	40	0/2
Shredded Wheat, Post, original, spoon size	1 c	6	0	40	0/2
Shredded Wheat, Post, vanilla almond, spoon size	1 c	5	11	43	11/3
Shredded Wheat, Post, wheat 'n bran, spoon size	1¼ c	8	0	49	0/3
Smart Start, Kellogg's, maple brown sugar	1¼ c	5	17	47	17/3
Smart Start, Kellogg's, original antioxidants	1 c	3	14	43	14/3
Smart Start, Kellogg's, strawberry oat bites	30 pcs	6	7	43	7/3
Smart Start, Kellogg's, toasted oat	1¼ c	5	17	48	17/3
Smorz, Kellogg's	1 c	0	13	25	13/2
Special K, Kellogg's, chocolatey delight	¾ c	1	9	25	9/2
Special K, Kellogg's, cinnamon pecan	¾ c	1	7	25	7/2
Special K, Kellogg's, original	1 c	1	4	23	4/2
Strawberry Crisp, Erewhon, gluten free	¾ c	1	6	28	6/2
Strawberry Fields, Kashi	1 c	1	9	27	9/2
Toasties, Post, corn flakes	1 c	1	2	24	2/2
Toasties, Post, frosted flakes	¾ c	0	11	27	11/2
Toasties, Post, O's	1 c	2	11	28	11/2
Total, General Mills, blueberry pomegranate	1 c	4	11	38	11/2
Total, General Mills, cinnamon crunch	1 c	4	9	40	9/2
Total, General Mills, cranberry crunch	1¼ c	4	16	44	16/3
Total, General Mills, raisin bran	1 c	5	17	40	17/2
Total, General Mills, whole grain	¾ c	3	5	23	5/2
Trail Mix Crunch, Post, cranberry vanilla	½ c	4	12	36	12/2
Trail Mix Crunch, Post, raisin & almond	½ c	5	10	37	10/2
Trix, General Mills	1 c	1	11	28	11/2
U, Kashi, black currants & walnuts	1 c	7	10	42	10/3
Ultima, Barbara's, organic flax & granola	1 c	4	9	43	9/3
Ultima, Barbara's, organic high fiber	1 c	11	9	44	9/3
Ultima, Barbara's, organic pomegranate	1 c	6	11	44	11/3
Uncle Sam, U.S. Mills, original	¾ c	10	0	38	0/2
Uncle Sam, U.S. Mills, w/ real mixed berries	1 c	10	2	39	2/2
Vive, Kashi, toasted graham & vanilla	1¼ c	12	10	43	10/3

CEREALS, cont'd.

FOOD	Svg Size	Fbr	Sgr	Cbs	S/C Val
Waffle Crisp, Post	1 c	0	12	25	12/2
Wheaties, General Mills	¾ c	3	4	22	4/2

HOT CEREALS

FOOD	Svg Size	Fbr	Sgr	Cbs	S/C Val
Barley Flakes, Bob's Red Mill, rolled, whole grain	¼ c	3	0	16	0/1
Barley Plus, Erewhon, organic	¼ c	4	0	37	0/2
Brown rice cream, Erewhon, organic	¼ c	1	0	36	0/2
Cracked wheat, Bob's Red Mill, whole grain	¼ c	5	0	29	0/2
Cracked wheat, Bob's Red Mill, whole grain, organic	¼ c	5	0	29	0/2
Cream of rice, Amy's	1 pkg	2	8	39	8/2
Cream of rice, B&G	1 pkt	0	0	36	0/2
Cream of rye, Roman Meal	⅓ c	6	2	27	2/2
Cream of Wheat	¼ c	2	0	31	0/2
Cream of Wheat, instant, B&G, cinnamon swirl	1 pkt	1	14	29	14/2
Cream of Wheat, instant, B&G, maple brown sugar	1 pkt	1	13	28	13/2
Cream of Wheat, instant, B&G, original	1 pkt	1	0	19	0/1
Cream of Wheat, instant, B&G, Healthy Grain, maple brown sugar	1 pkt	6	0	30	0/2
Cream of Wheat, instant, B&G, Healthy Grain, original	1 pkt	6	0	30	0/2
Cream of Wheat, instant, B&G, SpongeBob SquarePants, chocolate lagoon	1 pkt	1	10	27	10/2
Cream of Wheat, instant, B&G, SpongeBob SquarePants, maple brown sugar	1 pkt	1	10	27	10/2
Creamy buckwheat, Bob's Red Mill, whole grain, organic	¼ c	3	0	30	0/2
Creamy rice, Bob's Red Mill, brown rice farina	¼ c	2	0	32	0/2
Creamy rice, Bob's Red Mill, brown rice farina, organic	¼ c	2	0	32	0/2
Creamy rye flakes, Bob's Red Mill	¼ c	4	0	21	0/2
Creamy wheat, Bob's Red Mill	¼ c	1	0	33	0/2
8 Grain hot cereal, Bob's Red Mill, whole grain	¼ c	6	0	27	0/2
Golean, Kashi, honey & cinnamon	1 pkt	5	7	26	7/2
Golean, Kashi, truly vanilla	1 pkt	7	6	25	6/2
Grits, yellow & white	¼ c	1	0	31	0/2
Grits, instant, Quaker, cheddar cheese	1 pkt	1	1	20	1/1
Grits, instant, Quaker, country bacon	1 pkt	1	0	21	0/2
Grits, instant, Quaker, ham 'n cheese	1 pkt	1	1	20	1/1
Grits, instant, Quaker, original	1 pkt	1	0	22	0/2
Grits, quick, Quaker, original	¼ c	2	0	29	0/2
Healthy Elements, Roman Meal, apple	1 c	5	10	32	10/2
Healthy Elements, Roman Meal, honey	1 c	4	9	32	9/2
Healthy Elements, Roman Meal, maple	1 c	5	9	31	9/2
Healthy Elements, Roman Meal, original	1 c	5	5	28	5/2
Healthy Elements, Roman Meal, raisin	1 c	4	11	31	11/2
High Fiber hot cereal, Bob's Red Mill	⅓ c	10	0	27	0/2
Hot cereal, Roman Meal, original w/oats	1 c	5	5	28	5/2
Kamut, Bob's Red Mill, whole grain	¼ c	4	0	26	0/2
Maltex, Homestat Farm	⅓ c	5	1	37	1/2
Mighty Tasty gluten free hot cereal, Bob's Red Mill	¼ c	4	0	31	0/2
Multi-grain, Amy's	1 c	5	12	40	12/2

FOOD	Svg Size	Fbr	Sgr	Cbs	S/C Val
Oatmeal, instant, Erewhon, apple cinnamon, organic	1 pkt	3	4	24	4/2
Oatmeal, instant, Erewhon, cinnamon raisin & flax, organic	1 pkt	4	6	24	6/2
Oatmeal, instant, Erewhon, maple spice, organic	1 pkt	3	4	25	4/2
Oatmeal, instant, Erewhon, w/ added oat bran, organic	1 pkt	4	0	25	0/2
Oatmeal, instant, Kashi Heart to Heart, golden brown maple	1 pkt	5	12	33	12/2
Oatmeal, instant, Mother's	½ c	4	1	27	1/2
Oatmeal, instant, Quaker, apples & cinnamon	1 pkt	3	13	27	13/2
Oatmeal, instant, Quaker, apples & cinnamon, Lower Sugar	1 pkt	3	6	22	6/2
Oatmeal, instant, Quaker, banana bread, Weight Control	1 pkt	6	1	29	1/2
Oatmeal, instant, Quaker, cinnamon, Weight Control	1 pkt	6	1	29	1/2
Oatmeal, instant, Quaker, cinnamon & spice	1 pkt	3	15	35	15/2
Oatmeal, instant, Quaker, high fiber	1 pkt	10	7	34	7/2
Oatmeal, instant, Quaker, honey nut	1 pkt	3	12	31	12/2
Oatmeal, instant, Quaker, maple & brown sugar	1 pkt	3	13	33	13/2
Oatmeal, instant, Quaker, maple & brown sugar, Lower Sugar	1 pkt	3	4	24	4/2
Oatmeal, instant, Quaker, maple & brown sugar, Weight Control	1 pkt	6	1	29	1/2
Oatmeal, instant, Quaker, original	1 pkt	3	0	19	0/1
Oatmeal, instant, Quaker, peaches & cream	1 pkt	2	12	27	12/2
Oatmeal, instant, Quaker, raisins & spice	1 pkt	3	16	33	16/2
Oatmeal, instant, Quaker, strawberries & cream	1 pkt	2	12	27	12/2
Oatmeal, instant, Quaker, vanilla cinnamon	1 pkt	3	13	32	13/2
Oatmeal, instant, Uncle Sam	1 pkt	5	0	23	0/2
Oatmeal, old fashioned, Quaker	½ c	4	1	27	1/2
Oatmeal, quick oats, Quaker	½ c	4	1	27	1/2
Oatmeal, steel-cut, Amy's	1 pkt	5	15	42	15/3
Oatmeal, steel cut, John McCann's	¼ c	3	0	27	0/2
Oatmeal, steel cut, Quaker	¼ c	4	1	27	1/2
Peppy Kernels, Bob's Red Mill, whole grain	¼ c	4	0	18	0/1
Rolled oats, Amy's	1 pkg	5	14	42	14/3
Rolled spelt, Bob's Red Mill, whole grain	½ c	3	0	28	0/2
Rolled triticale, Bob's Red Mill	¼ c	4	0	22	0/2
Rolled wheat, Bob's Red Mill, whole grain	¼ c	3	0	14	0/1
7 Grain hot cereal, Bob's Red Mill	¼ c	6	1	28	1/2
Simple Harvest, Quaker, apples w/ cinnamon	1 pkt	4	12	33	12/2
Simple Harvest, Quaker, maple brown sugar w/ pecans	1 pkt	4	9	30	9/2
Simple Harvest, Quaker, vanilla, almond & honey	1 pkt	4	9	31	9/2
6 Grain hot cereal w/ flaxseed, Bob's Red Mill	¼ c	5	0	27	0/2
Soy grits, Bob's Red Mill, defatted	¼ c	7	4	14	4/1
Spice n' Nice w/ Cinnamon & Raisins, Bob's Red Mill	¼ c	4	3	28	3/2
Wheatena, Homestat Farm	⅓ c	5	0	33	0/2
Whole wheat farina, Bob's Red Mill, whole grain	¼ c	4	0	33	0/2

FOOD	Svg Size	Fbr	Sgr	Cbs	S/C Val
Alfalfa sprouts	1 c	1	0	1	0/0
Artichoke, medium	1	7	1	13	1/1
Artichoke, large	1	9	2	17	2/1
Artichoke hearts	½ c	5	1	9	1/1
Artichoke hearts, canned in oil	½ c	4	1	9	1/1
Arugula	1 c	0	0	1	0/0
Asparagus	1 c	3	3	5	3/1
Asparagus, spears, medium	4	1	1	2	1/0
Bamboo shoots	½ c	2	2	4	2/0
Bamboo shoots, canned	½ c	1	1	2	1/0
Basil, fresh	½ c	0	0	0	0/0
Bean sprouts, mung	1 c	2	4	6	4/1
Beet	½ c	2	5	7	5/1
Beet, whole, 2" diameter	1	2	6	8	6/1
Beet, pickled	½ c	3	15	18	15/1
Beet, pickled, Del Monte	½ c	2	16	19	16/1
Beet greens	½ c	1	0	1	0/0
Bok choy, sliced	1 c	1	1	2	1/0
Bok choy, baby, sliced	1 c	1	1	2	1/0
Broccoli, bunch, average	1	16	10	40	10/2
Broccoli, chopped	1 c	2	2	6	2/1
Broccoli, Chinese	1 c	2	1	3	1/0
Broccoli raab, chopped	1 c	1	0	1	0/0
Brussels sprout, average	1	1	0	2	0/0
Brussels sprouts	1 c	3	2	8	2/1
Burdock root, average	1	5	5	27	5/2
Burdock root, chopped	¼ c	1	1	5	1/1
Cabbage, leaf, large	1	1	1	2	1/0
Cabbage, shredded	1 c	2	2	4	2/0
Cabbage, Chinese, pak-choi, shredded	1 c	1	1	2	1/0
Cabbage, Chinese, pe-tsai, shredded	1 c	1	1	2	1/0
Cabbage, mustard	1 c	4	2	7	2/1
Cabbage, red, chopped	1 c	2	3	5	3/1
Cabbage, red, shredded	1 c	2	3	7	3/1
Cabbage, savoy, shredded	1 c	2	2	4	2/0
Carrot, small	1	1	2	5	2/1
Carrot, medium	1	2	3	6	3/1
Carrot, large	1	2	3	7	3/1
Carrots, baby	5	1	2	4	2/0
Carrots, chopped	½ c	2	3	6	3/1
Carrots, grated	½ c	2	3	5	3/1
Cassava, chopped	¼ c	1	1	20	1/1
Cauliflower, small (4" diameter head)	1	5	5	13	5/1
Cauliflower, medium (5"-6" diameter head)	1	12	11	29	11/2

FOOD	Svg Size	Fbr	Sgr	Cbs	S/C Val
Cauliflower, large (6"-7" diameter head)	1	17	16	42	16/3
Cauliflower, chopped	1 c	2	2	5	2/1
Cauliflower, green, small (4" diameter head)	1	10	10	20	10/1
Cauliflower, green, medium (5"-6" diameter head)	1	14	13	26	13/2
Cauliflower, green, large (6"-7" diameter head)	1	16	15	31	15/2
Cauliflower, green, chopped	1 c	2	2	4	2/0
Celeriac	½ c	1	1	7	1/1
Celery, small (5" long)	1	0	0	1	0/0
Celery, medium (7"-8" long)	1	1	1	1	1/0
Celery, large (11"-12" long)	1	1	1	2	1/0
Celery, chopped	1 c	2	2	3	2/0
Chard, Swiss, chopped	1 c	1	0	1	0/0
Chicory greens, chopped	1 c	1	0	1	0/0
Chicory root, average	1	1	5	11	5/1
Chicory root, chopped	½ c	1	4	8	4/1
Chives, fresh, chopped	2 T	0	0	0	0/0
Cilantro (coriander), fresh	¼ c	0	0	0	0/0
Collards	1 c	1	0	2	0/0
Corn, cream style, Del Monte, sweet, can	½ c	2	7	14	7/1
Corn, cream style, Del Monte, white, can	½ c	2	6	21	6/2
Corn, cream style, Green Giant, can	½ c	1	7	19	7/1
Corn, cream style, Green Giant, frozen	½ c	2	7	24	7/2
Corn, white, small ear (5.5"-6.5" long)	1	2	2	14	2/1
Corn, white, medium ear (6.75"-7.5" long)	1	2	3	17	3/1
Corn, white, large ear (7.75"-9" long)	1	4	5	27	5/2
Corn, white, hominy	1 c	4	3	24	3/2
Corn, white, kernels	½ c	2	2	15	2/1
Corn, yellow, small ear (5.5"-6.5" long)	1	2	5	14	5/1
Corn, yellow, medium ear (6.75"-7.5" long)	1	2	6	19	6/1
Corn, yellow, large ear (7.75"-9" long)	1	3	9	27	9/2
Corn, yellow, kernels	½ c	1	5	14	5/1
Cress, garden	1 c	0	2	3	2/0
Cucumber, 8" long	1	2	5	11	5/1
Cucumber, sliced	½ c	0	1	2	1/0
Dandelion greens	1 c	2	0	5	0/1
Dill weed, fresh, sprigs	¼ c	0	0	0	0/0
Eggplant, approx. 1.25 lb.	1	19	13	31	13/2
Eggplant, cubed	1 c	3	2	5	2/1
Endive, chopped	½ c	1	0	1	0/0
Fennel, bulb	1	7	0	17	0/1
Fennel, sliced	½ c	1	0	3	0/0
Garlic, chopped	1 T	0	0	3	0/0
Garlic, clove	1	0	0	1	0/0
Ginger, pickled	0.5 oz	0	0	1	0/0

FOOD	Svg Size	Fbr	Sgr	Cbs	S/C Val
Gingerroot	1 T	0	0	1	0/0
Green beans	1 c	2	2	4	2/0
Green beans	10	3	3	7	3/1
Jicama, average	1	32	12	58	12/3
Jicama, sliced	½ c	3	1	5	1/1
Kale, chopped	1 c	1	1	7	1/1
Leek, average	1	2	3	13	3/1
Lettuce, butterhead (incl. Boston & Bibb), average leaf	5	0	0	1	0/0
Lettuce, butterhead (incl. Boston & Bibb), chopped	1 c	1	1	1	1/0
Lettuce, iceberg, average leaf	5	1	1	1	1/0
Lettuce, iceberg, chopped	1 c	1	1	2	1/0
Lettuce, iceberg, shredded	1 c	1	1	2	1/0
Lettuce, red leaf, average leaf	5	1	0	1	0/0
Lettuce, red leaf, shredded	1 c	0	0	1	0/0
Lettuce, romaine, average leaf	5	2	1	3	1/0
Lettuce, romaine, shredded	1 c	1	1	2	1/0
Mixed, canned, Del Monte	½ c	2	3	8	3/1
Mixed, canned, Del Monte, homestyle vegetable medley	½ c	2	3	11	3/1
Mixed, canned, Ka-Me, stir-fry vegetables	1 can	2	2	4	2/0
Mixed, frozen, Big Valley, California blend	¾ c	3	6	6	6/1
Mixed, frozen, Big Valley, Italian blend	¾ c	2	3	5	3/1
Mixed, frozen, Big Valley, Oriental blend	¾ c	3	2	5	2/1
Mixed, frozen, Big Valley, stew vegetables	⅔ c	2	3	10	3/1
Mixed, frozen, Big Valley, winter blend	¾ c	2	1	4	1/0
Mixed, frozen, Birds Eye, California blend	1 c	1	2	4	2/0
Mixed, frozen, Birds Eye, classic	⅔ c	2	4	12	4/1
Mixed, frozen, Birds Eye, Normandy blend	1 c	1	2	4	2/0
Mixed, frozen, Birds Eye, Oriental stir-fry	1 c	2	5	9	5/1
Mixed, frozen, Birds Eye, teriyaki stir-fry	2 cs	3	11	33	11/2
Mixed, frozen, Birds Eye, Thai stir-fry	1 c	3	6	10	6/1
Mixed, frozen, Cascadian Farm, California-style blend	⅔ c	2	2	5	2/1
Mixed, frozen, Cascadian Farm, Chinese-style stirfry blend	1 c	2	2	5	2/1
Mixed, frozen, Cascadian Farm, gardener's blend	¾ c	3	3	11	3/1
Mixed, frozen, Cascadian Farm, garden vegetable medley	½ pkg	1	3	12	3/1
Mixed, frozen, Cascadian Farm, Thai-style stirfry blend	¾ c	2	2	5	2/1
Mixed, frozen, Green Giant, baby vegetable medley	½ c	2	4	9	4/1
Mixed, frozen, Green Giant, Digestive Health	½ c	5	2	14	2/1
Mixed, frozen, Green Giant, garden vegetable medley	½ c	1	3	11	3/1
Mixed, frozen, Green Giant, Healthy Heart	1 pkg	4	4	28	4/2
Mixed, frozen, Green Giant, Immunity Blend	1 c	2	7	11	7/1
Mixed, frozen, Green Giant, teriyaki vegetables	1¼ cs	3	1	11	1/1
Mixed, frozen, Green Giant, Valley Fresh Steamers	½ c	2	4	12	4/1
Mixed, frozen, Green Giant, Valley Fresh Steamers, Asian style medley	½ c	2	4	8	4/1
Mixed, frozen, Tree of Life, organic mixed vegetables	½ c	3	3	13	3/1

FOOD	Svg Size	Fbr	Sgr	Cbs	S/C Val
Mushrooms, brown, Italian, or crimini	2	0	1	2	1/0
Mushrooms, brown, Italian, or crimini, whole	1 c	1	2	4	2/0
Mushrooms, chanterelle	7	1	0	3	0/0
Mushrooms, chanterelle, chopped	1 c	2	0	4	0/0
Mushrooms, enoki	7	1	0	3	0/0
Mushrooms, enoki, sliced	1 c	2	0	5	0/1
Mushrooms, maitake	2	0	0	0	0/0
Mushrooms, maitake, diced	1 c	2	1	5	1/1
Mushrooms, morel	3	1	0	2	0/0
Mushrooms, morel, chopped	1 c	2	0	3	0/0
Mushrooms, oyster, small (0.5 oz)	2	1	0	2	0/0
Mushrooms, oyster, large (5 oz)	2	7	3	18	3/1
Mushrooms, oyster, sliced	1 c	2	1	5	1/1
Mushrooms, portobello	2	2	4	7	4/1
Mushrooms, portobello, diced	1 c	1	2	3	2/0
Mushrooms, shiitake	2	1	0	3	0/0
Mushrooms, white	2	0	1	1	1/0
Mushrooms, white, sliced	1 c	1	2	3	2/0
Mustard greens	1 c	2	1	3	1/0
Okra	1 c	3	1	7	1/1
Onion, average	½	1	2	5	2/1
Onion, chopped	1 c	3	7	15	7/1
Onion, sliced	1 c	2	5	11	5/1
Onion, spring (scallion), average	1	0	0	1	0/0
Onion, sweet, average	½	2	8	13	8/1
Parsley, fresh	½ c	1	0	2	0/0
Parsnips, sliced	1 c	3	3	12	3/1
Peas, edible pod	½ c	1	1	2	1/0
Peas, green	½ c	4	4	10	4/1
Peas, snow	⅔ c	2	3	6	3/1
Peas, sugar snap	⅔ c	2	3	7	3/1
Pepper, banana, medium	1	1	2	2	2/0
Pepper, chili, hot, green	1	1	2	4	2/0
Pepper, chili, hot, red	1	1	2	4	2/0
Pepper, jalapeño	2	1	1	2	1/0
Pepper, serrano	3	1	1	1	0/0
Pepper, sweet/bell, green, chopped	1 c	3	4	7	4/1
Pepper, sweet/bell, green, small	1	1	2	3	2/0
Pepper, sweet/bell, green, medium	1	2	3	6	3/1
Pepper, sweet/bell, green, large	1	3	4	8	4/1
Pepper, sweet/bell, red, chopped	1 c	3	6	9	6/1
Pepper, sweet/bell, red, small	1	2	3	4	3/0
Pepper, sweet/bell, red, medium	1	3	5	7	5/1
Pepper, sweet/bell, red, large	1	3	7	10	7/1

FOOD	Svg Size	Fbr	Sgr	Cbs	S/C Val
Peppermint, fresh	¼ c	1	0	2	0/0
Pickles, dill	½ c	1	1	2	1/0
Pickles, dill, Del Monte, hamburger chips	7	0	0	1	0/0
Pickles, dill, Del Monte, whole	1	0	0	1	0/0
Pickles, dill, Vlasic, Snack'mms, kosher	3	0	0	1	0/0
Pickles, sour	½ c	1	1	2	1/0
Pickles, sweet	½ c	1	14	16	14/1
Pickles, sweet, Del Monte, chips	6	0	10	10	10/1
Pickles, sweet, Del Monte, chips, bread & butter	4	0	7	8	7/1
Potato, small (up to 2.25" diameter)	1	4	1	30	1/2
Potato, medium (up to 3.25" diameter)	1	5	2	37	2/2
Potato, large (up to 4.25" diameter)	1	8	3	64	3/4
Potato, diced	1 c	3	1	26	1/2
Potato, red, small (up to 2.25" diameter)	1	3	2	27	2/2
Potato, red, medium (up to 3.25" diameter)	1	4	2	34	2/2
Potato, red, large (up to 4.25" diameter)	1	6	4	59	4/3
Potato, red, diced	½ c	1	1	12	1/1
Potato, frozen, fries, Ore-Ida, Golden Fries	16 pcs	1	0	20	0/1
Potato, frozen, fries, Ore-Ida, shoestrings	38 pcs	2	0	22	0/2
Potato, frozen, fries, Ore-Ida, steak	7 pcs	2	1	17	1/1
Potato, frozen, fries, Ore-Ida, waffle	15 pcs	2	0	22	0/2
Potato, frozen, hash browns, Ore-Ida, country style	1 c	1	0	13	0/1
Potato, frozen, hash browns, Ore-Ida, Golden Patties	1 pc	1	0	16	0/1
Potato, frozen, hash browns, Ore-Ida, Tater Tots	9 pcs	2	0	21	0/2
Potato, frozen, hash browns, Simply Potatoes, shredded	½ c	2	0	16	0/1
Potato, mix, au gratin, Betty Crocker, as prepared	½ c	1	1	22	1/2
Potato, mix, au gratin, Hungry Jack, as prepared	½ c	1	3	24	3/2
Potato, mix, cheddar & bacon, Betty Crocker, as prepared	½ c	1	2	21	2/2
Potato, mix, cheddar & bacon, Hungry Jack, as prepared	½ c	2	3	24	3/2
Potato, mix, mashed, Betty Crocker, roasted garlic, as prepared	½ c	1	2	19	2/1
Potato, mix, mashed, Betty Crocker, sour cream & chives, as prepared	½ c	1	2	21	2/2
Potato, mix, mashed, Hungry Jack, original	⅓ c	1	0	19	0/1
Potato, mix, mashed, Hungry Jack, Easy Mash'd, creamy butter	¼ c	1	1	19	1/1
Potato, mix, mashed, Hungry Jack, Easy Mash'd, roasted garlic 'n skins	¼ c	2	1	19	1/1
Potato, mix, mashed, Hungry Jack, Easy Mash'd, sour cream & chives	¼ c	1	0	20	0/1
Potato, mix, scalloped, Betty Crocker, as prepared	½ c	1	3	23	3/2
Potato, mix, scalloped, Betty Crocker, cheesy, as prepared	½ c	1	3	20	3/1
Potato, mix, scalloped, Hungry Jack, cheesy, as prepared	½ c	1	3	24	3/2
Potato, mix, scalloped, Hungry Jack, creamy, as prepared	½ c	2	3	24	3/2
Pumpkin, canned	½ c	4	4	10	4/1
Pumpkin, canned, Libby's, easy pumpkin pie mix	⅓ c	3	17	20	17/1
Pumpkin, canned, Libby's, 100% pure pumpkin	½ c	5	4	9	4/1
Pumpkin, cubed	½ c	0	1	4	1/0
Radicchio	1 c	0	0	2	0/0

VEGETABLES & FRESH HERBS, cont'd.

FOOD	Svg Size	Fbr	Sgr	Cbs	S/C Val
Radish, average	1	0	0	0	0/0
Radish, sliced	½ c	1	1	2	1/0
Radish, Oriental, 7" long	1	5	9	14	9/1
Rosemary, fresh	¼ c	1	0	1	0/0
Rutabaga, average	1	10	22	31	22/2
Rutabaga, cubed	½ c	2	4	6	4/1
Salad, Ready Pac, Bistro, chef	1 pkg	2	5	10	5/1
Salad, Ready Pac, Bistro, chicken Caesar	1 pkg	1	3	8	3/1
Salad, Ready Pac, Bistro, cobb	1 pkg	2	4	7	4/1
Salad, Ready Pac, Bistro, Santa Fe style Caesar	1 pkg	2	5	15	5/1
Salad, Ready Pac, Bistro, spinach bacon	1 pkg	3	8	19	8/1
Salad mix, Dole, Asian Island Crunch salad kit	1½ c	1	5	12	5/1
Salad mix, Dole, Caesar salad kit	1½ c	1	2	9	2/1
Salad mix, Dole, classic iceberg blend	1½ c	1	2	4	2/0
Salad mix, Dole, coleslaw, classic	1½ c	2	0	5	0/1
Salad mix, Dole, field greens blend	1½ c	2	1	4	1/0
Salad mix, Dole, Italian blend	1½ c	1	0	3	0/0
Salad mix, Dole, Southwest salad kit	1½ c	2	3	10	3/1
Salad mix, Fresh Express, American salad	1½ c	1	2	3	2/0
Salad mix, Fresh Express, Asian Supreme kit	2½ c	2	8	17	8/1
Salad mix, Fresh Express, Caesar salad kit	2½ c	2	2	8	2/1
Salad mix, Fresh Express, fancy greens	2½ c	1	1	3	1/0
Salad mix, Fresh Express, Italian salad	2 c	1	1	2	1/0
Salad mix, Fresh Express, lettuce trio	2½ c	1	1	3	1/0
Salad mix, Fresh Express, Mediterranean Supreme kit	3 c	5	6	16	6/1
Salad mix, Fresh Express, old fashioned coleslaw	2 c	2	3	5	3/1
Salad mix, Ready Pac, All American	2 c	1	2	3	2/0
Salad mix, Ready Pac, American blue cheese	1¾ c	1	2	8	2/1
Salad mix, Ready Pac, Asian	1½ c	1	9	14	9/1
Salad mix, Ready Pac, baby arugula	4 c	1	2	3	2/0
Salad mix, Ready Pac, baby spinach	2 c	2	12	24	12/2
Salad mix, Ready Pac, classic Caesar	2 c	1	2	8	2/1
Salad mix, Ready Pac, coleslaw	1 c	2	11	13	11/1
Salad mix, Ready Pac, Lafayette	3 c	0	1	3	1/0
Salad mix, Ready Pac, Parisian	2½ c	2	8	11	8/1
Salad mix, Ready Pac, Santa Barbara	3 c	0	1	3	1/0
Salad mix, Ready Pac, Santa Fe Caesar	1¾ c	1	3	7	3/1
Salad mix, Ready Pac, spring mix	4½ c	2	0	4	0/0
Salad mix, Ready Pac, veggie medley	2 c	1	2	4	2/0
Salad mix, Ready Pac, zesty baby greens	4½ c	2	0	4	0/0
Sauerkraut	½ c	2	1	3	1/0
Seaweed, agar, dried	2 T	1	0	8	0/1
Seaweed, agar, raw	2 T	0	0	1	0/0
Seaweed, Irish moss, raw	2 T	0	0	1	0/0

VEGETABLES & FRESH HERBS, cont'd.

FOOD	Svg Size	Fbr	Sgr	Cbs	S/C Val
Seaweed, kelp, raw	2 T	0	0	1	0/0
Seaweed, laver, raw	2 T	0	0	1	0/0
Seaweed, spirulina, dried	2 T	1	0	3	0/0
Seaweed, wakame, raw	2 T	0	0	1	0/0
Shallot, chopped	2 T	0	0	3	0/0
Snap beans, green	1 c	3	3	7	3/1
Spearmint, fresh	¼ c	2	0	2	0/0
Spinach	1 c	1	0	1	0/0
Spinach, average bunch	1	8	1	12	1/1
Spinach, creamed, Green Giant, frozen	½ c	1	4	9	4/1
Squash, butternut, cubed	1 c	3	3	16	3/1
Squash, crookneck, sliced	1 c	1	4	5	4/1
Squash, straightneck, sliced	1 c	1	4	5	4/1
Squash, summer, all varieties, sliced	1 c	1	2	4	2/0
Squash, winter, all varieties, cubed	1 c	2	3	10	3/1
Sweet potato, 5" long	1	4	5	26	5/2
Sweet potato, cubed	½ c	2	3	13	3/1
Thyme, fresh	2 T	1	0	1	0/0
Tomatillo, average	1	1	1	2	1/0
Tomatillo, chopped	½ c	1	3	4	3/0
Taro, sliced	½ c	2	0	14	0/1
Taro leaves	1 c	1	1	2	1/0
Tomato, cherry, average	½ c	1	2	3	2/0
Tomato, green, average	1	1	5	6	5/1
Tomato, green, chopped	½ c	1	4	5	4/1
Tomato, Italian, average	1	1	2	2	2/0
Tomato, plum, average	1	1	2	2	2/0
Tomato, red, average	1	2	3	5	3/1
Tomato, red, chopped	½ c	1	2	4	2/0
Tomato, sun dried, average	1 pc	0	1	1	1/0
Tomato, sun dried	2 T	1	3	4	3/0
Tomato, canned, crushed, Contadina	¼ c	1	2	4	2/0
Tomato, canned, crushed, Eden Organic	¼ c	1	2	3	2/0
Tomato, canned, crushed, Hunt's	½ c	2	5	7	5/1
Tomato, canned, crushed, Progresso	¼ c	1	2	4	2/0
Tomato, canned, diced, Del Monte	½ c	2	4	6	4/1
Tomato, canned, diced, Hunt's	½ c	2	6	7	6/1
Tomato, canned, diced, Muir Glen, organic	½ c	1	4	6	4/1
Tomato, canned, paste	2 T	1	4	6	4/1
Tomato, canned, paste, Contadina	2 T	1	3	6	3/1
Tomato, canned, petite diced, Contadina	½ c	2	4	6	4/1
Tomato, canned, petite diced, Del Monte	½ c	2	4	6	4/1
Tomato, canned, petite diced, Hunt's	½ c	1	3	5	3/1
Tomato, canned, puree, Contadina	¼ c	0	1	4	1/0

VEGETABLES & FRESH HERBS, cont'd.

FOOD	Svg Size	Fbr	Sgr	Cbs	S/C Val
Tomato, canned, puree, Progresso	¼ c	1	3	5	3/1
Tomato, canned, stewed, Del Monte, no salt added	½ c	2	7	9	7/1
Tomato, canned, stewed, Hunt's	½ c	2	6	7	6/1
Tomato, canned, whole, Hunt's	2	1	5	4	5/0
Tomato, canned, whole, Muir Glen, fire roasted, organic	½ c	1	3	5	3/1
Tomato, canned, whole, Muir Glen, peeled, organic	½ c	1	3	5	3/1
Tomato, canned, whole, Progresso, peeled, w/ basil	½ c	1	3	4	3/0
Turnip, average	1	2	5	8	5/1
Turnip, cubed	½ c	1	3	4	3/0
Turnip greens	1 c	2	0	4	0/0
Watercress	½ c	0	0	0	0/0
Yam, cubed	1 c	6	1	42	1/3
Zucchini, average	1	2	5	6	5/1
Zucchini, sliced	½ c	1	1	2	1/0

FRUITS

FOOD	Svg Size	Fbr	Sgr	Cbs	S/C Val
Acerola, average	1	0	0	0	0/0
Apple, extra small (2.5" diameter)	1	2	10	14	10/1
Apple, small (2.75" diameter)	1	3	15	21	15/2
Apple, medium (3" diameter)	1	4	19	25	19/2
Apple, large (3.25" diameter)	1	5	23	31	23/2
Apple, dried, w/o added sugar	1 c	5	34	39	34/2
Applesauce, chunky, Mott's	½ c	1	21	23	21/2
Applesauce, cinnamon, Mott's	½ c	1	25	29	25/2
Applesauce, original, Mott's	½ c	1	25	27	25/2
Applesauce, unsweetened	½ c	1	11	14	11/1
Applesauce, unsweetened, Tree of Life	½ c	2	13	19	13/1
Apricot, average	1	1	3	4	3/0
Apricot, dried halves, w/o added sugar	½ c	3	24	28	24/2
Avocado, all varieties, average	1	14	1	17	1/1
Avocado, California, average	1	9	0	12	0/1
Avocado, Florida, average	1	17	7	24	7/2
Banana, smaller than 6" long	1	2	10	19	10/1
Banana, 6"-7" long	1	3	12	23	12/2
Banana, 7"-8" long	1	3	14	27	14/2
Banana, 8"-9" long	1	4	17	31	17/2
Banana, 9" long or larger	1	4	19	35	19/2
Banana, dried	½ c	5	24	44	24/3
Blackberries	¼ c	2	2	3	2/0
Blueberries	¼ c	1	4	5	4/1
Cantaloupe, 5" diameter	⅛	1	5	6	5/1
Cantaloupe, cubed	½ c	1	6	7	6/1
Casaba melon, average	¼	4	23	27	23/2

FOOD	Svg Size	Fbr	Sgr	Cbs	S/C Val
Casaba melon, cubed	½ c	1	5	6	5/1
Cherries, sour	¼ c	0	2	3	2/0
Cherries, sweet	¼ c	1	4	6	4/1
Cherry, maraschino	1	0	2	2	2/0
Coconut, dried meat, unsweetened	1 oz	5	2	7	2/1
Coconut, raw meat, shredded	¼ c	2	1	3	1/0
Cranberries	¼ c	1	1	3	1/0
Cranberries, dried, sweetened, average	⅓ c	2	26	33	26/2
Cranberries, dried, Ocean Spray, Craisins	⅓ c	3	26	33	26/2
Cranberries, dried, Sun-Maid, Cape Cod	⅓ c	2	27	33	27/2
Cranberries, dried, Sun-Maid, tart	⅓ c	2	28	34	28/2
Date, deglet noor, average	1	1	5	5	5/1
Date, medjool, average	1	2	16	18	16/1
Fig, dried, uncooked	¼ c	4	18	24	18/2
Fig, raw, 1.5" diameter	1	1	7	8	7/1
Fig, raw, 2.5" diameter	1	2	10	12	10/1
Grapefruit, pink & red, average	½	2	8	13	8/1
Grapefruit, white, average	½	1	9	10	9/1
Grapes, American (slip skin)	1 c	1	15	16	15/1
Grapes, European (red or green)	1 c	1	23	27	23/2
Grapes, European (red or green)	10	0	8	9	8/1
Honeydew, 5.25" diameter	⅛	1	10	11	10/1
Honeydew, 7" diameter	⅛	1	13	15	13/1
Honeydew, diced	½ c	1	7	8	7/1
Kiwi, green, average	1	2	6	10	6/1
Kiwi, yellow, average	1	2	9	12	9/1
Kumquat, average	1	1	2	3	2/0
Lemon, average	½	1	1	3	1/0
Lime, average	1	2	1	7	1/1
Lychees	2	0	3	3	3/0
Lychees	½ c	1	14	16	14/1
Mango, average	1	4	31	35	31/2
Mango, dried, Philippine Brand	1.5 oz	1	32	39	32/2
Mango, sliced	½ c	2	12	14	12/1
Nectarine, average	1	2	11	15	11/1
Nectarine, sliced	½ c	1	6	8	6/1
Olives, black, average	2	0	0	0	0/0
Olives, green, average	2	0	0	1	0/0
Orange, all varieties, average	1	3	12	15	12/1
Orange, Florida, average	1	3	13	17	13/1
Orange, navel, average	1	3	12	18	12/1
Peach, average	1	2	12	14	12/1
Peach, dried, w/o added sugar	¼ c	2	11	13	11/1
Pear, Asian, small (up to 2.5" diameter)	1	4	9	13	9/1

FOOD	Svg Size	Fbr	Sgr	Cbs	S/C Val
Pear, Asian, large (up to 4" diameter)	1	10	19	29	19/2
Pear, small	1	5	15	23	15/2
Pear, medium	1	6	17	28	17/2
Pear, large	1	7	23	36	23/2
Pear, cubed	½ c	3	8	12	8/1
Pear, dried, w/o added sugar	¼ c	4	17	22	17/2
Persimmon, average	1	6	21	31	21/2
Pineapple, all varieties	½ c	1	8	11	8/1
Pineapple, extra sweet	½ c	1	9	11	9/1
Pineapple, traditional varieties	½ c	1	7	10	7/1
Plantain, green, fried	½ c	2	2	29	2/2
Plantain, raw or cooked, sliced	½ c	2	11	24	11/2
Plum, average	1	1	7	8	7/1
Plum, sliced	½ c	1	8	9	8/1
Preserves, jam	1 T	0	10	14	10/1
Preserves, jam, Nature's Hollow, all flavors	1 T	0	0	7	0/1
Preserves, jam, Smucker's, all flavors	1 T	0	12	13	12/1
Preserves, jam, Welch's, all flavors	1 T	0	13	13	13/1
Preserves, jelly, Smucker's, all flavors	1 T	0	12	13	12/1
Preserves, jelly, Smucker's, low sugar, all flavors	1 T	0	5	6	5/1
Preserves, jelly, Welch's, all flavors	1 T	0	13	13	13/1
Preserves, jelly, Welch's, reduced sugar, all flavors	1 T	0	6	6	6/1
Preserves, spread, Cascadian Farm, all flavors	1 T	0	10	10	10/1
Preserves, spread, Smucker's Simply Fruit, all flavors	1 T	0	8	10	8/1
Preserves, spread, Welch's, all flavors	1 T	0	13	13	13/1
Prunes, stewed, w/o added sugar	¼ c	2	15	17	15/1
Prunes, uncooked	¼ c	3	17	28	17/2
Raisins, seedless	¼ c	1	22	29	22/2
Raisins, seedless, golden	¼ c	1	22	29	22/2
Raspberries	¼ c	2	1	4	1/0
Rhubarb, average stalk	1	1	1	2	1/0
Rhubarb, diced	1 c	2	1	6	1/1
Star fruit, average	1	3	4	6	4/1
Star fruit, sliced	½ c	2	2	4	2/0
Strawberries, sliced	¼ c	1	2	3	2/0
Strawberries, small (1" diameter)	3	0	1	2	1/0
Strawberries, medium (1.25" diameter)	3	1	2	3	2/0
Strawberries, large (1.4" diameter)	3	1	3	4	3/0
Strawberries, extra large (1.6" diameter)	3	2	4	6	4/1
Strawberries, frozen, sweetened, thawed	1 c	5	48	54	48/3
Strawberries, frozen, unsweetened, thawed	1 c	4	10	20	10/1
Tamarind	10	1	11	13	11/1
Tamarind, pulp	½ c	3	34	38	34/2
Tangerine, average	1	2	10	13	10/1
Watermelon, diced	½ c	0	5	6	5/1

OILS & SWEETENERS

FOOD	Svg Size	Fbr	Sgr	Cbs	S/C Val
OILS					
Butter, all varieties	1 c	0	0	0	0/0
Canola oil	1 T	0	0	0	0/0
Coconut oil	1 T	0	0	0	0/0
Cooking oils, all varieties	1 T	0	0	0	0/0
Fish oil, all varieties	1 T	0	0	0	0/0
Fish oil, Barlean's Omega Swirl, lemon zest	2 t	0	0	4	0/0
Fish & flax oil blend, Barlean's Total Omega, orange cream	1 T	0	0	5	0/1
Flaxseed oil	1 T	0	0	0	0/0
Flax oil blend, Barlean's Essential Woman, chocolate raspberry	1 T	0	0	5	0/1
Flax oil blend, Barlean's Omega Swirl, strawberry banana	1 T	0	0	5	0/1
Flax oil blend, Barlean's Total Omega, pomegranate blueberry, vegan	1 T	0	0	5	0/1
Grapeseed oil	1 T	0	0	0	0/0
Hemp oil	1 T	0	0	0	0/0
Lard	1 T	0	0	0	0/0
Margarine, most varieties	1 T	0	0	0	0/0
Olive oil	1 T	0	0	0	0/0
Pam cooking spray (one-second spray)	1 spr	0	0	0	0/0
Peanut oil	1 T	0	0	0	0/0
Shortening	1 T	0	0	0	0/0
Soybean oil	1 T	0	0	0	0/0
Spread, Country Crock	1 T	0	0	0	0/0
Spread, Earth Balance	1 T	0	0	0	0/0
Spread, I Can't Believe It's Not Butter!	1 T	0	0	0	0/0
Spread, Smart Balance	1 T	0	0	0	0/0
Vegetable oil	1 T	0	0	0	0/0
SWEETENERS					
Agave nectar	1 T	0	16	16	16/1
Corn syrup, dark	1 T	0	5	16	5/1
Corn syrup, high fructose	1 T	0	5	14	5/1
Corn syrup, light	1 T	0	6	17	6/1
Equal (aspartame)	1 pkt	0	0	0	0/0
Honey	1 T	0	17	17	17/1
Honey, imitation, Nature's Hollow, Tastes Like Honey	1 T	0	0	7	0/1
Maltitol, Joseph's Maltitol Sweetener	¼ c	0	0	9	0/1
Molasses	1 T	0	11	15	11/1
NutraSweet (aspartame)	1 pkt	0	0	0	0/0
Splenda (sucralose)	1 pkt	0	0	0	0/0
Stevia, PureVia	1 pkt	0	0	2	0/0
Stevia, SweetLeaf Sweetener	1 pkt	0	0	0	0/0
Stevia blend, Truvia	1 pkt	0	0	3	0/0
Sugar, brown, packed	1 t	0	4	5	4/1
Sugar, brown, packed	¼ c	0	54	54	54/3

OILS & SWEETENERS, cont'd.

FOOD	Svg Size	Fbr	Sgr	Cbs	S/C Val
Sugar, brown, unpacked	1 t	0	3	3	3/0
Sugar, brown, unpacked	¼ c	0	35	36	35/2
Sugar, powdered, sifted	¼ c	0	24	25	24/2
Sugar, powdered, unsifted	1 t	0	2	2	2/0
Sugar, powdered, unsifted	¼ c	0	29	30	29/2
Sugar, turbinado	1 t	0	4	4	4/0
Sugar, turbinado	¼ c	0	50	50	50/3
Sugar, white, granulated	1 t	0	4	4	4/0
Sugar, white, granulated	¼ c	0	50	50	50/3
Sweet'N Low (saccharin)	1 pkt	0	0	0	0/0
Xylitol, XyloSweet	1 t	0	0	4	0/0

CHIPS, CRACKERS & SAVORY SNACKS

FOOD	Svg Size	Fbr	Sgr	Cbs	S/C Val
CHIPS					
Athenos, pita chips, original	11	0	0	19	0/1
Athenos, pita chips, roasted garlic & herb	11	0	0	19	0/1
Athenos, pita chips, whole wheat	11	2	0	18	0/1
Bugles, caramel	⅔ c	0	9	17	9/1
Bugles, nacho cheese	1⅓ c	0	1	18	1/1
Bugles, original	1⅓ c	0	1	18	1/1
Cheetos, crunchy	21	0	1	15	1/1
Cheetos, crunchy, Baked!	34	0	1	19	1/1
Cheetos, crunchy, Flamin' Hot	21	0	0	15	0/1
Cheetos, crunchy, Flamin' Hot, limon	28	0	0	15	0/1
Cheetos, Flamin' Hot, Baked!	34	0	0	19	0/1
Cheetos, puffs	13	0	0	15	0/1
Doritos, cool ranch	12	2	1	18	1/1
Doritos, cool ranch, reduced fat	12	2	1	19	1/1
Doritos, nacho cheese	12	1	1	17	1/1
Doritos, nacho cheese, Baked!	12	2	1	21	1/2
Doritos, nacho cheese, reduced fat	12	1	2	19	2/1
Doritos, spicy nacho	12	1	1	18	1/1
Doritos, spicy sweet chili	12	1	1	18	1/1
Doritos, toasted corn	12	1	0	18	0/1
El Sabroso, Guacachip	1 oz	2	0	14	0/1
El Sabroso, Salsitas	1 oz	2	0	15	0/1
Fritos, chili cheese	31	1	1	15	1/1
Fritos, Flamin' Hot	28	1	0	15	0/1
Fritos, honey BBQ	23	1	1	16	1/1
Fritos, lightly salted	34	1	0	16	0/1
Fritos, original	32	0	0	15	0/1
Fritos, Scoops!	10	1	0	16	0/1

FOOD	Svg Size	Fbr	Sgr	Cbs	S/C Val
Funyuns, onion flavored rings	13	1	1	18	1/1
Kettle Brand, backyard barbeque	13	2	1	15	1/1
Kettle Brand, Death Valley chipotle	13	2	0	16	0/1
Kettle Brand, fully loaded baked potato	13	1	1	16	1/1
Kettle Brand, honey dijon	13	1	2	16	2/1
Kettle Brand, jalapeño	13	1	1	16	1/1
Kettle Brand, lightly salted	13	1	0	16	0/1
Kettle Brand, New York cheddar	13	1	1	16	1/1
Kettle Brand, sea salt & vinegar	13	1	0	16	0/1
Kettle Brand, sour cream, onion & chive	13	1	1	16	1/1
Kettle Brand, spicy Thai	13	1	1	16	1/1
Kettle Brand, sweet onion	13	1	1	16	1/1
Kettle Brand, Tuscan three cheese	13	1	1	16	1/1
Kettle Brand, unsalted	13	2	0	16	0/1
Kettle Brand, yogurt & green onion	13	1	1	16	1/1
Kettle Brand, Baked, aged white cheddar	20	2	1	20	1/1
Kettle Brand, Baked, hickory honey barbeque	20	2	1	21	1/2
Kettle Brand, Baked, lightly salted	20	2	0	21	0/2
Kettle Brand, Baked, salt & fresh ground pepper	20	2	0	21	0/2
Kettle Brand, Baked, sea salt & vinegar	20	2	0	21	0/2
Kettle Brand, Krinkle Cut, Buffalo bleu	9	1	1	16	1/1
Kettle Brand, Krinkle Cut, cheddar & sour cream	9	1	1	16	1/1
Kettle Brand, Krinkle Cut, classic barbeque	9	2	1	15	1/1
Kettle Brand, Krinkle Cut, lightly salted	9	1	0	16	0/1
Kettle Brand, Krinkle Cut, salt & fresh ground pepper	9	2	0	16	0/1
Kettle Brand, tortilla chips, black bean	11	2	0	18	0/1
Kettle Brand, tortilla chips, blue corn	8	2	0	18	0/1
Kettle Brand, tortilla chips, chili lime	11	2	0	18	0/1
Kettle Brand, tortilla chips, multi grain	11	2	0	18	0/1
Kettle Brand, tortilla chips, yellow corn	8	2	0	18	0/1
Lay's, barbecue	15	1	2	15	2/1
Lay's, barbecue, Baked!	14	2	3	22	3/2
Lay's, cheddar & sour cream	15	0	0	15	0/1
Lay's, cheddar & sour cream, Baked!	10	2	3	21	3/2
Lay's, classic	15	1	0	15	0/1
Lay's, original, Baked!	15	2	2	23	2/2
Lay's, Parmesan & Tuscan herb, Baked!	14	2	2	21	2/2
Lay's, salt & vinegar	17	1	1	15	1/1
Lay's, sour cream & onion	11	1	1	15	1/1
Lay's, sour cream & onion, Baked!	14	2	3	21	3/2
Lay's, Southwestern ranch, Baked!	14	2	2	21	2/2
Lay's, Kettle Cooked, jalapeño	15	1	0	16	0/1
Lay's, Kettle Cooked, original	16	1	0	18	0/1
Lay's, Kettle Cooked, reduced fat	16	2	0	19	0/1

FOOD	Svg Size	Fbr	Sgr	Cbs	S/C Val
Lay's, Kettle Cooked, sharp cheddar	18	1	1	16	1/1
Lay's, Stax, cheddar	1 oz	1	1	15	1/1
Lay's, Stax, mesquite barbecue	1 oz	1	2	15	2/1
Lay's, Stax, original	1 oz	1	0	16	0/1
Lay's, Stax, ranch	1 oz	1	2	15	2/1
Lay's, Stax, sour cream & onion	1 oz	1	2	15	2/1
Lay's, Wavy, hickory barbeque	13	1	0	16	0/1
Lay's, Wavy, original	11	1	0	15	0/1
Lay's, Wavy, ranch	12	1	0	16	0/1
Mission, tortilla chips, stone ground	14	1	0	19	0/1
Mission, tortilla chips, stone ground, organic	14	1	0	19	0/1
Mission, tortilla chips, super thin, white corn	13	2	0	19	0/1
Mission, tortilla chips, tortilla rounds, yellow corn	10	1	0	17	0/1
Mission, tortilla chips, tortilla strips, white corn	12	1	0	17	0/1
Mission, tortilla chips, tortilla triangles	10	1	0	17	0/1
Mission, tortilla chips, tortilla triangles, premium white corn	8	1	0	17	0/1
New York Style, Bagel Crisps, cinnamon raisin	6	0	7	19	7/1
New York Style, Bagel Crisps, everything	6	0	1	17	1/1
New York Style, Bagel Crisps, jalapeño cheddar, mini	22	1	1	17	1/1
New York Style, Bagel Crisps, multigrain	6	2	2	17	2/1
New York Style, Bagel Crisps, plain	6	0	1	18	1/1
New York Style, Bagel Crisps, roasted garlic	6	0	1	17	1/1
New York Style, Bagel Crisps, roasted garlic, mini	22	0	1	17	1/1
New York Style, Bagel Crisps, sea salt	6	0	1	18	1/1
New York Style, Bagel Crisps, sesame	6	0	1	16	1/1
New York Style, pita chips, cinnamon sugar	7	0	3	17	3/1
New York Style, pita chips, garlic	7	0	1	16	1/1
New York Style, pita chips, lightly salted	7	0	1	16	1/1
New York Style, pita chips, spicy three pepper	7	1	1	16	1/1
New York Style, pita chips, whole wheat	7	2	1	17	1/1
Pirate Brands, Original Tings	1 oz	0	0	16	0/1
Pirate Brands, Potato Flyers, homestyle barbeque	1 oz	1	2	19	2/1
Pirate Brands, Potato Flyers, the original	1 oz	1	0	18	0/1
Pirate Brands, Potato Flyers, sea salt & vinegar	1 oz	1	1	18	1/1
Pirate Brands, Potato Flyers, sour cream & onion	1 oz	1	1	19	1/1
Pirate Brands, Smart Puffs	1 oz	0	1	17	1/1
Pringles, bacon ranch	16	1	1	15	1/1
Pringles, barbecue	16	1	1	15	1/1
Pringles, barbecue, light	16	1	1	15	1/1
Pringles, cheddar cheese	16	1	1	15	1/1
Pringles, cheesy cheddar, multigrain	16	1	1	16	1/1
Pringles, creamy ranch, multigrain	16	1	1	16	1/1
Pringles, jalapeño	16	1	1	15	1/1
Pringles, original	16	1	0	15	0/1

FOOD	Svg Size	Fbr	Sgr	Cbs	S/C Val
Pringles, original, light	15	1	1	15	1/1
Pringles, original, multigrain	16	1	1	16	1/1
Pringles, original, 100 calorie packs	1 pkg	0	0	13	0/1
Pringles, original, reduced fat	16	1	1	17	1/1
Pringles, pizza	16	1	1	15	1/1
Pringles, ranch	16	1	1	15	1/1
Pringles, salt & vinegar	16	1	1	15	1/1
Pringles, sour cream & onion	16	1	0	15	0/1
Ruffles, authentic barbecue	11	1	0	16	0/1
Ruffles, cheddar & sour cream	11	1	0	14	0/1
Ruffles, cheddar & sour cream, Baked!	10	2	2	21	2/2
Ruffles, original	12	1	0	14	0/1
Ruffles, original, Baked!	9	2	2	21	2/2
Ruffles, reduced fat	13	1	0	18	0/1
Ruffles, sea salted, reduced fat	11	1	0	17	0/1
Stacy's, Simply Naked, bagel chips	15	1	2	19	2/1
Stacy's, Simply Naked, pita chips	9	1	0	18	0/1
Stacy's, Simply Naked, pita chips, multigrain	9	2	0	19	0/1
Stacy's, Simply Naked, pita chips, Parmesan garlic & herb	9	1	0	18	0/1
Stacy's, Simply Naked, pita chips, Tuscan herb	7	2	2	28	2/2
SunChips, French onion	15	3	3	18	3/1
SunChips, garden salsa	15	3	2	19	2/1
SunChips, harvest cheddar	15	3	2	19	2/1
SunChips, original	15	3	2	19	2/1
Terra, potato chips, Kettles, most flavors	15	1	0	18	0/1
Terra, potato chips, Kettles, sea salt & pepper	15	1	0	15	0/1
Terra, potato chips, Kettles, sea salt & vinegar	15	1	0	15	0/1
Terra, potato chips, unsalted, au naturel	18	2	0	15	0/1
Terra, potato chips, unsalted, hickory BBQ	16	1	0	15	0/1
Terra, potato chips, unsalted, lemon pepper	16	1	0	15	0/1
Terra, sweet potato chips, plain	17	3	3	15	3/1
Terra, sweet potato chips, sea salt	17	3	3	15	3/1
Terra, sweet potato chips, spiced	17	2	3	14	3/1
Terra, sweet potato chips, sweets & beets	16	1	0	15	0/1
Terra, sweet potato chips, sweets & carrots	13	5	7	15	7/1
Terra, taro chips, original	1 oz	4	1	19	1/1
Terra, taro chips, spiced	1 oz	2	2	20	2/1
Terra, vegetable chips, most flavors	14	3	3	16	3/1
Terra, vegetable chips, Exotic Harvest, sea salt	16	3	5	16	5/1
Terra, vegetable chips, Exotic Harvest, sweet onion	16	3	5	18	5/1
Terra, vegetable chips, Stripes & Blues, barbecue	14	2	5	16	5/1
Terra, vegetable chips, Stripes & Blues, sea salt	14	2	5	16	5/1
Tostitos, tortilla chips, blue corn, restaurant style	7	2	0	19	0/1
Tostitos, tortilla chips, blue corn, restaurant style, Natural	7	1	0	19	0/1

FOOD	Svg Size	Fbr	Sgr	Cbs	S/C Val
Tostitos, tortilla chips, multigrain	8	2	1	18	1/1
Tostitos, tortilla chips, Scoops!, Baked!	1 oz	2	0	22	0/2
Tostitos, tortilla chips, white corn, bite size	24	2	0	18	0/1
Tostitos, tortilla chips, white corn, crispy rounds	13	2	0	18	0/1
Tostitos, tortilla chips, white corn, restaurant style	7	2	0	19	0/1
Tostitos, tortilla chips, white corn, Scoops!	12	2	0	19	0/1
Tostitos, tortilla chips, yellow corn, restaurant style, Natural	7	1	0	19	0/1
Veggie Stix, Good Health Natural Foods	1 oz	1	0	18	0/1

DIPS

FOOD	Svg Size	Fbr	Sgr	Cbs	S/C Val
Bean, Fritos	2 T	2	0	5	0/1
Cheddar, jalapeño, Fritos	2 T	0	0	3	0/0
Cheddar, jalapeño, Heluva Good!	2 T	0	2	2	2/0
Cheddar, mild, Fritos	2 T	0	0	4	0/0
Chili cheese, Fritos	2 T	0	1	3	1/0
French onion, Dean's	2 T	0	2	2	2/0
French onion, Dean's, lite	2 T	0	3	4	3/0
French onion, Dean's, no fat	2 T	0	4	5	4/1
French onion, Frito-Lay	2 T	0	1	4	1/0
French onion, Heluva Good!	2 T	0	1	2	1/0
French onion, Heluva Good!, fat free	2 T	0	2	3	2/0
French onion, Kraft Dip	2 T	0	1	3	1/0
French onion, Lay's	2 T	0	0	2	0/0
Green onion, Dean's	2 T	0	2	3	2/0
Green onion, Kraft Dip	2 T	0	1	3	1/0
Guacamole	2 T	2	0	2	0/0
Guacamole, Dean's	2 T	0	1	2	1/0
Guacamole, Kraft Dip	2 T	0	1	3	1/0
Guacamole, Mission	2 T	0	0	3	0/0
Guacamole, Ortega	2 T	0	1	4	1/0
Guacamole, Wholly Guacamole	2 T	2	0	2	0/0
Guacamole, Wholly Guacamole, pico de gallo style	2 T	2	0	2	0/0
Guacamole, Wholly Guacamole, spicy	2 T	2	1	2	1/0
Guacamole, Wholly Guacamole, w/ green salsa	2 T	1	1	2	1/0
Hummus	2 T	1	0	6	0/1
Hummus, Athenos, Greek style	2 T	1	1	5	1/1
Hummus, Athenos, original	2 T	0	0	5	0/1
Hummus, Athenos, roasted eggplant	2 T	0	0	4	0/0
Hummus, Athenos, roasted red pepper	2 T	0	0	5	0/1
Hummus, Baba Foods, fresh cilantro & jalapeño	2 T	2	1	6	1/1
Hummus, Casbah	1 T	1	0	5	0/1
Hummus, Sabra, classic	2 T	1	0	4	0/0
Hummus, Sabra, jalapeño	2 T	0	0	2	0/0
Hummus, Sabra, roasted garlic	2 T	0	0	3	0/0
Hummus, Sabra, roasted red pepper	2 T	1	0	3	0/0

FOOD	Svg Size	Fbr	Sgr	Cbs	S/C Val
Hummus, Tribe, all natural, classic	2 T	1	0	4	0/0
Hummus, Tribe, all natural, roasted red peppers	2 T	1	0	3	0/0
Ranch, Dean's	2 T	0	2	2	2/0
Ranch, Dean's, lite	2 T	1	2	3	2/0
Ranch, Heluva Good!	2 T	0	2	2	2/0
Ranch, Kraft Dip	2 T	0	1	3	1/0
Ranch, Lay's	2 T	0	0	1	0/0
Salsa	2 T	0	1	2	1/0
Salsa, Green Mountain Gringo	2 T	0	0	2	0/0
Salsa, La Victoria, suprema	2 T	0	0	1	0/0
Salsa, La Victoria, thick 'n chunky	2 T	0	1	2	1/0
Salsa, La Victoria, verde	2 T	0	1	2	1/0
Salsa, Muir Glen	2 T	0	1	3	1/0
Salsa, Muir Glen, black bean & corn	2 T	0	1	4	1/0
Salsa, Muir Glen, chipotle	2 T	0	1	2	1/0
Salsa, Newman's Own	2 T	0	1	2	1/0
Salsa, Newman's Own, black bean & corn	2 T	2	1	5	1/1
Salsa, Newman's Own, mango	2 T	0	3	5	3/1
Salsa, Newman's Own, peach	2 T	0	5	6	5/1
Salsa, Newman's Own, pineapple	2 T	0	3	3	3/0
Salsa, Newman's Own, tequila lime	2 T	0	2	3	2/0
Salsa, Old El Paso, Thick 'n Chunky	2 T	0	1	2	1/0
Salsa, Ortega	2 T	0	0	2	0/0
Salsa, Ortega, con queso	2 T	0	1	4	1/0
Salsa, Ortega, garden vegetable	2 T	0	1	2	1/0
Salsa, Ortega, thick & chunky	2 T	0	1	2	1/0
Salsa, Ortega, verde	2 T	0	1	2	1/0
Salsa, Pace	2 T	0	2	2	2/0
Salsa, Pace, black bean & corn	2 T	1	2	5	2/1
Salsa, Pace, con queso	2 T	0	2	5	2/1
Salsa, Pace, pico de gallo	2 T	0	2	3	2/0
Salsa, Pace, pineapple chipotle	2 T	0	4	4	4/0
Salsa, Pace, verde	2 T	0	2	2	2/0
Salsa, Tostitos, con queso	2 T	0	0	5	0/1
Spinach, Tostitos	2 T	0	0	2	0/0
CRACKERS					
Annie's Homegrown, Bunny Classics, buttery rich	10	0	1	10	1/1
Annie's Homegrown, Bunny Classics, cheddar	9	0	0	9	0/1
Annie's Homegrown, Bunny Classics, saltines	13	0	1	11	1/1
Annie's Homegrown, Cheddar Bunnies, organic	50	0	0	19	0/1
Annie's Homegrown, Cheddar Bunnies, original	50	1	0	19	0/1
Annie's Homegrown, Sour Cream & Onion Bunnies	55	0	1	18	1/1
Annie's Homegrown, White Cheddar Bunnies	55	1	1	18	1/1
Annie's Homegrown, Whole Wheat Bunnies	50	3	1	17	1/1

FOOD	Svg Size	Fbr	Sgr	Cbs	S/C Val
Better Cheddars, Nabisco	22	0	0	18	0/1
Breton, Dare, multigrain	3	1	1	10	1/1
Breton, Dare, original	3	0	2	8	2/1
Breton, Dare, reduced fat	7	1	3	22	3/2
Carr's, poppy & sesame crackers	4	0	0	9	0/1
Carr's, table water crackers	5	0	0	13	0/1
Carr's, whole wheat crackers	2	1	3	10	3/1
Cheese Nips, Nabisco, cheddar	29	0	0	19	0/1
Cheese Nips, Nabisco, cheddar, reduced fat	29	1	0	21	0/2
Cheez-It, Sunshine, big	13	0	0	17	0/1
Cheez-It, Sunshine, hot & spicy	25	0	0	18	0/1
Cheez-It, Sunshine, original	27	0	0	17	0/1
Cheez-It, Sunshine, Parmesan & garlic	25	0	0	19	0/1
Cheez-It, Sunshine, pepper Jack	25	0	0	19	0/1
Cheez-It, Sunshine, reduced fat	29	0	0	20	0/1
Cheez-It, Sunshine, white cheddar	25	0	0	19	0/1
Cheez-It, Sunshine, white cheddar, reduced fat	25	0	0	22	0/2
Chicken in a Biskit, Nabisco	12	1	2	19	2/1
Club, multi-grain	4	0	2	9	2/1
Club, original	4	0	1	9	1/1
Club, reduced fat	5	0	2	12	2/1
Combos, cheddar cheese cracker	1/3 c	0	4	18	4/1
Combos, pepperoni pizza cracker	1/3 c	0	3	18	3/1
Doctor Kracker, crackers, klassic 3 seed	8	4	0	13	0/1
Doctor Kracker, crackers, seeded spelt	8	4	0	12	0/1
Doctor Kracker, flatbread, klassic 3 seed	1	3	0	11	0/1
Doctor Kracker, flatbread, seeded spelt	1	3	0	10	0/1
Goldfish, Pepperidge Farm, cheddar	55	0	0	20	0/1
Goldfish, Pepperidge Farm, cheddar, baby	89	0	0	20	0/1
Goldfish, Pepperidge Farm, original	55	0	0	20	0/1
Goldfish, Pepperidge Farm, pretzel	43	0	0	24	0/2
Goldfish, Pepperidge Farm, ranch, Flavor Blasted	54	0	0	19	0/1
Goldfish, Pepperidge Farm, sour cream & onion, Flavor Blasted	57	0	0	18	0/1
Goldfish, Pepperidge Farm, whole grain	55	2	0	19	0/1
Grissol, melba toast, multifibre	5	3	1	17	1/1
Grissol, melba toast, plain	4	1	1	17	1/1
Grissol, melba toast, rye & sesame	4	1	1	16	1/1
Grissol, melba toast, sesame	4	1	1	15	1/1
Grissol, melba toast, 12 grains	4	2	1	16	1/1
Grissol, melba toast, whole wheat 60%	4	2	1	14	1/1
Handi-Snacks, breadsticks 'n cheez	1 pkg	0	4	14	4/1
Handi-Snacks, Ritz crackers 'n cheese dip	1 pkg	0	2	11	2/1
Honey Maid, Nabisco, cinnamon graham (full crackers)	2	1	10	28	10/2
Honey Maid, Nabisco, cinnamon graham, low fat (full crackers)	2	1	11	29	11/2

FOOD	Svg Size	Fbr	Sgr	Cbs	S/C Val
Honey Maid, Nabisco, honey graham (full crackers)	2	1	8	24	8/2
Honey Maid, Nabisco, honey graham, low fat (full crackers)	2	2	8	28	8/2
Keebler, cinnamon graham (full crackers)	2	1	8	23	8/2
Keebler, honey graham (full crackers)	2	0	7	23	7/2
Keebler, original graham (full crackers)	2	0	7	22	7/2
Krispy, Sunshine, saltine, original	5	0	0	11	0/1
Krispy, Sunshine, saltine, wheat	5	0	0	11	0/1
Krispy, Sunshine, soup & oyster crackers	16	0	0	11	0/1
Old London, melba toast, classic	3	0	0	13	0/1
Old London, melba toast, rye	3	1	0	12	0/1
Old London, melba toast, sesame	3	1	0	11	0/1
Old London, melba toast, sourdough	3	1	0	12	0/1
Old London, melba toast, wheat	3	1	0	13	0/1
Old London, melba toast, whole grain	3	2	0	12	0/1
Pepperidge Farm, cheese crisps	20	1	3	19	3/1
Pepperidge Farm, Entertaining Quartet	4	0	1	10	1/1
Pepperidge Farm, Entertaining Trio	4	1	1	11	1/1
Pepperidge Farm, golden butter	4	0	1	11	1/1
Pepperidge Farm, harvest wheat	3	0	2	11	2/1
Pepperidge Farm, pretzel thins	11	1	2	21	2/2
Pepperidge Farm, Snack Sticks, toasted sesame	12	2	0	20	0/1
Pepperidge Farm, wheat crisps	17	2	5	21	5/2
Premium, Nabisco, saltine, fat free	5	0	0	13	0/1
Premium, Nabisco, saltine, low sodium	5	0	0	11	0/1
Premium, Nabisco, saltine, multigrain	5	0	0	10	0/1
Premium, Nabisco, saltine, original	5	0	0	11	0/1
Premium, Nabisco, saltine, original, minis	17	0	0	11	0/1
Premium, Nabisco, soup & oyster crackers	22	0	0	11	0/1
Ritz, Nabisco, original	5	0	1	10	1/1
Ritz, Nabisco, reduced fat	5	0	1	11	1/1
Ritz, Nabisco, roasted vegetable	5	0	1	10	1/1
Ritz, Nabisco, whole wheat	5	0	2	11	2/1
Ritz Bits, Nabisco, cheese	13	0	4	17	4/1
Ritz Bits, Nabisco, peanut butter	12	1	3	16	3/1
Saltines	5	0	0	11	0/1
Sociables, Nabisco	5	0	0	9	0/1
Tree of Life, classic golden, low fat	5	0	1	12	1/1
Tree of Life, cracked pepper	10	0	1	23	1/2
Tree of Life, garden vegetable	10	0	1	22	1/2
Tree of Life, sesame & flax seed	10	1	1	23	1/2
Tree of Life, water crackers	4	0	0	12	0/1
Tree of Life, water crackers, cracked pepper	4	0	0	12	0/1
Tree of Life, water crackers, sesame	4	0	0	11	0/1
Triscuit, Nabisco, original	6	3	0	20	0/1

FOOD	Svg Size	Fbr	Sgr	Cbs	S/C Val
Triscuit, Nabisco, reduced fat	7	3	0	23	0/2
Triscuit, Nabisco, rye w/ caraway seeds	6	3	0	20	0/1
Triscuit, Nabisco, Thin Crisps, original	15	3	0	21	0/2
Triscuit, Nabisco, Thin Crisps, Parmesan garlic	14	3	0	20	0/1
Triscuit, Nabisco, Thin Crisps, quatro formaggio	15	3	0	22	0/2
Vegetable Thins, Nabisco	21	1	2	19	2/1
Wasa, crispbread, fiber	1	2	0	7	0/1
Wasa, crispbread, hearty	1	2	0	11	0/1
Wasa, crispbread, multigrain	1	2	0	10	0/1
Wasa, crispbread, rye, light	2	3	0	14	0/1
Wasa, crispbread, rye, mild	3	2	1	16	1/1
Wasa, crispbread, sesame	1	0	0	9	0/1
Wasa, crispbread, 7 grain	3	1	0	13	0/1
Wasa, crispbread, sourdough	1	2	0	9	0/1
Wasa, crispbread, whole grain	1	2	0	10	0/1
Wasa, crispbread, whole wheat	1	1	0	10	0/1
Wheatables, original golden wheat	17	1	4	20	4/1
Wheatables, toasted honey wheat	17	1	4	20	4/1
Wheatables, Nut Crisps, roasted almond	16	1	4	20	4/1
Wheatables, Nut Crisps, toasted pecan	16	1	3	20	3/1
Wheatsworth, Nabisco	4	0	1	9	1/1
Wheat Thins, Nabisco, big	11	2	4	22	4/2
Wheat Thins, Nabisco, multigrain	16	2	4	22	4/2
Wheat Thins, Nabisco, 100% whole grain	16	2	3	21	3/2
Wheat Thins, Nabisco, original	16	2	4	22	4/2
Wheat Thins, Nabisco, ranch	15	2	4	21	4/2
Wheat Thins, Nabisco, reduced fat	16	2	4	22	4/2
Wheat Thins, Nabisco, sundried tomato & basil	16	2	4	21	4/2
Wheat Thins, Nabisco, Artisan, Vermont white cheddar	12	1	4	21	4/2
Wheat Thins, Nabisco, Artisan, Wisconsin Colby	14	1	4	22	4/2
Wheat Thins, Nabisco, Fiber Selects, 5-grain	13	5	4	22	4/2
Wheat Thins, Nabisco, Fiber Selects, garden vegetable	15	5	3	22	3/2
Wheat Thins, Nabisco, Flatbread, garlic & parsley	2	0	2	12	2/1
Wheat Thins, Nabisco, Flatbread, Tuscan herb	2	0	2	12	2/1

ENERGY BARS & GRANOLA BARS

FOOD	Svg Size	Fbr	Sgr	Cbs	S/C Val
Balance, almond brownie	1 bar	2	17	22	17/2
Balance, chocolate	1 bar	1	18	23	18/2
Balance, chocolate raspberry fudge	1 bar	2	19	22	19/2
Balance, cookie dough	1 bar	1	17	22	17/2
Balance, honey peanut	1 bar	1	17	21	17/2
Balance, mocha chip	1 bar	1	18	21	18/2
Balance, peanut butter	1 bar	1	17	21	17/2
Balance, yogurt honey peanut	1 bar	1	17	21	17/2
Balance Bare, chocolate almond	1 bar	3	12	23	12/2

FOOD	Svg Size	Fbr	Sgr	Cbs	S/C Val
Balance Bare, peanut butter	1 bar	3	11	22	11/2
Balance Bare, trail mix chocolate chip	1 bar	3	14	22	14/2
Balance CarbWell, caramel 'n chocolate	1 bar	1	1	23	1/2
Balance CarbWell, chocolate peanut butter	1 bar	1	1	22	1/2
Balance Gold, caramel nut blast	1 bar	1	14	23	14/2
Balance Gold, chocolate mint cookie crunch	1 bar	1	14	23	14/2
Balance Gold, chocolate peanut butter	1 bar	1	14	23	14/2
Balance Gold, triple chocolate chaos	1 bar	1	15	23	15/2
Balance Pure, banana cashew	1 bar	2	18	23	18/2
Balance Pure, cherry pecan	1 bar	2	18	22	18/2
Balance Pure, chocolate cashew	1 bar	4	16	23	16/2
Clif Bar, apricot	1 bar	5	21	45	21/3
Clif Bar, banana nut bread	1 bar	4	22	42	22/3
Clif Bar, black cherry almond	1 bar	5	20	44	20/3
Clif Bar, blueberry crisp	1 bar	5	21	43	21/3
Clif Bar, carrot cake	1 bar	5	21	46	21/3
Clif Bar, chocolate brownie	1 bar	5	22	44	22/3
Clif Bar, chocolate chip	1 bar	5	22	44	22/3
Clif Bar, chocolate chip peanut crunch	1 bar	5	21	42	21/3
Clif Bar, cool mint chocolate	1 bar	5	17	43	17/3
Clif Bar, cranberry apple cherry	1 bar	5	21	45	21/3
Clif Bar, cranberry orange nut bread	1 bar	4	23	42	23/3
Clif Bar, crunchy peanut butter	1 bar	5	20	42	20/3
Clif Bar, iced gingerbread	1 bar	4	22	43	22/3
Clif Bar, maple nut	1 bar	5	20	42	20/3
Clif Bar, oatmeal raisin walnut	1 bar	5	20	43	20/3
Clif Bar, peanut toffee buzz	1 bar	5	20	42	20/3
Clif Bar, spiced pumpkin pie	1 bar	5	23	45	23/3
Clif Bar, white chocolate macadamia	1 bar	4	21	41	21/3
Clif Builder's, chocolate	1 bar	4	20	30	20/2
Clif Builder's, chocolate mint	1 bar	4	20	31	20/2
Clif Builder's, cookies 'n cream	1 bar	4	20	30	20/2
Clif Builder's, lemon	1 bar	1	23	31	23/2
Clif Builder's, peanut butter	1 bar	4	20	30	20/2
Clif Builder's, vanilla almond	1 bar	3	22	30	22/2
Clif C, apple	1 bar	4	17	25	17/2
Clif C, blueberry	1 bar	4	17	26	17/2
Clif C, cherry pomegranate	1 bar	4	18	25	18/2
Clif C, raspberry	1 bar	4	17	25	17/2
Clif Kid Organic ZBar, apple cinnamon	1 bar	3	11	23	11/2
Clif Kid Organic ZBar, blueberry	1 bar	3	11	23	11/2
Clif Kid Organic ZBar, chocolate brownie	1 bar	3	10	23	10/2
Clif Kid Organic ZBar, chocolate chip	1 bar	3	11	24	11/2
Clif Kid Organic ZBar, honey graham	1 bar	3	10	26	10/2

FOOD	Svg Size	Fbr	Sgr	Cbs	S/C Val
Clif Kid Organic ZBar, peanut butter	1 bar	3	11	20	11/1
Clif Kid Organic ZBar, spooky s'mores	1 bar	3	11	24	11/2
Clif Mojo, honey roasted peanut	1 bar	2	9	20	9/1
Clif Mojo, mixed nuts	1 bar	2	8	19	8/1
Clif Mojo, mountain mix	1 bar	2	12	21	12/2
Clif Mojo, peanut butter pretzel	1 bar	2	9	21	9/2
Fiber One, chocolate mocha	1 bar	9	10	29	10/2
Fiber One, oats & apple streusel	1 bar	9	11	31	11/2
Fiber One, oats & caramel	1 bar	9	9	30	9/2
Fiber One, oats & chocolate	1 bar	9	10	29	10/2
Fiber One, oats & peanut butter	1 bar	9	9	28	9/2
Fiber One, oats & strawberry	1 bar	9	9	29	9/2
Fiber One, 90 Calorie, chocolate	1 bar	5	5	17	5/1
Fiber One, 90 Calorie, chocolate peanut butter	1 bar	5	5	17	5/1
Kashi Golean Chewy, chocolate almond toffee	1 bar	6	31	45	31/3
Kashi Golean Chewy, cookies n' cream	1 bar	6	35	50	35/3
Kashi Golean Chewy, malted chocolate crisp	1 bar	6	35	49	35/3
Kashi Golean Chewy, oatmeal raisin cookie	1 bar	6	33	49	33/3
Kashi Golean Chewy, peanut butter & chocolate	1 bar	6	31	48	31/3
Kashi Golean Crunchy!, chocolate almond	1 bar	5	13	27	13/2
Kashi Golean Crunchy!, chocolate caramel	1 bar	6	14	28	14/2
Kashi Golean Crunchy!, chocolate peanut	1 bar	6	13	30	13/2
Kashi Golean Crunchy!, chocolate pretzel	1 bar	5	13	28	13/2
Kashi Golean Crunchy!, cinnamon coffee cake	1 bar	5	13	26	13/2
Kashi Golean Roll!, caramel peanut	1 bar	6	14	27	14/2
Kashi Golean Roll!, chocolate peanut	1 bar	6	14	27	14/2
Kashi Golean Roll!, chocolate turtle	1 bar	6	14	27	14/2
Kashi Golean Roll!, fudge sundae	1 bar	6	13	27	13/2
Kashi Golean Roll!, oatmeal walnut	1 bar	6	13	27	13/2
Kashi TLC, baked apple spice	1 bar	3	9	21	9/2
Kashi TLC, blackberry graham	1 bar	3	9	21	9/2
Kashi TLC, cherry dark chocolate	1 bar	4	8	24	8/2
Kashi TLC, dark chocolate coconut	1 bar	4	7	21	7/2
Kashi TLC, dark mocha almond	1 bar	4	6	21	6/2
Kashi TLC, honey almond flax	1 bar	4	5	19	5/1
Kashi TLC, honey toasted 7 grain	1 bar	4	8	26	8/2
Kashi TLC, peanut peanut butter	1 bar	4	5	19	5/1
Kashi TLC, pumpkin pie	1 bar	4	8	22	8/2
Kashi TLC, pumpkin spice flax	1 bar	4	8	26	8/2
Kashi TLC, raspberry chocolate	1 bar	4	7	21	7/2
Kashi TLC, ripe strawberry	1 bar	3	9	21	9/2
Kashi TLC, roasted almond crunch	1 bar	4	8	26	8/2
Kashi TLC, trail mix	1 bar	4	6	20	6/1
Kudos, chocolate chip	1 bar	1	11	20	11/1

FOOD	Svg Size	Fbr	Sgr	Cbs	S/C Val
Kudos, M&M's	1 bar	1	9	17	9/1
Kudos, peanut butter	1 bar	1	10	18	10/1
Kudos, Snickers	1 bar	1	9	16	9/1
Luna, berry almond	1 bar	3	11	29	11/2
Luna, blueberry bliss	1 bar	3	13	27	13/2
Luna, caramel nut brownie	1 bar	3	12	27	12/2
Luna, caramel nut brownie, mini	1 bar	1	5	11	5/1
Luna, chai tea	1 bar	3	12	26	12/2
Luna, chocolate peppermint stick	1 bar	4	12	28	12/2
Luna, chocolate raspberry	1 bar	5	13	27	13/2
Luna, cookies 'n cream delight	1 bar	3	13	27	13/2
Luna, dulce de leche	1 bar	3	13	27	13/2
Luna, iced oatmeal raisin	1 bar	3	13	27	13/2
Luna, LemonZest	1 bar	3	13	27	13/2
Luna, LemonZest, mini	1 bar	1	5	11	5/1
Luna, nutz over chocolate	1 bar	4	10	25	10/2
Luna, nutz over chocolate, mini	1 bar	1	5	11	5/1
Luna, peanut butter cookie	1 bar	4	11	26	11/2
Luna, peanut butter cookie, mini	1 bar	1	5	11	5/1
Luna, s'mores	1 bar	3	13	27	13/2
Luna, s'mores, mini	1 bar	1	5	11	5/1
Luna, toasted nuts & cranberry	1 bar	3	11	26	11/2
Luna, vanilla almond	1 bar	3	11	25	11/2
Luna, white chocolate macadamia	1 bar	3	11	25	11/2
Luna, white chocolate macadamia, mini	1 bar	1	5	11	5/1
Nature Valley, apple crisp	2 bars	2	11	26	11/2
Nature Valley, cinnamon	2 bars	2	12	29	12/2
Nature Valley, maple brown sugar	2 bars	2	12	29	12/2
Nature Valley, oats 'n dark chocolate	2 bars	3	12	28	12/2
Nature Valley, oats 'n honey	2 bars	2	12	29	12/2
Nature Valley, peanut butter	2 bars	2	11	28	11/2
Nature Valley, pecan dark crunch	2 bars	2	12	28	12/2
Nature Valley, roasted almond	2 bars	2	11	28	11/2
Nature Valley, Chewy Trail Mix, cranberry & pomegranate	1 bar	1	13	24	13/2
Nature Valley, Chewy Trail Mix, dark chocolate & nut	1 bar	1	14	25	14/2
Nature Valley, Chewy Trail Mix, fruit & nut	1 bar	1	12	25	12/2
Nature Valley, Roasted Nut Crunch, almond crunch	1 bar	2	6	13	6/1
Nature Valley, Roasted Nut Crunch, peanut crunch	1 bar	2	6	13	6/1
Nature Valley, Sweet & Salty Nut, almond	1 bar	2	12	22	12/2
Nature Valley, Sweet & Salty Nut, cashew	1 bar	1	12	22	12/2
Nature Valley, Sweet & Salty Nut, dark chocolate, peanut & almond	1 bar	2	12	21	12/2
Nature Valley, Sweet & Salty Nut, peanut	1 bar	2	11	19	11/1
Nature Valley, Sweet & Salty Nut, roasted mixed nut	1 bar	1	12	21	12/2
Nature Valley, Yogurt, strawberry	1 bar	1	14	26	14/2

FOOD	Svg Size	Fbr	Sgr	Cbs	S/C Val
Nature Valley, Yogurt, vanilla	1 bar	1	14	26	14/2
Nutri-Grain, apple cinnamon	1 bar	2	12	24	12/2
Nutri-Grain, blackberry	1 bar	2	11	24	11/2
Nutri-Grain, blueberry	1 bar	2	12	24	12/2
Nutri-Grain, cherry	1 bar	2	12	24	12/2
Nutri-Grain, mixed berry	1 bar	2	12	23	12/2
Nutri-Grain, raspberry	1 bar	2	12	24	12/2
Nutri-Grain, strawberry	1 bar	2	12	24	12/2
Nutri-Grain, strawberry yogurt	1 bar	2	13	25	13/2
PowerBar, Fruit Smoothie Energy, berry blast	1 bar	1	27	43	27/3
PowerBar, Fruit Smoothie Energy, creamy citrus	1 bar	1	29	43	29/3
PowerBar, Fruit Smoothie Energy, tangy tropical	1 bar	1	30	43	30/3
PowerBar, Harvest Energy, apple cinnamon crisp	1 bar	5	20	42	20/3
PowerBar, Harvest Energy, double chocolate crisp	1 bar	5	21	42	21/3
PowerBar, Harvest Energy, oatmeal raisin cookie	1 bar	5	22	43	22/3
PowerBar, Harvest Energy, peanut butter chocolate chip	1 bar	5	18	42	18/3
PowerBar, Harvest Energy, strawberry crunch	1 bar	5	20	42	20/3
PowerBar, Harvest Energy, toffee chocolate chip	1 bar	5	20	42	20/3
PowerBar, Nut Naturals Energy, fruit and nuts	1 bar	3	9	20	9/1
PowerBar, Nut Naturals Energy, mixed nuts	1 bar	2	7	21	7/2
PowerBar, Nut Naturals Energy, trail mix	1 bar	2	10	21	10/2
PowerBar, Performance Energy, apple cinnamon	1 bar	2	25	45	25/3
PowerBar, Performance Energy, banana	1 bar	1	26	46	26/3
PowerBar, Performance Energy, caramel cookie	1 bar	1	24	45	24/3
PowerBar, Performance Energy, chocolate	1 bar	1	12	20	12/1
PowerBar, Performance Energy, chocolate peanut butter	1 bar	1	26	44	26/3
PowerBar, Performance Energy, cookies & cream	1 bar	1	26	45	26/3
PowerBar, Performance Energy, honey roasted nut	1 bar	2	24	45	24/3
PowerBar, Performance Energy, milk chocolate brownie	1 bar	1	26	45	26/3
PowerBar, Performance Energy, oatmeal raisin	1 bar	2	26	45	26/3
PowerBar, Performance Energy, peanut butter	1 bar	1	12	20	12/1
PowerBar, Performance Energy, vanilla crisp	1 bar	1	25	45	25/3
PowerBar, Performance Energy, wild berry	1 bar	1	25	45	25/3
PowerBar, Pria 110 Plus, double chocolate cookie	1 bar	1	10	16	10/1
PowerBar, Pria 110 Plus, French vanilla crisp	1 bar	1	9	17	9/1
PowerBar, Pria 110 Plus, mint chocolate cookie	1 bar	1	9	15	9/1
PowerBar, ProteinPlus, chocolate crisp	1 bar	2	18	37	18/2
PowerBar, ProteinPlus, chocolate peanut butter	1 bar	1	19	39	19/2
PowerBar, ProteinPlus, chocolate peanut butter, reduced sugar	1 bar	2	1	30	1/2
PowerBar, ProteinPlus, cinnamon roll	1 bar	0	20	38	20/2
PowerBar, ProteinPlus, cookies n cream	1 bar	1	18	38	18/2
PowerBar, ProteinPlus, dark chocolate toffee nut	1 bar	1	17	35	17/2
PowerBar, ProteinPlus, dulce de leche	1 bar	1	32	35	32/2
PowerBar, ProteinPlus, vanilla yogurt	1 bar	1	19	38	19/2

FOOD	Svg Size	Fbr	Sgr	Cbs	S/C Val
PowerBar, Pure & Simple Energy, cranberry oatmeal cookie	1 bar	2	10	23	10/2
PowerBar, Pure & Simple Energy, roasted peanut butter	1 bar	2	10	22	10/2
PowerBar, Recovery, cookies & cream caramel crisp	1 bar	0	19	30	19/2
PowerBar, Recovery, peanut butter caramel crisp	1 bar	0	19	30	19/2
PowerBar, Triple Threat Energy, caramel peanut fusion	1 bar	3	15	31	15/2
PowerBar, Triple Threat Energy, chocolate caramel fusion	1 bar	3	15	30	15/2
PowerBar, Triple Threat Energy, chocolate peanut butter crisp	1 bar	4	13	32	13/2
PowerBar, Triple Threat Energy, chocolate toffee almond	1 bar	3	16	31	16/2
PowerBar, Triple Threat Energy, s'mores	1 bar	3	16	31	16/2
Quaker Chewy, chocolate chip	1 bar	1	7	18	7/1
Quaker Chewy, peanut butter chocolate chip	1 bar	1	7	17	7/1
Quaker Chewy, s'mores	1 bar	1	8	19	8/1
Quaker Chewy, Dipps, caramel nut	1 bar	1	13	21	13/2
Quaker Chewy, Dipps, chocolate chip	1 bar	1	12	22	12/2
Quaker Chewy, Dipps, peanut butter	1 bar	1	10	19	10/1
Quaker Chewy, 90 Calories, chocolate chunk	1 bar	1	7	19	7/1
Quaker Chewy, 90 Calories, dark chocolate cherry	1 bar	1	7	19	7/1
Quaker Chewy, 90 Calories, honey nut	1 bar	1	6	19	6/1
Quaker Chewy, 90 Calories, oatmeal raisin	1 bar	1	7	19	7/1
Quaker Chewy, 90 Calories, peanut butter	1 bar	1	7	18	7/1
Quaker Chewy, 90 Calories, strawberry vanilla	1 bar	1	7	19	7/1
Quaker Chewy, Protein, chocolate & peanut butter	1 bar	1	7	18	7/1
Quaker Chewy, Protein, nutty peanut butter	1 bar	1	6	17	6/1
Quaker Chewy, 25% Less Sugar, chocolate chip	1 bar	3	5	17	5/1
Quaker Chewy, 25% Less Sugar, cookies & cream	1 bar	2	5	18	5/1
Quaker Chewy, 25% Less Sugar, honey graham	1 bar	2	5	18	5/1
Quaker Chewy, 25% Less Sugar, peanut butter chocolate chip	1 bar	3	5	17	5/1
Quaker Fiber & Omega-3, dark chocolate chunk	1 bar	9	7	26	7/2
Quaker Fiber & Omega-3, peanut butter chocolate	1 bar	9	7	25	7/2
Quaker Oatmeal to Go, apples & cinnamon	1 bar	5	22	44	22/3
Quaker Oatmeal to Go, banana bread	1 bar	5	19	43	19/3
Quaker Oatmeal to Go, brown sugar cinnamon	1 bar	5	19	43	19/3
Quaker Oatmeal to Go, maple brown sugar, high fiber	1 bar	10	13	43	13/3
Quaker Oatmeal to Go, oatmeal raisin	1 bar	5	19	43	19/3
Quaker Oatmeal to Go, raspberry streusel	1 bar	5	19	43	19/3
Quaker Simple Harvest, dark chocolate chunk	1 bar	2	10	26	10/2
Quaker Simple Harvest, trail mix	1 bar	2	9	25	9/2
Quaker Sweet & Salty Crunch, oats, nuts & honey	1 bar	2	8	24	8/2
Quaker Sweet & Salty Crunch, toffee almond	1 bar	2	9	25	9/2
Quaker True Delights, dark chocolate raspberry almond	1 bar	3	8	23	8/2
Quaker True Delights, honey roasted cashew mixed berry	1 bar	3	10	24	10/2
Quaker True Delights, toasted coconut banana macadamia nut	1 bar	3	8	23	8/2
Slim-Fast!, meal bar, chewy chocolate crisp	1 bar	5	10	26	10/2
Slim-Fast!, meal bar, chocolate peanut caramel	1 bar	5	12	23	12/2

FOOD	Svg Size	Fbr	Sgr	Cbs	S/C Val
Slim-Fast!, meal bar, fruit & yogurt trail mix	1 bar	5	10	24	10/2
Slim-Fast!, meal bar, oatmeal cinnamon raisin	1 bar	5	12	27	12/2
Slim-Fast!, meal bar, sweet & salty chocolate almond	1 bar	5	9	23	9/2
Slim-Fast!, snack bar, chocolate nougat gone nuts	1 bar	1	7	14	7/1
Slim-Fast!, snack bar, chocolatey vanilla blitz	1 bar	1	6	17	6/1
Slim-Fast!, snack bar, double-Dutch chocolate	1 bar	2	7	16	7/1
Slim-Fast!, snack bar, nutty chocolate chew	1 bar	0	7	15	7/1
Slim-Fast!, snack bar, peanut butter crunch time	1 bar	0	13	16	13/1
SoyJoy, apple walnut	1 bar	3	12	16	12/1
SoyJoy, berry	1 bar	3	12	17	12/1
SoyJoy, blueberry	1 bar	4	12	17	12/1
SoyJoy, mango coconut	1 bar	3	11	16	11/1
SoyJoy, peanut chocolate chip	1 bar	3	12	16	12/1
SoyJoy, raisin almond	1 bar	3	11	16	11/1
SoyJoy, strawberry	1 bar	3	11	17	11/1
Tiger's Milk, peanut butter	1 bar	1	13	18	13/1
Tiger's Milk, peanut butter, king size	1 bar	1	20	28	20/2
Tiger's Milk, peanut butter & honey	1 bar	1	13	19	13/1
Tiger's Milk, peanut butter crunch	1 bar	1	13	18	13/1
Tiger's Milk, protein rich	1 bar	1	13	18	13/1
Tiger's Milk, protein rich, king size	1 bar	1	21	28	21/2

OTHER SAVORY SNACKS

FOOD	Svg Size	Fbr	Sgr	Cbs	S/C Val
CornNuts, barbecue	⅓ c	1	1	20	1/1
CornNuts, original	⅓ c	1	0	20	0/1
CornNuts, ranch	⅓ c	1	0	20	0/1
Granola snack, Nature Valley, Nut Clusters, honey roasted peanut	7 pcs	1	8	15	8/1
Granola snack, Nature Valley, Nut Clusters, nut lovers	6 pcs	1	6	14	6/1
Granola snack, Nature Valley, Nut Clusters, roasted almond	7 pcs	2	7	15	7/1
Granola snack, Nature Valley, Nut Clusters, roasted cashew	7 pcs	1	7	18	7/1
Granola snack, Quaker, Granola Bites, all flavors	1 pkt	2	6	14	6/1
Pirate's Booty, aged white cheddar	1 oz	0	0	19	0/1
Pirate's Booty, barbeque	1 oz	0	0	21	0/2
Pirate's Booty, sea salt & vinegar	1 oz	0	0	20	0/1
Pirate's Booty, sour cream & onion	1 oz	1	1	18	1/1
Pirate's Booty, veggie	1 oz	1	0	19	0/1
Popcorn, air popped	1 c	1	0	6	0/1
Popcorn, caramel	1 oz	2	15	22	15/2
Popcorn, cheese	1 c	1	0	6	0/1
Popcorn, microwave, oil popped	1 c	1	0	5	0/1
Popcorn, Cracker Jack	½ c	1	15	23	15/2
Popcorn, Newman's Own, butter	3½ c	1	0	17	0/1
Popcorn, Newman's Own, light butter	3½ c	1	0	22	0/2
Popcorn, Orville Redenbacher, butter	1 c	0	0	3	0/0
Popcorn, Orville Redenbacher, kettle	1 c	0	0	3	0/0

FOOD	Svg Size	Fbr	Sgr	Cbs	S/C Val
Popcorn, Orville Redenbacher, movie theater butter	1 c	0	0	4	0/0
Popcorn, Pop Secret, butter	1 c	0	0	3	0/0
Popcorn, Pop Secret, kettle	1 c	0	0	3	0/0
Popcorn cakes, average	3	1	0	24	0/2
Pork skins, fried, plain	any	0	0	0	0/0
Pretzels, Combos, cheddar cheese	⅓ c	0	5	19	5/1
Pretzels, Combos, nacho cheese	⅓ c	0	5	19	5/1
Pretzels, Combos, pizzeria	⅓ c	0	4	19	4/1
Pretzels, Pepperidge Farm, pretzel thins	11	1	2	21	2/2
Pretzels, Pretzel Crisps, most flavors	11	1	2	23	2/2
Pretzels, Pretzel Crisps, cinnamon toast	10	1	4	23	4/2
Pretzels, Pretzel Crisps, Tuscan three cheese	10	1	3	22	3/2
Pretzels, Rold Gold, braided twists, honey wheat	8	1	3	23	3/2
Pretzels, Rold Gold, rods, classic	3	1	1	22	1/2
Pretzels, Rold Gold, thins, classic	9	1	0	23	0/2
Pretzels, Rold Gold, tiny twists, cheddar	20	1	0	22	0/2
Pretzels, Rold Gold, tiny twists, classic style	17	1	0	23	0/2
Pretzels, Rold Gold, tiny twists, honey mustard	20	1	1	23	1/2
Pretzels, Snyder's, hard, sourdough	1	1	0	22	0/2
Pretzels, Snyder's, mini	20	1	0	25	0/2
Pretzels, Snyder's, nibblers, sourdough	16	1	0	25	0/2
Pretzels, Snyder's, rods	3	1	0	24	0/2
Pretzels, Snyder's, snaps	24	1	0	25	0/2
Pretzels, Snyder's, sticks	28	0	0	23	0/2
Pretzels, Snyder's, sticks, honey wheat	6	2	4	24	4/2
Rice cakes, brown rice, plain, average	2	1	0	15	0/1
Rice cakes, Quaker, apple cinnamon	1	0	3	11	3/1
Rice cakes, Quaker, butter popped corn	1	0	0	8	0/1
Rice cakes, Quaker, caramel corn	1	0	3	11	3/1
Rice cakes, Quaker, lightly salted	1	0	0	7	0/1
Rice cakes, Quaker, white cheddar	1	0	1	8	1/1
Rice cakes, Quaker Mini Delights, chocolatey mint	1 pkg	1	7	14	7/1
Rice cakes, Quaker Mini Delights, cinnamon streusel	1 pkg	1	6	14	6/1
Rice cakes, Quaker Quakes, apple cinnamon	8	0	4	13	4/1
Rice cakes, Quaker Quakes, cheddar cheese	9	0	0	11	0/1
Rice cakes, Quaker Quakes, kettle	15	1	7	26	7/2
Rice cakes, Quaker Quakes, ranch	10	0	0	10	0/1
Rice cakes, Quaker True Delights, blackberry pomegranate	13	5	6	23	6/2
Rice cakes, Quaker True Delights, wild blueberry	13	5	6	23	6/2
Snack mix, Annie's Homegrown, Snack Mix Bunnies	45 pcs	0	1	20	1/1
Snack mix, Annie's Homegrown, Snack Mix Bunnies, cheddar	40 pcs	0	1	20	1/1
Snack mix, Chex Mix, barbecue	½ c	0	2	19	2/1
Snack mix, Chex Mix, bold party blend	½ c	0	2	20	2/1
Snack mix, Chex Mix, cheddar	⅔ c	0	2	22	2/2

FOOD	Svg Size	Fbr	Sgr	Cbs	S/C Val
Snack mix, Chex Mix, dark chocolate	⅔ c	0	8	23	8/2
Snack mix, Chex Mix, honey nut, sweet 'n salty	⅔ c	0	5	22	5/2
Snack mix, Chex Mix, peanut butter chocolate	⅔ c	0	9	24	9/2
Snack mix, Chex Mix, peanut lovers	½ c	1	2	19	2/1
Snack mix, Chex Mix, sour cream & onion	½ c	0	2	19	2/1
Snack mix, Chex Mix, traditional	⅔ c	1	2	22	2/2
Snack mix, Gardettos, Italian cheese	½ c	0	2	20	2/1
Snack mix, Gardettos, original	½ c	1	0	18	0/1
Snack mix, Gardettos, original, reduced fat	½ c	1	0	20	0/1
Snack mix, Himalania, goji berries almonds crunch	1 oz	3	5	9	5/1
Trail mix, Chex Mix, sweet 'n salty	½ c	1	7	22	7/2
Trail mix, Emerald, berry blend	¼ c	2	11	16	11/1
Trail mix, Emerald, breakfast blend	¼ c	2	14	19	14/1
Trail mix, Good Sense, dietary snack mix	3 T	2	5	8	5/1
Trail mix, Good Sense, feel'n healthy mix	¼ c	3	9	14	9/1
Trail mix, Good Sense, milk chocolate crunch	3 T	1	7	13	7/1
Trail mix, Good Sense, tropical	⅓ c	2	18	23	18/2
Trail mix, Himalania, raw vitality, goji berry mix	1 oz	3	5	10	5/1
Trail mix, Planters, Daybreak Blend, berry almond	1 pkt	3	17	27	17/2
Trail mix, Planters, fruit & nut	3 T	2	10	13	10/1
Trail mix, Planters, nut & chocolate	3 T	2	13	16	13/1
Trail mix, Planters, nuts, seeds & raisins	3 T	2	7	11	7/1
Trail mix, Planters, spicy nuts & Cajun sticks	¼ c	2	1	10	1/1

SWEET TREATS

FOOD	Svg Size	Fbr	Sgr	Cbs	S/C Val
CAKES, PASTRIES & BAKED GOODS					
Brownie, average	2 oz	1	10	18	10/1
Brownie, Entenmann's, fudge, single serve	1	2	34	50	34/3
Brownie, Little Debbie, Cosmic brownies	1 pc	1	26	43	26/3
Cake, angel food	1 slc	0	9	16	9/1
Cake, Boston cream pie	1 slc	0	10	12	10/1
Cake, chocolate	1 slc	1	11	21	11/2
Cake, fruitcake	1 slc	1	8	17	8/1
Cake, German chocolate	1 slc	1	14	23	14/2
Cake, marble	1 slc	1	16	22	16/2
Cake, pound	1 slc	0	10	15	10/1
Cake, sponge	1 slc	0	10	17	10/1
Cake, white	1 slc	0	10	16	10/1
Cake, yellow	1 slc	0	12	22	12/2
Cake, Entenmann's, all butter, crumb	⅛ pkg	0	16	29	16/2
Cake, Entenmann's, all butter, loaf	⅙ pkg	0	18	30	18/2
Cake, Entenmann's, angel food, loaf	⅙ pkg	0	20	35	20/2

FOOD	Svg Size	Fbr	Sgr	Cbs	S/C Val
Cake, Entenmann's, chocolate chip crumb, loaf	⅛ pkg	0	19	33	19/2
Cake, Entenmann's, coffee, crumb	⅒ pkg	1	13	34	13/2
Cake, Entenmann's, crumb, single serve	1	1	24	51	24/3
Cake, Entenmann's, crumb, ultimate	⅒ pkg	0	15	33	15/2
Cake, Entenmann's, marble, loaf	⅛ pkg	0	15	26	15/2
Cake, Entenmann's, marble, single serve	1	0	21	39	21/2
Cake, Entenmann's, pound, single serve	1	0	22	39	22/2
Cake, Entenmann's, raisin, loaf	⅛ pkg	1	21	33	21/2
Cake, Entenmann's, sour cream, loaf	⅛ pkg	0	13	24	13/2
Cake, Little Debbie, chocolate chip	2 pcs	1	33	42	33/3
Cake, Sara Lee, chocolate lava cake, Simple Singles	1 pc	2	27	42	27/3
Cake, Sara Lee, coffee cake, butter streusel	⅙ pkg	0	11	24	11/2
Cake, Sara Lee, coffee cake, pecan	⅙ pkg	0	9	22	9/2
Cake, Sara Lee, pound cake, all butter	1 oz	0	20	35	20/2
Cheesecake, Entenmann's, French	⅙ pkg	0	25	39	25/2
Cheesecake, Jell-O, no bake, homestyle	⅙ pkg	1	28	44	28/3
Cheesecake, Jell-O, no bake, real	⅛ pkg	2	27	39	27/2
Cheesecake, Sara Lee, cherry	¼ pkg	1	32	50	32/3
Cheesecake, Sara Lee, classic	¼ pkg	0	24	35	24/2
Cheesecake, Sara Lee, classic, New York style	⅙ pkg	1	31	47	31/3
Cheesecake, Sara Lee, strawberry, French	⅙ pkg	0	24	37	24/2
Cupcake, Hostess, Cup Cakes, frosted chocolate	1	1	20	29	20/2
Cupcake, Little Debbie, strawberry	1	0	21	29	21/2
Doughnut, chocolate, glazed, average	1	1	13	24	13/2
Doughnut, plain, chocolate frosting, average	1	1	11	22	11/2
Doughnut, plain, glazed, average	1	1	11	23	11/2
Doughnut, plain, no glaze, average	1	1	9	25	9/2
Doughnut, Entenmann's, buttermilk, glazed	1	1	23	37	23/2
Doughnut, Entenmann's, crumb	1	0	21	36	21/2
Doughnut, Entenmann's, Devil's food, frosted	1	2	24	36	24/2
Doughnut, Entenmann's, frosted, mini	1	1	9	15	9/1
Doughnut, Entenmann's, glazed	1	0	12	25	12/2
Doughnut, Entenmann's, plain, Softee	1	0	7	21	7/2
Doughnut, Entenmann's, rich frosted	1	1	17	30	17/2
Doughnuts, Hostess, Donettes, crunch	6	1	33	62	33/4
Doughnuts, Hostess, Donettes, frosted	6	1	22	38	22/2
Doughnuts, Hostess, Donettes, powdered	6	0	23	43	23/3
Doughnuts, Little Debbie, frosted, mini	4	1	18	32	18/2
Doughnut holes, Entenmann's, frosted Pop'ems	4	1	16	28	16/2
Doughnut holes, Entenmann's, glazed Pop'ems	4	0	19	30	19/2
Ice cream cone, cake, average	1	0	1	3	1/0
Ice cream cone, Keebler Fudge Shoppe, cup	1	0	2	6	2/1
Ice cream cone, Oreo	1	0	6	12	6/1
Ice cream cone, sugar, average	1	1	3	8	3/1

SWEET TREATS, cont'd.

FOOD	Svg Size	Fbr	Sgr	Cbs	S/C Val
Ice cream cone, waffle, average	1	1	2	23	2/2
Muffin, Fiber One, apple cinnamon bun	1	7	18	34	18/2
Muffin, Fiber One, banana chocolate chip	1	7	19	36	19/2
Muffin, Fiber One, mixed fruits, nuts & honey	1	7	16	34	16/2
Muffin, Fiber One, wild blueberry & oats	1	7	16	34	16/2
Muffin, Little Debbie, banana nut	1	1	19	30	19/2
Muffin, Vitalicious VitaMuffin, banana nut, sugar free	1	5	0	21	0/2
Muffin, Vitalicious VitaMuffin, velvety chocolate, sugar free	1	6	0	23	0/2
Muffin, Vitalicious VitaTop, banana nut, sugar free	1	5	0	21	0/2
Muffin, Vitalicious VitaTop, velvety chocolate, sugar free	1	9	0	23	0/2
Pastry, Entenmann's, apple puff	1	1	20	39	20/2
Pastry, Entenmann's, cheese topped bun	1	1	19	40	19/2
Pastry, Entenmann's, cinnamon bun, single serve	1	2	36	72	36/4
Pastry, Entenmann's, cinnamon bun, super	1	1	23	49	23/3
Pastry, Entenmann's, cinnamon raisin swirl bun	1	2	22	45	22/3
Pastry, Entenmann's, cinnamon twists	2	0	4	11	4/1
Pastry, Entenmann's, Danish, cheese, single serve	1	1	28	52	28/3
Pastry, Entenmann's, Danish, cherry cheese, single serve	1	1	21	52	21/3
Pastry, Entenmann's, Danish, cinnamon, single serve	1	2	33	61	33/4
Pastry, Entenmann's, Danish, raspberry, single serve	1	2	31	61	31/4
Pastry, Entenmann's, eclair	1	3	27	46	27/3
Pastry, Entenmann's, honey bun, jumbo, single serve	1	1	28	68	28/4
Pastry, Hostess, Ding Dongs	2	1	36	47	36/3
Pastry, Hostess, Sno Balls	2	2	46	61	46/4
Pastry, Hostess, Suzy Q's	2	2	49	70	49/4
Pastry, Hostess, Twinkies	2	0	35	54	35/3
Pastry, Hostess, Zingers	3	3	51	71	51/4
Pastry, Little Debbie, honey bun	1	1	15	32	15/2
Pie, apple, 9" diameter	⅛ pie	2	20	43	20/3
Pie, banana cream, 9" diameter	⅛ pie	1	17	47	17/3
Pie, blueberry, 9" diameter	⅛ pie	1	12	44	12/3
Pie, cherry, 9" diameter	⅛ pie	1	18	50	18/3
Pie, coconut creme, 7" diameter	⅛ pie	1	17	18	17/1
Pie, Dutch apple, 9" diameter	⅛ pie	2	29	59	29/3
Pie, egg custard, 6" diameter	⅙ pie	2	12	22	12/2
Pie, lemon meringue, 8" diameter	⅙ pie	1	27	53	27/3
Pie, mince, 9" diameter	⅛ pie	4	47	79	47/4
Pie, peach, 8" diameter	⅙ pie	1	7	38	7/2
Pie, pecan, 9" diameter	⅛ pie	3	33	79	33/4
Pie, pumpkin, 9" diameter	⅛ pie	2	25	46	25/3
Pie, vanilla cream, 9" diameter	⅛ pie	1	16	41	16/3
Pie, Entenmann's, apple, single serve	1	2	13	43	13/3
Pie, Entenmann's, cherry, single serve	1	2	25	57	25/3
Pie, Entenmann's, cherry, snack size	1	0	27	50	27/3

FOOD	Svg Size	Fbr	Sgr	Cbs	S/C Val
Pie, Entenmann's, lemon, snack size	1	0	26	50	26/3
Pie, Hostess, apple	1	2	40	70	40/4
Pie, Sara Lee, apple	⅛ pie	2	17	47	17/3
Pie, Sara Lee, cherry	⅛ pie	2	14	45	14/3
Pie, Sara Lee, Dutch apple	⅛ pie	2	18	52	18/3
Pie, Sara Lee, French silk	⅕ pie	2	30	51	30/3
Pie, Sara Lee, Key West lime	⅛ pie	0	37	50	37/3
Pie, Sara Lee, lemon grove meringue	⅐ pie	0	41	51	41/3
Pie, Sara Lee, pumpkin	⅛ pie	2	20	39	20/2
Pie, Sara Lee, raspberry	⅛ pie	2	14	49	14/3
Toaster pastry, Fiber One, blueberry	1	5	15	36	15/2
Toaster pastry, Fiber One, brown sugar cinnamon	1	5	15	36	15/2
Toaster pastry, Fiber One, chocolate fudge	1	5	16	35	16/2
Toaster pastry, Fiber One, strawberry	1	5	15	36	15/2
Toaster pastry, Pillsbury Toaster Strudel, apple	1	0	9	27	9/2
Toaster pastry, Pillsbury Toaster Strudel, blueberry	1	0	8	27	8/2
Toaster pastry, Pillsbury Toaster Strudel, cherry	1	0	9	27	9/2
Toaster pastry, Pillsbury Toaster Strudel, Danish style cream cheese	1	0	8	24	8/2
Toaster pastry, Pillsbury Toaster Strudel, strawberry	1	0	9	27	9/2
Toaster pastry, Pop-Tarts, frosted brown sugar cinnamon	1	0	16	34	16/2
Toaster pastry, Pop-Tarts, frosted brown sugar cinnamon, low fat	1	0	19	38	19/2
Toaster pastry, Pop-Tarts, frosted brown sugar cinnamon, 20% DV Fiber	1	5	12	34	12/2
Toaster pastry, Pop-Tarts, frosted chocolate fudge	1	1	20	37	20/2
Toaster pastry, Pop-Tarts, frosted chocolate fudge, 20% DV Fiber	1	5	14	34	14/2
Toaster pastry, Pop-Tarts, frosted strawberry	1	0	17	38	17/2
Toaster pastry, Pop-Tarts, frosted strawberry, low fat	1	0	21	39	21/2
Toaster pastry, Pop-Tarts, frosted strawberry, 20% DV Fiber	1	5	13	35	13/2
Toaster pastry, Pop-Tarts, unfrosted brown sugar cinnamon	1	0	13	34	13/2
Toaster pastry, Pop-Tarts, unfrosted strawberry	1	0	16	37	16/2
GELATIN & PUDDING					
Gelatin, Jell-O, box mix, all regular flavors, as prepared	½ c	0	19	19	19/1
Gelatin, Jell-O, box mix, all sugar-free flavors, as prepared	½ c	0	0	0	0/0
Gelatin, Jell-O, snack cup, all regular flavors	1 pkg	0	17	17	17/1
Gelatin, Jell-O, snack cup, all sugar-free flavors	1 pkg	0	0	0	0/0
Pudding, Jell-O, cheesecake, instant, as prepared	½ c	0	20	24	20/2
Pudding, Jell-O, cheesecake, instant, sugar free, as prepared	½ c	0	0	6	0/1
Pudding, Jell-O, chocolate, cook & serve, as prepared	½ c	0	15	22	15/2
Pudding, Jell-O, chocolate, cook & serve, sugar free, as prepared	½ c	1	0	7	0/1
Pudding, Jell-O, chocolate, instant, as prepared	½ c	1	18	25	18/2
Pudding, Jell-O, chocolate, instant, sugar free, as prepared	½ c	1	0	8	0/1
Pudding, Jell-O, chocolate, snack cup	1 pkg	0	19	25	19/2
Pudding, Jell-O, chocolate, snack cup, fat free	1 pkg	1	17	23	17/2
Pudding, Jell-O, chocolate, snack cup, sugar free	1 pkg	1	0	13	0/1
Pudding, Jell-O, chocolate vanilla swirl, snack cup	1 pkg	1	19	24	19/2

FOOD	Svg Size	Fbr	Sgr	Cbs	S/C Val
Pudding, Jell-O, chocolate vanilla swirl, snack cup, fat free	1 pkg	1	17	23	17/2
Pudding, Jell-O, chocolate vanilla swirl, snack cup, sugar free	1 pkg	1	0	12	0/1
Pudding, Jell-O, tapioca, snack cup	1 pkg	0	19	25	19/2
Pudding, Jell-O, tapioca, snack cup, fat free	1 pkg	0	17	23	17/2
Pudding, Jell-O, vanilla, cook & serve, as prepared	½ c	0	16	21	16/2
Pudding, Jell-O, vanilla, cook & serve, sugar free, as prepared	½ c	0	0	5	0/1
Pudding, Jell-O, vanilla, instant, as prepared	½ c	0	19	23	19/2
Pudding, Jell-O, vanilla, instant, sugar free, as prepared	½ c	0	0	6	0/1
Pudding, Jell-O, vanilla, snack cup	1 pkg	0	18	23	18/2
Pudding, Jell-O, vanilla, snack cup, fat free	1 pkg	0	17	24	17/2
Pudding, Jell-O, vanilla, snack cup, sugar free	1 pkg	0	0	13	0/1
Pudding, Snack Pack, butterscotch	1 pkg	0	16	21	16/2
Pudding, Snack Pack, chocolate	1 pkg	0	16	23	16/2
Pudding, Snack Pack, chocolate, fat free	1 pkg	0	15	20	15/1
Pudding, Snack Pack, chocolate, sugar free	1 pkg	1	0	15	0/1
Pudding, Snack Pack, tapioca	1 pkg	0	15	20	15/1
Pudding, Snack Pack, vanilla	1 pkg	1	14	21	14/2
Pudding, Snack Pack, vanilla, sugar free	1 pkg	0	0	11	0/1

CANDY, GUM & MINTS

FOOD	Svg Size	Fbr	Sgr	Cbs	S/C Val
Black licorice twist stix, Perfectly Sweet, sugar free	7 pcs	0	0	25	0/2
Blow Pop	1	0	5	16	5/1
Boston Baked Beans	11 pcs	1	9	11	9/1
Candy corn	22 pcs	0	28	36	28/2
Caramels, Judy's Candy Company, sugar-free vanilla	1 pc	0	0	13	0/1
Cinna cubs, Perfectly Sweet, sugar free	9 pcs	0	0	37	0/2
Creme Savers, strawberries & creme	3 pcs	0	10	11	10/1
Dots	11 pcs	0	21	33	21/2
Everlasting Gobstopper, Wonka	9 pcs	0	14	14	14/1
Good & Fruity	43 pcs	0	30	37	30/2
Good & Plenty	33 pcs	0	25	35	25/2
Gum, Altoids	2 pcs	0	0	2	0/0
Gum, Big Red, Wrigley's	1 pc	0	2	2	2/0
Gum, Bubble Yum, cotton candy	1 pc	0	5	6	5/1
Gum, Bubble Yum, original	1 pc	0	5	6	5/1
Gum, Bubble Yum, original, sugarless	1 pc	0	0	3	0/0
Gum, Chiclets, peppermint	2 pcs	0	2	2	2/0
Gum, Chiclets, sugarless	2 pcs	0	0	2	0/0
Gum, Dentyne	1 pc	0	1	1	1/0
Gum, Doublemint, Wrigley's	1 pc	0	2	2	2/0
Gum, Eclipse	2 pcs	0	0	2	0/0
Gum, Extra, classic	1 pc	0	0	1	0/0
Gum, Extra, most flavors	1 pc	0	0	2	0/0
Gum, Extra Fruit Sensations, all flavors	1 pc	0	0	2	0/0
Gum, 5	1 pc	0	0	2	0/0

FOOD	Svg Size	Fbr	Sgr	Cbs	S/C Val
Gum, Freedent	1 pc	0	2	2	2/0
Gum, Ice Breakers, all flavors	1 pc	0	0	2	0/0
Gum, Ice Breakers, Ice Cubes, all flavors	1 pc	0	0	2	0/0
Gum, Ice Breakers, Ice Cubes, White, all flavors	1 pc	0	0	3	0/0
Gum, Juicy Fruit, Wrigley's	1 pc	0	2	2	2/0
Gum, Orbit, all flavors	1 pc	0	0	1	0/0
Gum, Orbit, Mist, all flavors	1 pc	0	0	1	0/0
Gum, Orbit, White, all flavors	2 pcs	0	0	2	0/0
Gum, Spearmint, Wrigley's	1 pc	0	2	2	2/0
Gum, Spry	1 pc	0	0	1	0/0
Gum, Stride, all flavors	1 pc	0	0	1	0/0
Gum, Trident, original, all flavors	1 pc	0	0	1	0/0
Gum, Trident Layers, all flavors	1 pc	0	0	2	0/0
Gum, Trident Splash, all flavors	1 pc	0	0	2	0/0
Gum, Trident White, all flavors	2 pcs	0	0	2	0/0
Gum, Trident Xtra Care, all flavors	1 pc	0	0	1	0/0
Gum, Winterfresh, Wrigley's	1 pc	0	2	2	2/0
Gummy bears, average	10 pcs	0	13	22	13/2
Gummy bears, Haribo Gold-Bears	17 pcs	0	21	31	21/2
Hot Tamales	20 pcs	0	23	36	23/2
Jelly beans	1 oz	0	19	26	19/2
Jelly beans, Jelly Belly, 30 Flavor	35 pcs	0	28	37	28/2
Jelly beans, Jolly Rancher	30 pcs	0	26	36	26/2
Jolly Rancher, gummies	9 pcs	0	22	28	22/2
Jolly Rancher, hard candy	3 pcs	0	11	17	11/1
Jujyfruits	16 pcs	0	22	32	22/2
Laffy Taffy, all flavors	1 pc	0	19	29	19/2
Laffy Taffy, mini, all flavors	5 pcs	0	21	33	21/2
Life Savers, butter rum	4 pcs	0	13	15	13/1
Life Savers, butter toffee, sugar free	5 pcs	0	0	13	0/1
Life Savers, cherry lemonade	4 pcs	0	14	14	14/1
Life Savers, five flavors	4 pcs	0	9	11	9/1
Life Savers, five flavors, sugar free	4 pcs	0	0	14	0/1
Life Savers, gummies	10 pcs	0	25	30	25/2
Life Savers, wild berries	4 pcs	0	13	16	13/1
Life Savers, wild cherry	4 pcs	0	13	16	13/1
Mike and Ike	23 pcs	0	23	36	23/2
Mints, Altoids, regular, all flavors	3 pcs	0	2	2	2/0
Mints, Altoids, chocolate dipped, all flavors	2 pcs	0	2	2	2/0
Mints, Altoids, Smalls, sugar free	1 pc	0	0	0	0/0
Mints, Breath Savers, all flavors	1 pc	0	0	2	0/0
Mints, Doublemint	4 pcs	0	2	2	2/0
Mints, Eclipse	3 pcs	0	0	2	0/0
Mints, Ice Breakers, all flavors	1 pc	0	0	0	0/0

FOOD	Svg Size	Fbr	Sgr	Cbs	S/C Val
Mints, Life Savers, Pep-O-Mint	4 pcs	0	15	16	15/1
Mints, Life Savers, Pep-O-Mint, sugar free	4 pcs	0	0	14	0/1
Mints, Life Savers, Wint-O-Green	4 pcs	0	15	16	15/1
Mints, Life Savers, Wint-O-Green, sugar free	4 pcs	0	0	14	0/1
Mints, Mentos	1 pc	0	2	3	2/0
Nerds, Wonka, all flavors	1 T	0	14	14	14/1
PayDay	1 bar	2	21	27	21/2
Peanut brittle	1 oz	1	15	20	15/1
Peanut brittle, Judy's Candy Company, sugar free	¾ c	0	0	16	0/1
Pez	1 pkg	0	9	9	9/1
Red Vines, black licorice twists	4 pcs	0	16	33	16/2
Red Vines, original red twists	4 pcs	0	16	34	16/2
Red Vines, Sugar Free Vines, all flavors	7 pcs	0	0	25	0/2
Reese's Pieces	51 pcs	1	21	25	21/2
Runts	12 pcs	0	13	14	13/1
Skittles	¼ c	0	32	39	32/2
Sour Patch, watermelon	11 pcs	0	25	35	25/2
Sour Patch Kids	16 pcs	0	25	36	25/2
Sour Punch Straws, all flavors	6 pcs	1	18	34	18/2
Spree, Wonka	8 pcs	0	13	13	13/1
Starburst, fruit chews, all flavors	8 pcs	0	23	33	23/2
Starburst, jelly beans	¼ c	0	29	37	29/2
Swedish Fish	7 pcs	0	30	38	30/2
SweeTarts, Wonka	8 pcs	0	13	13	13/1
SweeTarts, Wonka, giant chewy	1 pc	0	7	9	7/1
Tootsie Pop	1	0	10	15	10/1
Tootsie Roll, midgees	6 pcs	0	19	28	19/2
Twizzlers, cherry bites	17 pcs	0	16	32	16/2
Twizzlers, cherry twists	4 pcs	0	19	36	19/2
Twizzlers, licorice bites	17 pcs	0	16	31	16/2
Twizzlers, licorice twists	4 pcs	0	18	35	18/2
Twizzlers, strawberry twists	4 pcs	0	19	36	19/2
Werther's Originals, caramels	6 pcs	1	15	28	15/2
Werther's Originals, hard candies	3 pcs	0	10	14	10/1
Werther's Originals, hard candies, sugar free	3 pcs	0	0	15	0/1
COOKIES					
Entenmann's, black & white cookie	1	0	48	60	48/3
Entenmann's, chocolate chip, chocolate chunk	1	0	13	25	13/2
Entenmann's, chocolate chip, milk chocolate	3	0	11	20	11/1
Entenmann's, chocolate chip, original recipe	3	0	11	20	11/1
Entenmann's, ultimate black & white cookies	1	0	16	20	16/1
Entenmann's, ultimate madeleines	1	0	16	26	16/2
Famous Amos, chocolate	3	1	14	25	14/2
Famous Amos, chocolate chip	4	0	9	20	9/1

FOOD	Svg Size	Fbr	Sgr	Cbs	S/C Val
Famous Amos, chocolate chip & pecans	4	1	9	18	9/1
Famous Amos, vanilla	3	1	13	25	13/2
Girl Scouts, Caramel deLites	2	1	13	19	13/1
Girl Scouts, Do-Si-Dos	2	0	7	16	7/1
Girl Scouts, Lemon Chalet Cremes	3	0	13	26	13/2
Girl Scouts, Peanut Butter Patties	2	0	10	17	10/1
Girl Scouts, Peanut Butter Sandwich	3	0	8	26	8/2
Girl Scouts, Samoas	2	0	11	19	11/1
Girl Scouts, Shortbread	4	0	4	19	4/1
Girl Scouts, Tagalongs	4	0	8	13	8/1
Girl Scouts, Thin Mints	2	0	10	21	10/2
Girl Scouts, Trefoils	5	0	7	22	7/2
Grandma's, chocolate chip	1	0	15	25	15/2
Grandma's, fudge chocolate chip	1	1	10	27	10/2
Grandma's, oatmeal raisin	1	1	15	30	15/2
Grandma's, peanut butter	1	1	13	24	13/2
Grandma's, peanut butter sandwich creme	5	2	14	28	14/2
Grandma's, rich 'n chewy, chocolate chip	6	2	23	38	23/2
Grandma's, vanilla sandwich creme	5	1	14	30	14/2
Handi-Snacks, Oreo cookies 'n creme	1 pkg	1	13	20	13/1
Jennies, coconut macaroons, unsweetened coconut	2	1	1	13	1/1
Joseph's, sugar-free cookies, almond	4	1	0	13	0/1
Joseph's, sugar-free cookies, chocolate chip	4	1	0	13	0/1
Joseph's, sugar-free cookies, chocolate mint	4	1	0	14	0/1
Joseph's, sugar-free cookies, chocolate peanut butter	4	1	0	13	0/1
Joseph's, sugar-free cookies, chocolate walnut	4	1	0	14	0/1
Joseph's, sugar-free cookies, coconut	4	1	0	14	0/1
Joseph's, sugar-free cookies, lemon	4	1	0	15	0/1
Joseph's, sugar-free cookies, oatmeal	4	1	0	15	0/1
Joseph's, sugar-free cookies, oatmeal chocolate chip w/ pecans	4	1	0	14	0/1
Joseph's, sugar-free cookies, peanut butter	4	1	0	14	0/1
Joseph's, sugar-free cookies, pecan chocolate chip	4	1	0	13	0/1
Joseph's, sugar-free cookies, pecan shortbread	4	1	0	14	0/1
Kashi, happy trail mix	1	4	8	21	8/2
Kashi, oatmeal dark chocolate	1	4	8	20	8/1
Kashi, oatmeal raisin flax	1	4	7	20	7/1
Keebler, Chips Deluxe, oatmeal chocolate chip	1	0	5	10	5/1
Keebler, Chips Deluxe, original	2	1	9	19	9/1
Keebler, Chips Deluxe, soft 'n chewy	2	1	10	22	10/2
Keebler, E.L. Fudge, double stuffed	2	1	13	24	13/2
Keebler, E.L. Fudge, original	1	1	6	13	6/1
Keebler, Fudge Shoppe, Fudge Stripes	3	0	10	21	10/2
Keebler, Fudge Shoppe, Grasshopper	4	0	12	20	12/1
Keebler, Sandies, cashew shortbread	2	0	7	18	7/1

FOOD	Svg Size	Fbr	Sgr	Cbs	S/C Val
Keebler, Sandies, chocolate chips & pecans shortbread	2	0	8	18	8/1
Keebler, Sandies, pecan shortbread	2	0	7	18	7/1
Keebler, Sandies, simply shortbread	2	0	7	19	7/1
Keebler, Soft Batch, chocolate chip	1	0	6	11	6/1
Keebler, Vienna Fingers	2	0	10	23	10/2
Keebler, Vienna Fingers, reduced fat	2	0	12	24	12/2
Little Debbie, chocolate chip creme pies	1	0	13	23	13/2
Little Debbie, chocolate cremes	1	1	12	21	12/2
Little Debbie, fudge rounds	1	2	30	47	30/3
Little Debbie, PB&J oatmeal pies	1	1	13	22	13/2
LU, cinnamon sugar spice	2	0	10	18	10/1
LU, le petit beurre	4	0	8	24	8/2
LU, Petit Écolier	2	0	10	17	10/1
LU, Pim's	2	0	13	17	13/1
LU, rich tea	4	0	8	22	8/2
LU, shortbread	2	0	5	16	5/1
Mother's, Circus Animal	6	0	13	20	13/1
Mother's, English tea	2	0	12	27	12/2
Mother's, macaroons	2	1	8	17	8/1
Mother's, oatmeal	2	0	8	19	8/1
Mother's, vanilla creme	2	0	11	26	11/2
Murray, butter cookies	8	0	7	22	7/2
Murray, chocolate cremes	3	1	11	21	11/2
Murray, chocolatey chip	8	0	7	22	7/2
Murray, ginger snaps	5	0	9	22	9/2
Murray, lemon cremes	3	1	11	21	11/2
Murray, sugar wafers	5	0	11	20	11/1
Murray, vanilla cremes	3	1	11	21	11/2
Murray Sugar Free, chocolate	3	1	0	18	0/1
Murray Sugar Free, chocolate bites	1 pkt	3	0	16	0/1
Murray Sugar Free, chocolate chip	3	2	0	20	0/1
Murray Sugar Free, creme	3	0	0	20	0/1
Murray Sugar Free, fudge dipped vanilla wafers	4	4	0	19	0/1
Murray Sugar Free, oatmeal	3	3	0	21	0/2
Murray Sugar Free, peanut butter	3	1	0	16	0/1
Murray Sugar Free, shortbread	8	2	0	21	0/2
Nabisco, Barnum's Animal Crackers	8	1	7	22	7/2
Nabisco, Chips Ahoy!	3	0	11	22	11/2
Nabisco, Chips Ahoy!, chewy	2	0	10	18	10/1
Nabisco, Chips Ahoy!, chunky	1	0	6	11	6/1
Nabisco, Chips Ahoy!, mini	5	0	9	21	9/2
Nabisco, Chips Ahoy!, oatmeal chewy	2	1	8	18	8/1
Nabisco, Chips Ahoy!, peanut butter chunky	1	0	5	10	5/1
Nabisco, Chips Ahoy!, reduced fat	3	0	11	23	11/2

FOOD	Svg Size	Fbr	Sgr	Cbs	S/C Val
Nabisco, Fig Newtons	2	1	12	22	12/2
Nabisco, Fig Newtons, fat free	2	1	12	22	12/2
Nabisco, Fig Newtons, 100% whole grains	2	2	13	22	13/2
Nabisco, Ginger Snaps	4	0	11	23	11/2
Nabisco, Lorna Doone, shortbread	2	0	3	10	3/1
Nabisco, Nilla Wafers	8	0	11	21	11/2
Nabisco, Nilla Wafers, mini	20	0	11	21	11/2
Nabisco, Nilla Wafers, reduced fat	8	0	12	24	12/2
Nabisco, Nutter Butter	2	0	8	19	8/1
Nabisco, Nutter Butter, bites	10	0	9	21	9/2
Nabisco, Nutter Butter, creme patties	5	1	8	19	8/1
Nabisco, Oreo	3	1	14	25	14/2
Nabisco, Oreo, Double Stuf	2	0	13	21	13/2
Nabisco, Oreo, golden	3	0	12	25	12/2
Nabisco, Oreo, mini	9	1	11	21	11/2
Nabisco, Oreo, reduced fat	3	1	14	27	14/2
Nabisco, Oreo, sugar free	3	3	0	16	0/1
Nabisco, SnackWell's, creme sandwich	2	0	9	20	9/1
Nabisco, SnackWell's, devil's food	1	0	7	12	7/1
Nabisco, Teddy Grahams, chocolate	24	2	8	22	8/2
Nabisco, Teddy Grahams, cinnamon	24	1	7	23	7/2
Nabisco, Teddy Grahams, honey	24	1	8	23	8/2
Nabisco Classics, French vanilla creme	1	0	7	14	7/1
Nabisco Classics, iced animal cookies	5	0	15	23	15/2
Nabisco Classics, iced lemon shortbread	2	0	11	26	11/2
Nabisco Classics, oatmeal	1	0	7	14	7/1
Nabisco Classics, snickerdoodle	1	0	8	14	8/1
Nabisco Classics, soft oatmeal raisin	1	0	8	17	8/1
Pepperidge Farm, Bordeaux	4	0	12	19	12/1
Pepperidge Farm, Brussels	3	1	11	20	11/1
Pepperidge Farm, Chessmen	3	0	5	18	5/1
Pepperidge Farm, chewy granola, fruit & nut	1	2	8	20	8/1
Pepperidge Farm, chocolate chunk, Chesapeake	1	0	7	15	7/1
Pepperidge Farm, chocolate chunk, Sausalito	1	0	9	16	9/1
Pepperidge Farm, chocolate chunk, Tahoe	1	0	6	17	6/1
Pepperidge Farm, crunchy granola, dark chocolate almond	1	2	8	16	8/1
Pepperidge Farm, Geneva	3	1	8	19	8/1
Pepperidge Farm, gingerman	4	0	11	21	11/2
Pepperidge Farm, lemon	4	0	8	21	8/2
Pepperidge Farm, Milano	3	0	11	21	11/2
Pepperidge Farm, Milano, double chocolate	2	0	10	17	10/1
Pepperidge Farm, Milano, milk chocolate	3	0	13	21	13/2
Pepperidge Farm, Milano, mint	2	0	8	16	8/1
Pepperidge Farm, Milano, orange	2	0	8	16	8/1

FOOD	Svg Size	Fbr	Sgr	Cbs	S/C Val
Pepperidge Farm, Montieri, raspberry tart	2	0	12	23	12/2
Pepperidge Farm, oatmeal	3	0	9	22	9/2
Pepperidge Farm, Pirouette, chocolate fudge	2	1	12	18	12/1
Pepperidge Farm, Pirouette, chocolate hazelnut	2	1	13	19	13/1
Pepperidge Farm, Pirouette, French vanilla	2	0	12	18	12/1
Pepperidge Farm, Pirouette, mint chocolate	2	0	14	18	14/1
Pepperidge Farm, shortbread	2	0	5	16	5/1
Pepperidge Farm, soft baked, dark chocolate brownie	1	1	13	22	13/2
Pepperidge Farm, soft baked, oatmeal	1	1	9	22	9/2
Pepperidge Farm, soft baked, oatmeal raisin	1	2	13	23	13/2
Pepperidge Farm, soft baked, snickerdoodle	1	0	9	22	9/2
Pepperidge Farm, sugar	3	0	10	20	10/1
Pepperidge Farm, Verona, blueberry	3	0	11	23	11/2
Pepperidge Farm, Verona, strawberry	3	0	10	22	10/2
Walkers, almond shortbread	1	0	3	10	3/1
Walkers, Belgian chocolate cookies	1	0	7	12	7/1
Walkers, butter digestive biscuits	2	1	5	15	5/1
Walkers, shortbread rounds	1	0	3	10	3/1
Walkers, shortbread rounds, homebake	1	0	4	12	4/1
Walkers, shortbread thins	3	0	6	18	6/1
Walkers, shortbread triangles, homebake	1	0	3	11	3/1
Walkers, vanilla shortbread	2	0	5	14	5/1

CHOCOLATE & COCOA

FOOD	Svg Size	Fbr	Sgr	Cbs	S/C Val
Baking bar, Baker's, bittersweet	0.5 oz	1	5	7	5/1
Baking bar, Baker's, German's sweet chocolate	0.5 oz	1	7	8	7/1
Baking bar, Baker's, semi-sweet	0.5 oz	1	6	8	6/1
Baking bar, Baker's, unsweetened	0.5 oz	2	0	4	0/0
Baking bar, Baker's, white chocolate	0.5 oz	0	9	9	9/1
Baking bar, Ghirardelli, bittersweet, 60% cacao	0.5 oz	3	16	23	16/2
Baking bar, Ghirardelli, semi-sweet	0.5 oz	3	20	26	20/2
Baking bar, Ghirardelli, unsweetened, 100% cacao	0.5 oz	7	0	14	0/1
Baking bar, Ghirardelli, white	0.5 oz	0	26	26	26/2
Baking bar, Hershey's, semi-sweet	0.5 oz	0	8	9	8/1
Baking bar, Hershey's, unsweetened	0.5 oz	2	0	4	0/0
Baking bar, Nestlé Toll House, bittersweet, 62% cacao	0.5 oz	1	5	7	5/1
Baking bar, Nestlé Toll House, dark, 53% cacao	0.5 oz	1	6	8	6/1
Baking bar, Nestlé Toll House, semi-sweet	0.5 oz	0	8	9	8/1
Baking bar, Nestlé Toll House, white	0.5 oz	0	9	9	9/1
Candy, Andes Creme de Menthe	8 pcs	1	20	22	20/2
Candy, Buncha Crunch	1/3 c	0	20	26	20/2
Candy, Cadbury Creme Egg	1	0	25	28	25/2
Candy, Dove Promises, dark chocolate	5 pcs	2	17	21	17/2
Candy, Dove Promises, dark chocolate, almond	5 pcs	3	9	14	9/1
Candy, Dove Promises, dark chocolate, tiramisu	5 pcs	2	18	24	18/2

FOOD	Svg Size	Fbr	Sgr	Cbs	S/C Val
Candy, Dove Promises, milk chocolate	5 pcs	1	22	24	22/2
Candy, Dove Promises, milk chocolate, almond	5 pcs	2	19	21	19/2
Candy, Dove Promises, milk chocolate, caramel	5 pcs	1	21	24	21/2
Candy, Dove Promises, milk chocolate, peanut butter	5 pcs	1	18	20	18/1
Candy, Dove Sugar Free, all flavors	5 pcs	3	0	22	0/2
Candy, Ferrero Rocher	1 pc	0	5	5	5/1
Candy, Ferrero Rondnoir	1 pc	0	5	7	5/1
Candy, Goobers, Nestlé	¼ c	2	18	22	18/2
Candy, Guylian La Trufflina	1 pc	0	5	5	5/1
Candy, Guylian seashells	1 pc	0	6	6	6/1
Candy, Guylian seashells, extra dark	1 pc	0	4	5	4/1
Candy, Hershey's Kisses, milk chocolate	9 pcs	1	23	25	23/2
Candy, Hershey's Kisses, special dark	9 pcs	3	21	25	21/2
Candy, Hershey's Kisses, w/ almonds	9 pcs	1	19	21	19/2
Candy, Junior Mints	8 pcs	0	16	17	16/1
Candy, La Nouba, chocolate-covered marshmallows	1 pc	0	0	9	0/1
Candy, Lindt Lindor Truffles, dark	1 pc	1	5	6	5/1
Candy, Lindt Lindor Truffles, dark 60% cacao	1 pc	0	4	5	4/1
Candy, Lindt Lindor Truffles, milk	1 pc	0	5	6	5/1
Candy, Lindt Lindor Truffles, peanut butter	1 pc	0	4	5	4/1
Candy, M&M's, almond	¼ c	2	21	25	21/2
Candy, M&M's, dark chocolate	¼ c	2	24	29	24/2
Candy, M&M's, milk chocolate	¼ c	1	27	30	27/2
Candy, M&M's, peanut	¼ c	1	22	26	22/2
Candy, M&M's, peanut butter	¼ c	2	20	24	20/2
Candy, Milk Duds	13 pcs	0	20	28	20/2
Candy, Raisinets, dark chocolate	¼ c	2	26	32	26/2
Candy, Raisinets, milk chocolate	¼ c	2	27	32	27/2
Candy, Reese's Big Cup	1 pkg	1	19	22	19/2
Candy, Reese's Peanut Butter Cups	1 pkg	1	21	24	21/2
Candy, Reese's Peanut Butter Cups, miniatures, sugar free	5 pcs	6	0	27	0/2
Candy, Reese's Peanut Butter Cups, white chocolate	1 pkg	1	18	22	18/2
Candy, Riesen	4 pcs	0	15	28	15/2
Candy, Rolo	1 pkg	0	29	33	29/2
Candy, Sno-Caps	¼ c	2	24	30	24/2
Candy, Whoppers	18 pcs	0	26	31	26/2
Candy, Whoppers, peanut butter	17 pcs	0	18	25	18/2
Candy, Whoppers, strawberry	18 pcs	0	27	31	27/2
Candy, York Peppermint Patties	1 pc	0	25	31	25/2
Candy, York Peppermint Patties, miniature	3 pcs	0	27	33	27/2
Candy, York Peppermint Patties, sugar free	3 pcs	2	0	24	0/2
Candy bar, Almond Joy	1 pkg	2	20	26	20/2
Candy bar, Baby Ruth	1 bar	1	33	39	33/2
Candy bar, Butterfinger	1 bar	1	29	43	29/3

FOOD	Svg Size	Fbr	Sgr	Cbs	S/C Val
Candy bar, Cadbury, Caramello (1.6 oz bar)	1 bar	0	25	29	25/2
Candy bar, Cadbury, Caramello	6 pcs	0	24	28	24/2
Candy bar, Cadbury, dairy milk	7 pcs	0	22	23	22/2
Candy bar, Cadbury, fruit & nut	7 pcs	1	21	23	21/2
Candy bar, Cadbury, roast almond	7 pcs	1	19	21	19/2
Candy bar, ChocoPerfection, LowCarb Specialties, dark	1 bar	14	0	16	0/1
Candy bar, ChocoPerfection, LowCarb Specialties, milk	1 bar	14	0	16	0/1
Candy bar, Crunch, Nestlé	1 bar	1	24	29	24/2
Candy bar, Dove, dark chocolate	1 bar	3	15	20	15/1
Candy bar, Dove, dark chocolate, 63% cacao	1 bar	3	12	17	12/1
Candy bar, Dove, dark chocolate, 71% cacao	1 bar	3	9	14	9/1
Candy bar, Dove, dark chocolate, roasted almond	1 bar	2	15	18	15/1
Candy bar, Dove, milk chocolate	1 bar	1	18	20	18/1
Candy bar, Dove, milk chocolate, extra creamy	1 bar	2	16	20	16/1
Candy bar, Dove, milk chocolate, roasted almond	1 bar	1	16	18	16/1
Candy bar, Dove, milk chocolate, roasted hazelnut	1 bar	1	16	18	16/1
Candy bar, Endangered Species, all natural, 72% supreme dark	1.5 oz	5	12	18	12/1
Candy bar, Endangered Species, all natural, 88% extreme dark	1.5 oz	6	5	17	5/1
Candy bar, 5th Avenue	1 bar	1	29	38	29/2
Candy bar, Ghirardelli, dark & mint	3 pcs	2	20	24	20/2
Candy bar, Ghirardelli, dark & raspberry	3 pcs	2	20	24	20/2
Candy bar, Ghirardelli, milk & caramel	3 pcs	0	20	23	20/2
Candy bar, Ghirardelli, milk & peanut butter	4 pcs	1	20	22	20/2
Candy bar, Ghirardelli, Intense Dark, evening dream, 60% cacao	3 pcs	3	14	20	14/1
Candy bar, Ghirardelli, Intense Dark, midnight reverie, 86% cacao	4 pcs	5	5	15	5/1
Candy bar, Ghirardelli, Intense Dark, twilight delight, 72% cacao	3 pcs	4	10	17	10/1
Candy bar, Ghirardelli, Luxe Milk, almond	4 pcs	1	21	23	21/2
Candy bar, Ghirardelli, Luxe Milk, hazelnut	4 pcs	1	21	23	21/2
Candy bar, Ghirardelli, Luxe Milk, milk	4 pcs	0	24	26	24/2
Candy bar, Godiva, dark chocolate raspberry	1 bar	4	20	28	20/2
Candy bar, Godiva, milk chocolate	1 bar	1	23	24	23/2
Candy bar, Green & Black's, organic, dark 70%	3.5 oz	5	12	19	12/1
Candy bar, Green & Black's, organic, dark 85%	3.5 oz	4	5	10	5/1
Candy bar, Heath	1 bar	0	23	24	23/2
Candy bar, Hershey's, cookies 'n' creme	1 bar	0	19	27	19/2
Candy bar, Hershey's, milk chocolate	1 bar	1	24	26	24/2
Candy bar, Hershey's, milk chocolate, miniatures, sugar free	5 pcs	3	0	24	0/2
Candy bar, Hershey's, milk chocolate w/ almonds	1 bar	2	19	21	19/2
Candy bar, Hershey's, special dark	1 bar	3	21	25	21/2
Candy bar, Hershey's, special dark w/ almonds	1 bar	3	18	22	18/2
Candy bar, Hershey's Symphony	1 bar	0	20	21	20/2
Candy bar, Hershey's Symphony, almonds & toffee	1 bar	0	22	23	22/2
Candy bar, Kit Kat, milk chocolate	1 pkg	0	22	28	22/2
Candy bar, Kit Kat, white	1 pkg	0	18	26	18/2

FOOD	Svg Size	Fbr	Sgr	Cbs	S/C Val
Candy bar, La Nouba, Belgian milk chocolate, no sugar, most flavors	1 bar	4	0	4	0/0
Candy bar, La Nouba, Belgian milk chocolate, no sugar, dark	1 bar	4	0	1	0/0
Candy bar, Lindt Excellence, dark, 70% cacao	3 pcs	2	8	10	8/1
Candy bar, Lindt Excellence, dark, 85% cacao	3 pcs	2	4	6	4/1
Candy bar, Lindt Excellence, dark, 90% cacao	3 pcs	2	3	4	3/0
Candy bar, Lindt Excellence, dark, 99% cacao	1 bar	3	1	4	1/0
Candy bar, Lindt Lindor, dark	6 pcs	2	13	14	13/1
Candy bar, Milky Way	1 bar	1	35	41	35/3
Candy bar, Mounds	1 pkg	3	21	29	21/2
Candy bar, Mr. Goodbar	1 bar	2	23	26	23/2
Candy bar, 100 Grand	1 pkg	1	27	30	27/2
Candy bar, Reese's Fast Break	1 pkg	2	30	35	30/2
Candy bar, Reese's NutRageous	1 bar	2	22	28	22/2
Candy bar, ReeseSticks	1 pkg	1	17	23	17/2
Candy bar, Skor	1 pkg	0	24	25	24/2
Candy bar, Snickers	1 bar	1	30	35	30/2
Candy bar, Snickers, almond	1 bar	1	27	32	27/2
Candy bar, Snickers, dark	1 bar	2	24	31	24/2
Candy bar, Take 5	1 bar	1	18	25	18/2
Candy bar, 3 Musketeers	1 bar	1	40	46	40/3
Candy bar, Twix	1 pc	0	12	17	12/1
Candy bar, Whatchamacallit	1 bar	0	21	28	21/2
Chips, Baker's, semi-sweet chunks	1 T	1	8	9	8/1
Chips, Ghirardelli, bittersweet, 60% cacao	16 pcs	1	6	8	6/1
Chips, Ghirardelli, milk chocolate	16 pcs	0	10	10	10/1
Chips, Ghirardelli, semi-sweet	16 pcs	0	4	5	4/1
Chips, Hershey's, dark	1 T	1	8	9	8/1
Chips, Hershey's, milk chocolate	1 T	0	8	9	8/1
Chips, Hershey's, semi-sweet	1 T	0	8	10	8/1
Chips, Hershey's, sugar free	1 T	1	0	9	0/1
Chips, Nestlé Toll House, milk chocolate morsels	1 T	0	8	9	8/1
Chips, Nestlé Toll House, semi-sweet chunks	1 T	0	6	8	6/1
Chips, Nestlé Toll House, semi-sweet morsels	1 T	0	8	9	8/1
Chips, Nestlé Toll House, white morsels	1 T	0	9	9	9/1
Cocoa, Ghirardelli, sweet ground chocolate	2 T	1	16	17	16/1
Cocoa, Ghirardelli, unsweetened	1 T	1	0	3	0/0
Cocoa, Hershey's, natural unsweetened	1 T	2	0	3	0/0
Cocoa, Hershey's, special dark	1 T	2	0	3	0/0
Cocoa, Nestlé, dark chocolate	1 pkt	2	15	19	15/1
Cocoa, Nestlé, fat free	1 pkt	0	4	4	4/0
Cocoa, Nestlé, no sugar added	1 pkt	0	8	9	8/1
Cocoa, Nestlé, rich milk chocolate	1 pkt	0	12	14	12/1
Cocoa, Nestlé Toll House	1 T	1	0	3	0/0
Cocoa, Ovaltine, chocolate malt mix	4 T	0	15	18	15/1

FOOD	Svg Size	Fbr	Sgr	Cbs	S/C Val
Cocoa, Ovaltine, classic malt mix	4 T	0	14	18	14/1
Cocoa, Ovaltine, rich chocolate mix	4 T	0	18	19	18/1
Cocoa, Swiss Miss, diet	1 pkt	1	2	4	2/0
Cocoa, Swiss Miss, fat free	1 pkt	0	7	10	7/1
Cocoa, Swiss Miss, milk chocolate	1 pkt	0	16	23	16/2
Cocoa, Swiss Miss, no sugar added	1 pkt	0	7	10	7/1
Dipping, Baker's, dark semi-sweet	6 pcs	0	8	9	8/1
Dipping, Baker's, milk	6 pcs	0	8	9	8/1
Dipping, Dolci Frutta	10 pcs	1	17	18	17/1
Spread, Nutella	2 T	1	21	22	21/2

FROZEN DESSERTS

FOOD	Svg Size	Fbr	Sgr	Cbs	S/C Val
Bar, Ben & Jerry's, Cherry Garcia	1	1	23	28	23/2
Bar, Ben & Jerry's, Half Baked	1	2	33	46	33/3
Bar, Ben & Jerry's, vanilla	1	1	23	26	23/2
Bar, Blue Bunny, Bomb Pops	1	0	8	10	8/1
Bar, Blue Bunny, Bomb Pops, sugar free	1	1	0	7	0/1
Bar, Blue Bunny, FrozFruit, chunky strawberry	1	1	19	25	19/2
Bar, Blue Bunny, FrozFruit, chunky strawberry, no sugar added	1	3	2	15	2/1
Bar, Blue Bunny, FrozFruit, creamy coconut	1	1	13	14	13/1
Bar, Blue Bunny, 100 Calorie, butter pecan	1	2	2	10	2/1
Bar, Blue Bunny, 100 Calorie, English toffee	1	2	4	10	4/1
Bar, Blue Bunny, 100 Calorie, fudge	1	4	13	21	13/2
Bar, Blue Bunny, 100 Calorie, orange creme	1	0	14	19	14/1
Bar, Blue Bunny, 100 Calorie, raspberry creme	1	0	14	19	14/1
Bar, Blue Bunny, 100 Calorie, vanilla fudge	1	4	13	21	13/2
Bar, Blue Bunny, Sweet Freedom, almond, no sugar added	1	2	3	16	3/1
Bar, Blue Bunny, Sweet Freedom, black raspberry	1	2	2	11	2/1
Bar, Blue Bunny, Sweet Freedom, Caramel Lites, no sugar added	1	1	2	10	2/1
Bar, Blue Bunny, Sweet Freedom, fudge, no sugar added	1	2	4	16	4/1
Bar, Blue Bunny, Sweet Freedom, Fudge Lites, no sugar added	2	2	5	23	5/2
Bar, Blue Bunny, Sweet Freedom, Ice Cream Lites, no sugar added	1	1	3	11	3/1
Bar, Blue Bunny, Sweet Freedom, Krunch Lites	1	1	2	11	2/1
Bar, Blue Bunny, Yogurt Smoothie, all flavors	1	0	6	11	6/1
Bar, Breyers, Carb Smart, almond	1	2	5	9	5/1
Bar, Breyers, Carb Smart, fudge	1	1	3	9	3/1
Bar, Breyers, Carb Smart, vanilla	1	2	5	9	5/1
Bar, Breyers, Double Churn, creamy vanilla	1	3	15	21	15/2
Bar, Breyers, Double Churn, creamy vanilla, no sugar added	1	3	6	18	6/1
Bar, Breyers, Double Churn, Krunch, no sugar added	1	3	6	18	6/1
Bar, Breyers, Double Churn, rocky road	1	3	16	23	16/2
Bar, Breyers, Double Churn, vanilla & almond	1	3	15	21	15/2
Bar, Breyers, Pure Fruit, berry swirls	1	0	9	10	9/1
Bar, Breyers, Pure Fruit, pomegranate blends	1	0	9	10	9/1
Bar, Breyers, Pure Fruit, strawberry/orange/raspberry	1	0	9	10	9/1

FOOD	Svg Size	Fbr	Sgr	Cbs	S/C Val
Bar, Breyers, Pure Fruit, strawberry/tropical/raspberry, no sugar added	1	0	2	5	2/1
Bar, Coconut Bliss, dark chocolate	1	3	11	17	11/1
Bar, Coconut Bliss, naked coconut	1	2	9	14	9/1
Bar, Dreyer's/Edy's, Fruit Bars, acai blueberry	1	0	16	16	16/1
Bar, Dreyer's/Edy's, Fruit Bars, creamy coconut	1	1	15	21	15/2
Bar, Dreyer's/Edy's, Fruit Bars, grape	1	0	20	20	20/1
Bar, Dreyer's/Edy's, Fruit Bars, lemonade	1	0	19	20	19/1
Bar, Dreyer's/Edy's, Fruit Bars, lime	1	0	19	20	19/1
Bar, Dreyer's/Edy's, Fruit Bars, orange & cream	1	0	15	16	15/1
Bar, Dreyer's/Edy's, Fruit Bars, pineapple	1	0	18	19	18/1
Bar, Dreyer's/Edy's, Fruit Bars, pomegranate	1	0	16	17	16/1
Bar, Dreyer's/Edy's, Fruit Bars, strawberry	1	1	20	21	20/2
Bar, Dreyer's/Edy's, Fruit Bars, tangerine	1	0	19	19	19/1
Bar, Good Humor, chocolate eclair	1	1	4	30	4/2
Bar, Good Humor, original	1	0	13	17	13/1
Bar, Good Humor, strawberry shortcake	1	1	17	31	17/2
Bar, Good Humor, toasted almond	1	1	23	30	23/2
Bar, Häagen-Dazs, chocolate dark chocolate	1	2	20	24	20/2
Bar, Häagen-Dazs, vanilla dark chocolate	1	0	21	23	21/2
Bar, Häagen-Dazs, vanilla milk chocolate	1	0	21	22	21/2
Bar, Häagen-Dazs, vanilla milk chocolate almond	1	0	20	22	20/2
Bar, Healthy Choice, fudge	1	4	2	13	2/1
Bar, Healthy Choice, mocha swirl	1	1	14	17	14/1
Bar, Healthy Choice, sorbet & cream	1	1	12	17	12/1
Bar, Klondike, chocolate fudge, 100 calorie	1	4	5	20	5/1
Bar, Klondike, dark chocolate	1	1	23	29	23/2
Bar, Klondike, English toffee, 100 calorie	1	2	8	12	8/1
Bar, Klondike, French vanilla, 100 calorie	1	2	9	12	9/1
Bar, Klondike, krunch	1	1	23	30	23/2
Bar, Klondike, krunch, no sugar added	1	4	7	22	7/2
Bar, Klondike, Neapolitan	1	1	24	29	24/2
Bar, Klondike, original	1	1	23	29	23/2
Bar, Klondike, vanilla, no sugar added	1	4	7	21	7/2
Bar, Klondike, vanilla, 100 calorie	1	2	8	11	8/1
Bar, Popsicle, all flavors	1	0	8	11	8/1
Bar, Popsicle, all flavors, sugar free	1	0	0	4	0/0
Bar, Popsicle, Big Stick	1	0	13	17	13/1
Bar, Popsicle, Creamsicle, all flavors	1	0	8	13	8/1
Bar, Popsicle, Creamsicle, all flavors, no sugar added	1	0	1	5	1/1
Bar, Popsicle, Creamsicle, all flavors, 100 calories	1	0	12	20	12/1
Bar, Popsicle, Firecracker	1	0	7	9	7/1
Bar, Popsicle, Fudgsicle	1	0	9	12	9/1
Bar, Popsicle, Fudgsicle, fat free	1	1	10	13	10/1
Bar, Popsicle, Fudgsicle, no sugar added	1	2	2	10	2/1

SWEET TREATS, cont'd.

FOOD	Svg Size	Fbr	Sgr	Cbs	S/C Val
Bar, Popsicle, Fudgsicle, 100 calories	1	0	14	17	14/1
Bar, Popsicle, Pop-Ups, all flavors	1	0	10	18	10/1
Bar, Popsicle, Snow Cone	1	0	5	8	5/1
Bar, Popsicle, Super Twin, all flavors	1	0	9	14	9/1
Bar, Rice Dream, vanilla	1	0	16	24	16/2
Bar, Rice Dream, vanilla nutty	1	2	15	27	15/2
Bar, Skinny Cow, caramel truffle	1	3	12	19	12/1
Bar, Skinny Cow, chocolate truffle	1	3	12	19	12/1
Bar, Skinny Cow, French vanilla truffle	1	3	12	18	12/1
Bar, Skinny Cow, fudge	1	4	13	22	13/2
Bar, Skinny Cow, fudge pop minis	2	1	14	19	14/1
Bar, Skinny Cow, vanilla & caramel Skinny Dippers	1	2	7	11	7/1
Bar, Skinny Cow, vanilla & mint Skinny Dippers	1	2	7	11	7/1
Bar, Skinny Cow, white mint truffle	1	3	12	19	12/1
Bar, So Delicious, dairy free, sugar free, fudge	1	6	0	12	0/1
Bar, So Delicious, dairy free, sugar free, vanilla	1	6	0	15	0/1
Bar, Toffuti, milk free, chocolate dipped Mint by Mintz!, no sugar added	1	0	0	7	0/1
Bar, Toffuti, milk free, chocolate fudge treats, no sugar added	1	0	0	6	0/1
Bar, Toffuti, milk free, coffee break treats, no sugar added	1	0	0	6	0/1
Bar, Toffuti, milk free, Hooray! Hooray!, no sugar added	1	0	0	10	0/1
Bar, Toffuti, milk free, Marry Me	1	0	18	22	18/2
Bar, Toffuti, milk free, Totally Fudge	1	0	14	19	14/1
Cone, Blue Bunny, Durango, vanilla dark chocolate	1	3	20	31	20/2
Cone, Blue Bunny, Durango, vanilla raspberry	1	4	17	30	17/2
Cone, Blue Bunny, Sweet Freedom, chocolate, no sugar added	1	3	4	28	4/2
Cone, Blue Bunny, vanilla sundae, no sugar added	1	3	4	30	4/2
Cone, Good Humor, King Cone	1	1	19	30	19/2
Cone, Good Humor, King Cone, vanilla chocolate	1	2	30	44	30/3
Cone, Good Humor, sundae	1	1	18	29	18/2
Cone, Skinny Cow, chocolate w/ fudge	1	3	17	29	17/2
Cone, Skinny Cow, mint w/ fudge	1	3	17	29	17/2
Cone, Skinny Cow, vanilla w/ caramel	1	3	18	29	18/2
Frozen yogurt, Ben & Jerry's, Cherry Garcia	½ c	0	30	31	30/2
Frozen yogurt, Ben & Jerry's, chocolate fudge brownie	½ c	2	26	35	26/2
Frozen yogurt, Ben & Jerry's, Half Baked	½ c	1	23	35	23/2
Frozen yogurt, Ben & Jerry's, strawberry banana	½ c	0	23	32	23/2
Frozen yogurt, Blue Bunny, brownie fudge fantasy, fat free	½ c	0	16	24	16/2
Frozen yogurt, Blue Bunny, double raspberry	½ c	2	18	21	18/2
Frozen yogurt, Blue Bunny, homemade vanilla, fat free	½ c	0	17	19	17/1
Frozen yogurt, Blue Bunny, strawberry banana	½ c	2	16	19	16/1
Frozen yogurt, Blue Bunny, strawberry cheesecake, fat free	½ c	0	18	21	18/2
Frozen yogurt, Häagen-Dazs, coffee	½ c	0	20	31	20/2
Frozen yogurt, Häagen-Dazs, dulce de leche	½ c	0	25	35	25/2
Frozen yogurt, Häagen-Dazs, peach	½ c	0	23	31	23/2

FOOD	Svg Size	Fbr	Sgr	Cbs	S/C Val
Frozen yogurt, Häagen-Dazs, tart natural	½ c	0	21	30	21/2
Frozen yogurt, Häagen-Dazs, vanilla	½ c	0	21	31	21/2
Frozen yogurt, Häagen-Dazs, vanilla raspberry swirl	½ c	0	24	32	24/2
Frozen yogurt, Häagen-Dazs, wildberry	½ c	0	27	34	27/2
Frozen yogurt, Hood, chocolate, fat free	½ c	0	16	19	16/1
Frozen yogurt, Hood, chocolate chip cookie dough, low fat	½ c	0	17	23	17/2
Frozen yogurt, Hood, cookies & cream, low fat	½ c	0	16	22	16/2
Frozen yogurt, Hood, mocha fudge, fat free	½ c	0	17	22	17/2
Frozen yogurt, Hood, strawberry, fat free	½ c	0	12	18	12/1
Frozen yogurt, Hood, vanilla, fat free	½ c	0	14	19	14/1
Frozen yogurt, Hood, Frozen Tangy, blueberry	½ c	0	19	24	19/2
Frozen yogurt, Hood, Frozen Tangy, mango peach	½ c	0	19	24	19/2
Frozen yogurt, Hood, Frozen Tangy, pomegranate blueberry	½ c	0	18	23	18/2
Frozen yogurt, Hood, Frozen Tangy, strawberry	½ c	0	18	24	18/2
Frozen yogurt, Hood, Frozen Tangy, vanilla	½ c	0	18	23	18/2
Ice cream, Ben & Jerry's, banana split	½ c	1	27	30	27/2
Ice cream, Ben & Jerry's, brownie batter	½ c	1	26	33	26/2
Ice cream, Ben & Jerry's, cake batter	½ c	1	24	28	24/2
Ice cream, Ben & Jerry's, cheesecake brownie	½ c	0	23	26	23/2
Ice cream, Ben & Jerry's, Cherry Garcia	½ c	0	23	28	23/2
Ice cream, Ben & Jerry's, chocolate	½ c	2	22	25	22/2
Ice cream, Ben & Jerry's, chocolate chip cookie dough	½ c	0	24	32	24/2
Ice cream, Ben & Jerry's, chocolate fudge brownie	½ c	2	25	31	25/2
Ice cream, Ben & Jerry's, Chubby Hubby	½ c	1	25	31	25/2
Ice cream, Ben & Jerry's, Chunky Monkey	½ c	1	28	30	28/2
Ice cream, Ben & Jerry's, cinnamon buns	½ c	0	28	36	28/2
Ice cream, Ben & Jerry's, coffee Heath Bar crunch	½ c	0	26	29	26/2
Ice cream, Ben & Jerry's, crème brûlée	½ c	0	31	36	31/2
Ice cream, Ben & Jerry's, Dublin mudslide	½ c	0	23	29	23/2
Ice cream, Ben & Jerry's, Everything But The...	½ c	1	27	31	27/2
Ice cream, Ben & Jerry's, Fossil Fuel	½ c	1	25	32	25/2
Ice cream, Ben & Jerry's, Half Baked	½ c	1	25	33	25/2
Ice cream, Ben & Jerry's, Imagine Whirled Peace	½ c	0	25	28	25/2
Ice cream, Ben & Jerry's, Karamel Sutra	½ c	1	27	32	27/2
Ice cream, Ben & Jerry's, mint chocolate chunk	½ c	1	24	26	24/2
Ice cream, Ben & Jerry's, mint chocolate cookie	½ c	0	21	26	21/2
Ice cream, Ben & Jerry's, Mission to Marzipan	½ c	0	25	32	25/2
Ice cream, Ben & Jerry's, New York Super Fudge Chunk	½ c	2	24	29	24/2
Ice cream, Ben & Jerry's, oatmeal cookie chunk	½ c	1	23	30	23/2
Ice cream, Ben & Jerry's, peach cobbler	½ c	0	26	28	26/2
Ice cream, Ben & Jerry's, peanut butter cup	½ c	2	24	28	24/2
Ice cream, Ben & Jerry's, Phish Food	½ c	1	22	37	22/2
Ice cream, Ben & Jerry's, Pistachio Pistachio	½ c	1	18	22	18/2
Ice cream, Ben & Jerry's, s'mores	½ c	1	25	33	25/2

FOOD	Svg Size	Fbr	Sgr	Cbs	S/C Val
Ice cream, Ben & Jerry's, strawberry cheesecake	½ c	0	24	30	24/2
Ice cream, Ben & Jerry's, triple caramel chunk	½ c	0	25	32	25/2
Ice cream, Ben & Jerry's, Turtle Soup	½ c	1	25	30	25/2
Ice cream, Ben & Jerry's, vanilla	½ c	0	19	22	19/2
Ice cream, Ben & Jerry's, vanilla caramel fudge	½ c	0	25	31	25/2
Ice cream, Ben & Jerry's, vanilla Heath Bar crunch	½ c	0	26	29	26/2
Ice cream, Blue Bunny, banana split, premium	½ c	0	18	22	18/2
Ice cream, Blue Bunny, banana split, reduced fat, no sugar added	½ c	2	3	20	3/1
Ice cream, Blue Bunny, brownie sundae, fat free, no sugar added	½ c	5	4	23	4/2
Ice cream, Blue Bunny, butter pecan, light	½ c	3	8	16	8/1
Ice cream, Blue Bunny, butter pecan, premium	½ c	0	13	15	13/1
Ice cream, Blue Bunny, butter pecan, reduced fat, no sugar added	½ c	3	4	16	4/1
Ice cream, Blue Bunny, caramel toffee crunch, fat free, no sugar added	½ c	5	4	24	4/2
Ice cream, Blue Bunny, cherry vanilla, reduced fat, no sugar added	½ c	2	4	18	4/1
Ice cream, Blue Bunny, chocolate, reduced fat, no sugar added	½ c	3	6	16	6/1
Ice cream, Blue Bunny, double strawberry, premium	½ c	0	18	20	18/1
Ice cream, Blue Bunny, double strawberry, reduced fat, no sugar added	½ c	2	4	18	4/1
Ice cream, Blue Bunny, mint chocolate chip, premium	½ c	0	16	18	16/1
Ice cream, Blue Bunny, mint chocolate chip, reduced fat, no sugar added	½ c	3	5	17	5/1
Ice cream, Blue Bunny, rocky road, premium	½ c	0	16	21	16/2
Ice cream, Blue Bunny, rocky road, reduced fat, no sugar added	½ c	2	3	21	3/2
Ice cream, Blue Bunny, vanilla, fat free, no sugar added	½ c	5	5	20	5/1
Ice cream, Blue Bunny, vanilla, premium	½ c	0	15	16	15/1
Ice cream, Blue Bunny, vanilla, reduced fat, no sugar added	½ c	2	4	16	4/1
Ice cream, Breyers, butter pecan	½ c	0	14	14	14/1
Ice cream, Breyers, chocolate	½ c	1	16	17	16/1
Ice cream, Breyers, chocolate chip	½ c	1	16	17	16/1
Ice cream, Breyers, chocolate chip cookie dough	½ c	0	17	20	17/1
Ice cream, Breyers, coffee	½ c	0	15	15	15/1
Ice cream, Breyers, cookies & cream	½ c	0	16	19	16/1
Ice cream, Breyers, dulce de leche	½ c	0	19	21	19/2
Ice cream, Breyers, French vanilla	½ c	0	14	14	14/1
Ice cream, Breyers, homemade vanilla	½ c	0	13	16	13/1
Ice cream, Breyers, lactose free vanilla	½ c	0	14	14	14/1
Ice cream, Breyers, mint chocolate chip	½ c	0	17	17	17/1
Ice cream, Breyers, natural vanilla	½ c	0	14	14	14/1
Ice cream, Breyers, rocky road	½ c	1	17	20	17/1
Ice cream, Breyers, strawberry	½ c	0	15	15	15/1
Ice cream, Breyers, Carb Smart, chocolate	½ c	4	4	13	4/1
Ice cream, Breyers, Carb Smart, vanilla	½ c	4	4	13	4/1
Ice cream, Breyers, Smooth & Dreamy, butter pecan	½ c	0	16	16	16/1
Ice cream, Breyers, Smooth & Dreamy, butter pecan, no sugar added	½ c	4	4	14	4/1
Ice cream, Breyers, Smooth & Dreamy, chocolate cookies & cream, fat free	½ c	3	14	25	14/2
Ice cream, Breyers, Smooth & Dreamy, chocolate fudge brownie, fat free	½ c	4	15	25	15/2

FOOD	Svg Size	Fbr	Sgr	Cbs	S/C Val
Ice cream, Breyers, Smooth & Dreamy, chocolate fudge brownie, no sugar added	½ c	4	4	20	4/1
Ice cream, Breyers, Smooth & Dreamy, cookies & cream	½ c	0	18	20	18/1
Ice cream, Breyers, Smooth & Dreamy, creamy chocolate	½ c	1	16	17	16/1
Ice cream, Breyers, Smooth & Dreamy, creamy vanilla	½ c	0	16	16	16/1
Ice cream, Breyers, Smooth & Dreamy, creamy vanilla, fat free	½ c	3	12	21	12/2
Ice cream, Breyers, Smooth & Dreamy, French chocolate, fat free	½ c	4	13	22	13/2
Ice cream, Breyers, Smooth & Dreamy, French vanilla, no sugar added	½ c	4	4	14	4/1
Ice cream, Breyers, Smooth & Dreamy, mint chocolate chip	½ c	0	18	18	18/1
Ice cream, Breyers, Smooth & Dreamy, rocky road	½ c	1	19	23	19/2
Ice cream, Breyers, Smooth & Dreamy, strawberry, fat free	½ c	3	13	20	13/1
Ice cream, Breyers, Smooth & Dreamy, triple chocolate, no sugar added	½ c	4	4	17	4/1
Ice cream, Breyers, Smooth & Dreamy, vanilla, no sugar added	½ c	4	4	14	4/1
Ice cream, Breyers, Smooth & Dreamy, vanilla bean	½ c	0	16	16	16/1
Ice cream, Clemmy's, butter pecan	½ c	4	0	13	0/1
Ice cream, Clemmy's, chocolate	½ c	3	0	19	0/1
Ice cream, Clemmy's, chocolate chip	½ c	4	0	14	0/1
Ice cream, Clemmy's, chocolate mint swirl	½ c	3	0	20	0/1
Ice cream, Clemmy's, coffee	½ c	4	0	19	0/1
Ice cream, Clemmy's, toasted almond	½ c	4	0	20	0/1
Ice cream, Clemmy's, vanilla bean	½ c	4	0	18	0/1
Ice cream, Coconut Bliss, cappuccino	½ c	0	13	18	13/1
Ice cream, Coconut Bliss, chocolate hazelnut fudge	½ c	2	18	26	18/2
Ice cream, Coconut Bliss, dark chocolate	½ c	1	15	22	15/2
Ice cream, Coconut Bliss, mint galactica	½ c	0	13	18	13/1
Ice cream, Coconut Bliss, naked almond fudge	½ c	4	15	22	15/2
Ice cream, Coconut Bliss, naked coconut	½ c	0	12	17	12/1
Ice cream, Coconut Bliss, vanilla island	½ c	0	13	18	13/1
Ice cream, Dreyer's/Edy's, Grand, chocolate	½ c	1	15	17	15/1
Ice cream, Dreyer's/Edy's, Grand, chocolate chip	½ c	0	15	18	15/1
Ice cream, Dreyer's/Edy's, Grand, coffee	½ c	0	15	18	15/1
Ice cream, Dreyer's/Edy's, Grand, fudge swirl	½ c	0	11	16	11/1
Ice cream, Dreyer's/Edy's, Grand, mint chocolate chip	½ c	0	15	18	15/1
Ice cream, Dreyer's/Edy's, Grand, Neapolitan	½ c	0	14	16	14/1
Ice cream, Dreyer's/Edy's, Grand, real strawberry	½ c	0	15	16	15/1
Ice cream, Dreyer's/Edy's, Grand, rocky road	½ c	1	14	19	14/1
Ice cream, Dreyer's/Edy's, Grand, vanilla	½ c	0	13	15	13/1
Ice cream, Dreyer's/Edy's, Slow Churned, butter pecan	½ c	0	12	16	12/1
Ice cream, Dreyer's/Edy's, Slow Churned, butter pecan, no sugar added	½ c	2	3	15	3/1
Ice cream, Dreyer's/Edy's, Slow Churned, chocolate	½ c	0	13	15	13/1
Ice cream, Dreyer's/Edy's, Slow Churned, chocolate chip	½ c	0	13	17	13/1
Ice cream, Dreyer's/Edy's, Slow Churned, coffee	½ c	0	11	15	11/1
Ice cream, Dreyer's/Edy's, Slow Churned, French vanilla	½ c	0	11	15	11/1
Ice cream, Dreyer's/Edy's, Slow Churned, French vanilla, no sugar added	½ c	2	3	15	3/1
Ice cream, Dreyer's/Edy's, Slow Churned, fudge tracks	½ c	0	13	18	13/1

FOOD	Svg Size	Fbr	Sgr	Cbs	S/C Val
Ice cream, Dreyer's/Edy's, Slow Churned, fudge tracks, no sugar added	½ c	2	3	16	3/1
Ice cream, Dreyer's/Edy's, Slow Churned, mint chocolate chip	½ c	0	13	17	13/1
Ice cream, Dreyer's/Edy's, Slow Churned, mint chocolate chip, no sugar added	½ c	2	3	15	3/1
Ice cream, Dreyer's/Edy's, Slow Churned, Neapolitan	½ c	0	12	15	12/1
Ice cream, Dreyer's/Edy's, Slow Churned, Neapolitan, no sugar added	½ c	2	4	13	4/1
Ice cream, Dreyer's/Edy's, Slow Churned, rocky road	½ c	0	14	17	14/1
Ice cream, Dreyer's/Edy's, Slow Churned, strawberry	½ c	0	13	18	13/1
Ice cream, Dreyer's/Edy's, Slow Churned, triple chocolate, no sugar added	½ c	2	3	17	3/1
Ice cream, Dreyer's/Edy's, Slow Churned, vanilla	½ c	0	11	15	11/1
Ice cream, Dreyer's/Edy's, Slow Churned, vanilla, no sugar added	½ c	2	4	13	4/1
Ice cream, Dreyer's/Edy's, Slow Churned, vanilla bean	½ c	0	11	15	11/1
Ice cream, Dreyer's/Edy's, Slow Churned, vanilla bean, no sugar added	½ c	2	4	13	4/1
Ice cream, Dreyer's/Edy's, Slow Churned, Yogurt Blends, peach	½ c	0	14	17	14/1
Ice cream, Dreyer's/Edy's, Slow Churned, Yogurt Blends, strawberry	½ c	0	13	17	13/1
Ice cream, Dreyer's/Edy's, Slow Churned, Yogurt Blends, tart mango	½ c	0	15	19	15/1
Ice cream, Dreyer's/Edy's, Slow Churned, Yogurt Blends, vanilla	½ c	0	13	17	13/1
Ice cream, Dreyer's/Edy's, Slow Churned, Yogurt Blends, vanilla, fat free	½ c	0	14	20	14/1
Ice cream, Häagen-Dazs, banana split	½ c	0	27	31	27/2
Ice cream, Häagen-Dazs, butter pecan	½ c	0	18	21	18/2
Ice cream, Häagen-Dazs, caramel cone	½ c	0	27	32	27/2
Ice cream, Häagen-Dazs, cherry vanilla	½ c	0	22	23	22/2
Ice cream, Häagen-Dazs, chocolate	½ c	0	21	22	21/2
Ice cream, Häagen-Dazs, chocolate chip cookie dough	½ c	0	24	29	24/2
Ice cream, Häagen-Dazs, chocolate chocolate chip	½ c	2	24	26	24/2
Ice cream, Häagen-Dazs, chocolate peanut butter	½ c	2	24	27	24/2
Ice cream, Häagen-Dazs, coffee	½ c	0	21	21	21/2
Ice cream, Häagen-Dazs, cookies & cream	½ c	0	21	23	21/2
Ice cream, Häagen-Dazs, crème brûlée	½ c	0	22	23	22/2
Ice cream, Häagen-Dazs, dark chocolate	½ c	0	16	21	16/2
Ice cream, Häagen-Dazs, dulce de leche	½ c	0	28	28	28/2
Ice cream, Häagen-Dazs, green tea	½ c	0	19	20	19/1
Ice cream, Häagen-Dazs, mango	½ c	0	27	28	27/2
Ice cream, Häagen-Dazs, mint chip	½ c	0	23	26	23/2
Ice cream, Häagen-Dazs, pineapple coconut	½ c	0	24	25	24/2
Ice cream, Häagen-Dazs, pistachio	½ c	0	19	22	19/2
Ice cream, Häagen-Dazs, rocky road	½ c	1	24	29	24/2
Ice cream, Häagen-Dazs, rum raisin	½ c	0	21	22	21/2
Ice cream, Häagen-Dazs, strawberry	½ c	0	22	23	22/2
Ice cream, Häagen-Dazs, vanilla	½ c	0	21	21	21/2
Ice cream, Häagen-Dazs, white chocolate raspberry truffle	½ c	1	28	32	28/2
Ice cream, Häagen-Dazs, Five, coffee	½ c	0	21	23	21/2
Ice cream, Häagen-Dazs, Five, ginger	½ c	0	22	25	22/2
Ice cream, Häagen-Dazs, Five, lemon	½ c	0	24	26	24/2
Ice cream, Häagen-Dazs, Five, milk chocolate	½ c	0	20	22	20/2

FOOD	Svg Size	Fbr	Sgr	Cbs	S/C Val
Ice cream, Häagen-Dazs, Five, mint	½ c	0	23	24	23/2
Ice cream, Häagen-Dazs, Five, passion fruit	½ c	0	24	25	24/2
Ice cream, Häagen-Dazs, Five, vanilla bean	½ c	0	22	24	22/2
Ice cream, It's Soy Delicious, fruit sweetened, almond pecan	½ c	3	12	24	12/2
Ice cream, It's Soy Delicious, fruit sweetened, awesome chocolate	½ c	2	12	24	12/2
Ice cream, It's Soy Delicious, fruit sweetened, carob peppermint	½ c	2	11	24	11/2
Ice cream, It's Soy Delicious, fruit sweetened, chocolate peanut butter	½ c	3	11	24	11/2
Ice cream, It's Soy Delicious, fruit sweetened, espresso	½ c	2	9	23	9/2
Ice cream, It's Soy Delicious, fruit sweetened, green tea	½ c	2	9	24	9/2
Ice cream, It's Soy Delicious, fruit sweetened, pistachio almond	½ c	3	8	23	8/2
Ice cream, It's Soy Delicious, fruit sweetened, raspberry	½ c	2	8	25	8/2
Ice cream, It's Soy Delicious, fruit sweetened, vanilla	½ c	2	9	24	9/2
Ice cream, Purely Decadent, coconut milk, chocolate	½ c	6	12	20	12/1
Ice cream, Purely Decadent, coconut milk, coconut	½ c	6	11	19	11/1
Ice cream, Purely Decadent, coconut milk, cookie dough	½ c	5	15	24	15/2
Ice cream, Purely Decadent, coconut milk, mint chip	½ c	6	13	20	13/1
Ice cream, Purely Decadent, coconut milk, mocha almond fudge	½ c	5	14	21	14/2
Ice cream, Purely Decadent, coconut milk, passionate mango	½ c	5	13	19	13/1
Ice cream, Purely Decadent, coconut milk, vanilla bean	½ c	6	12	19	12/1
Ice cream, Purely Decadent, dairy free, Belgian chocolate	½ c	4	25	30	25/2
Ice cream, Purely Decadent, dairy free, chocolate obsession	½ c	5	20	36	20/2
Ice cream, Purely Decadent, dairy free, cookie dough	½ c	5	27	36	27/2
Ice cream, Purely Decadent, dairy free, dulce de leche	½ c	5	21	34	21/2
Ice cream, Purely Decadent, dairy free, mint chip	½ c	5	21	27	21/2
Ice cream, Purely Decadent, dairy free, praline pecan	½ c	5	15	33	15/2
Ice cream, Purely Decadent, dairy free, purely vanilla	½ c	6	18	29	18/2
Ice cream, Purely Decadent, dairy free, rocky road	½ c	5	21	31	21/2
Ice cream, Purely Decadent, dairy free, so very strawberry	½ c	4	22	33	22/2
Ice cream, Rice Dream, carob almond, gluten free	½ c	2	2	26	2/2
Ice cream, Rice Dream, cocoa marble fudge, organic, gluten free	½ c	1	17	31	17/2
Ice cream, Rice Dream, Cookies n' Dream	½ c	2	3	27	3/2
Ice cream, Rice Dream, mint carob chip	½ c	0	16	28	16/2
Ice cream, Rice Dream, Neapolitan, organic, gluten free	½ c	0	13	26	13/2
Ice cream, Rice Dream, orange vanilla, organic	½ c	0	14	26	14/2
Ice cream, Rice Dream, strawberry, organic, gluten free	½ c	2	2	25	2/2
Ice cream, Rice Dream, vanilla, organic, gluten free	½ c	2	2	26	2/2
Ice cream, Rice Dream, vanilla Swiss almond	½ c	2	3	27	3/2
Ice cream, Skinny Cow, caramel cone	1 pkg	4	24	33	24/2
Ice cream, Skinny Cow, chocolate fudge brownie	1 pkg	4	17	29	17/2
Ice cream, Skinny Cow, cookies 'n cream	1 pkg	4	18	29	18/2
Ice cream, Skinny Cow, dulce de leche	1 pkg	4	22	32	22/2
Ice cream, Skinny Cow, strawberry cheesecake	1 pkg	4	21	32	21/2
Ice cream, Soy Dream, butter pecan	½ c	1	14	23	14/2
Ice cream, Soy Dream, chocolate fudge brownie	½ c	1	13	21	13/2

SWEET TREATS, cont'd.

FOOD	Svg Size	Fbr	Sgr	Cbs	S/C Val
Ice cream, Soy Dream, French vanilla	½ c	0	11	17	11/1
Ice cream, Soy Dream, green tea	½ c	1	13	21	13/2
Ice cream, Soy Dream, mocha fudge	½ c	0	14	21	14/2
Ice cream, Soy Dream, vanilla	½ c	0	11	17	11/1
Ice cream, Soy Dream, vanilla fudge swirl	½ c	1	16	23	16/2
Ice cream, Starbucks, caramel maccchiato	½ c	0	21	27	21/2
Ice cream, Starbucks, coffee	½ c	0	19	21	19/2
Ice cream, Starbucks, java chip Frappuccino	½ c	0	22	25	22/2
Ice cream, Starbucks, mocha Frappuccino	½ c	0	20	23	20/2
Ice cream, Starbucks, signature hot chocolate	½ c	1	23	25	23/2
Ice cream, Starbucks, strawberries & crème Frappuccino	½ c	0	21	23	21/2
Ice cream, Starbucks, vanilla bean Frappuccino	½ c	0	20	22	20/2
Sandwich, Blue Bunny, Sedona, double chocolate	1	3	16	34	16/2
Sandwich, Blue Bunny, Sedona, double strawberry	1	3	16	34	16/2
Sandwich, Blue Bunny, Sweet Freedom, vanilla, no sugar added	1	4	4	32	4/2
Sandwich, Breyers, chocolate caramel brownie	1	3	16	31	16/2
Sandwich, Breyers, chocolate chip cookie dough	1	2	15	30	15/2
Sandwich, Breyers, vanilla fudge brownie	1	2	15	30	15/2
Sandwich, Breyers, Double Churn, all flavors	1	3	13	28	13/2
Sandwich, Good Humor, chocolate chip cookie sandwich	1	1	25	44	25/3
Sandwich, Good Humor, Neapolitan, giant	1	1	21	38	21/2
Sandwich, Good Humor, vanilla	1	0	13	26	13/2
Sandwich, Good Humor, vanilla, low fat	1	2	12	26	12/2
Sandwich, Healthy Choice, caramel swirl	1	1	16	30	16/2
Sandwich, Healthy Choice, ice cream	1	2	12	25	12/2
Sandwich, Klondike, peanut butter chocolate	1	1	17	33	17/2
Sandwich, Klondike, vanilla	1	0	16	31	16/2
Sandwich, Klondike, vanilla, no sugar added	1	2	3	20	3/1
Sandwich, Klondike, vanilla, 100 calorie	1	2	10	21	10/2
Sandwich, Rice Dream, chocolate pie	1	2	14	40	14/2
Sandwich, Rice Dream, mint pie	1	2	14	40	14/2
Sandwich, Rice Dream, mocha pie	1	2	14	40	14/2
Sandwich, Rice Dream, vanilla pie	1	1	12	40	12/2
Sandwich, Skinny Cow, chocolate peanut butter	1	3	15	30	15/2
Sandwich, Skinny Cow, cookies & cream	1	3	15	31	15/2
Sandwich, Skinny Cow, mint	1	3	15	30	15/2
Sandwich, Skinny Cow, strawberry shortcake	1	3	15	30	15/2
Sandwich, Skinny Cow, vanilla	1	3	15	30	15/2
Sandwich, Skinny Cow, vanilla, no sugar added	1	5	5	30	5/2
Sandwich, Toffuti, Cuties, nondairy, chocolate	1	0	9	16	9/1
Sandwich, Toffuti, Cuties, nondairy, cookies 'n cream	1	0	9	11	9/1
Sandwich, Toffuti, Cuties, nondairy, mint chocolate chip	1	0	10	19	10/1
Sandwich, Toffuti, Cuties, nondairy, peanut butter	1	0	10	20	10/1
Sandwich, Toffuti, Cuties, nondairy, totally vanilla	1	0	9	17	9/1

FOOD	Svg Size	Fbr	Sgr	Cbs	S/C Val
Sandwich, Toffuti, Cuties, nondairy, vanilla	1	0	9	17	9/1
Sherbet, Dreyer's/Edy's, berry rainbow	½ c	0	22	29	22/2
Sherbet, Dreyer's/Edy's, orange cream	½ c	0	19	23	19/2
Sherbet, Dreyer's/Edy's, tropical rainbow	½ c	0	24	29	24/2
Sorbet, Ben & Jerry's, Berried Treasure	½ c	1	24	29	24/2
Sorbet, Ben & Jerry's, Jamaican Me Crazy	½ c	1	29	33	29/2
Sorbet, Del Monte, Fruit Chillers, cup, all flavors	1	2	26	45	26/3
Sorbet, Del Monte, Fruit Chillers, tube, all flavors	1	0	11	13	11/1
Sorbet, Häagen-Dazs, chocolate	½ c	2	20	28	20/2
Sorbet, Häagen-Dazs, cranberry blueberry	½ c	1	20	25	20/2
Sorbet, Häagen-Dazs, mango	½ c	0	36	37	36/2
Sorbet, Häagen-Dazs, orchard peach	½ c	0	29	33	29/2
Sorbet, Häagen-Dazs, raspberry	½ c	2	26	30	26/2
Sorbet, Häagen-Dazs, strawberry	½ c	1	28	31	28/2
Sorbet, Häagen-Dazs, zesty lemon	½ c	0	29	28	29/2

BEVERAGES & POWDERED DRINK MIXES

FOOD	Svg Size	Fbr	Sgr	Cbs	S/C Val
COFFEE, TEA, WATER & FLAVORED DRINKS					
Amazing Grass, Green SuperFood, mix, berry	1 scp	2	0	4	0/0
Amazing Grass, Green SuperFood, mix, chocolate	1 scp	2	0	4	0/0
Amazing Grass, Kidz SuperFood, mix, outrageous chocolate	1 scp	1	1	4	1/0
AriZona, Arnold Palmer, lite	8 oz	0	13	14	13/1
AriZona, Arnold Palmer, zero	8 oz	0	0	1	0/0
AriZona, black & white iced tea	8 oz	0	14	14	14/1
AriZona, black tea, lemon	8 oz	0	24	25	24/2
AriZona, black tea, peach	8 oz	0	17	18	17/1
AriZona, black tea, raspberry	8 oz	0	22	23	22/2
AriZona, black tea, w/ ginseng & honey	8 oz	0	14	14	14/1
AriZona, black tea, w/ lemon flavor, diet	8 oz	0	0	0	0/0
AriZona, black tea, w/ peach flavor, diet	8 oz	0	0	0	0/0
AriZona, green tea, blueberry, diet	8 oz	0	0	2	0/0
AriZona, green tea, extra sweet	8 oz	0	23	23	23/2
AriZona, green tea, pomegranate	8 oz	0	18	19	18/1
AriZona, green tea, pomegranate, organic	8 oz	0	13	13	13/1
AriZona, green tea, white cranberry apple, diet	8 oz	0	0	2	0/0
AriZona, green tea, w/ ginseng & honey	8 oz	0	17	18	17/1
AriZona, green tea, w/ ginseng & honey, diet	8 oz	0	0	0	0/0
AriZona, green tea, w/ ginseng & honey, organic	8 oz	0	13	14	13/1
AriZona, Rx Energy, herbal tonic	8 oz	0	26	27	26/2
AriZona, Rx Stress, herbal iced tea	8 oz	0	18	19	18/1
AriZona, Southern style, sweet tea	8 oz	0	23	23	23/2
AriZona, Southern style, unsweetened brewed tea	8 oz	0	0	0	0/0

FOOD	Svg Size	Fbr	Sgr	Cbs	S/C Val
AriZona, white tea, blueberry	8 oz	0	18	19	18/1
Capri Sun, original, most flavors	6 oz	0	16	16	16/1
Capri Sun, original, lemonade	6 oz	0	16	17	16/1
Capri Sun, 100% Juice, apple splash	6 oz	0	22	23	22/2
Capri Sun, 100% Juice, berry breeze	6 oz	0	19	24	19/2
Capri Sun, 100% Juice, citrus wave	6 oz	0	21	23	21/2
Capri Sun, 100% Juice, fruit dive	6 oz	0	20	25	20/2
Capri Sun, 100% Juice, grape tide	6 oz	0	23	25	23/2
Capri Sun, Roarin' Waters, all flavors	6 oz	0	7	7	7/1
Capri Sun, Sunrise, all flavors	6 oz	0	15	15	15/1
Clearly Canadian, all flavors	8 oz	0	6	6	6/1
Club soda	8 oz	0	0	0	0/0
Coffee, brewed, unflavored, hot or iced	8 oz	0	0	0	0/0
Coffee, instant, as prepared	8 oz	0	0	1	0/0
Crystal Light, most flavors	1 pkt	0	0	0	0/0
Crystal Light, Fiber, raspberry peach	1 pkt	3	0	3	0/0
Crystal Light, Green Tea, all varieties	1 pkt	0	0	2	0/0
Crystal Light, Hunger Satisfaction, strawberry banana	1 pkt	5	0	6	0/1
Crystal Light, Immunity, cherry pomegranate	1 pkt	0	0	2	0/0
Crystal Light, Pure Fitness, all flavors	1 pkt	0	6	6	6/1
Emergen-C, most flavors	1 pkt	0	6	6	6/1
Emergen-C, berry blue	1 pkt	0	5	5	5/1
Emergen-C, cranberry pomegranate	1 pkt	0	5	5	5/1
Emergen-C, Heart Health	1 pkt	0	4	5	4/1
Emergen-C, Immune+, packet	1	0	4	5	4/1
Emergen-C, Immune+, shot	1	0	7	7	7/1
Emergen-C, Joint Health	1 pkt	0	5	5	5/1
Emergen-C, Kidz	1 pkt	0	6	7	6/1
Emergen-C, lite	1 pkt	0	1	1	1/0
Emergen-C, MSM, lite	1 pkt	0	0	1	0/0
Emergen-C, Multi-Vitamin	1 pkt	0	6	6	6/1
Emergen-C, orange, shot	1	0	7	7	7/1
Emergen-C, super orange	1 pkt	0	5	6	5/1
Emergen-C, tangerine	1 pkt	0	5	5	5/1
Emergen-C, vitamin D & calcium	1 pkt	0	5	5	5/1
Gatorade, G2, all flavors	8 oz	0	5	5	5/1
Gatorade, original, all flavors	8 oz	0	14	14	14/1
Gatorade, mix, G2, all flavors	½ pkt	0	5	5	5/1
Gatorade, mix, original, all flavors	1 T	0	14	14	14/1
Hi-C, juice box, flashin' fruit punch	6.75 oz	0	24	25	24/2
Hi-C, juice box, poppin' lemonade	6.75 oz	0	26	27	26/2
Jay Robb, whey protein, all flavored mixes	1 scp	0	0	1	0/0
Jay Robb, whey protein, unflavored	1 scp	0	0	0	0/0
Kool-Aid, mix, Singles, all flavors	1 pkt	0	14	14	14/1

FOOD	Svg Size	Fbr	Sgr	Cbs	S/C Val
Kool-Aid, mix, sweetened, all flavors	2 T	0	16	16	16/1
Kool-Aid, mix, unsweetened, all flavors	1 pkt	0	0	0	0/0
Kool-Aid Jammers, blue raspberry	6 oz	0	19	19	19/1
Kool-Aid Jammers, cherry	6 oz	0	20	20	20/1
Kool-Aid Jammers, tropical punch	6 oz	0	19	19	19/1
Kool-Aid Jammers 10, all flavors	6.75 oz	0	2	2	2/0
Lipton, iced tea, mix, honey & lemon green tea	1½ T	0	16	18	16/1
Lipton, iced tea, mix, mango	1½ T	0	19	19	19/1
Lipton, iced tea, mix, natural lemon	1⅓ T	0	18	18	18/1
Lipton, iced tea, mix, summer peach	1½ T	0	19	19	19/1
Lipton, iced tea, mix, unsweetened	1½ T	0	0	0	0/0
Lipton, iced tea, mix, wild raspberry	1½ T	0	19	19	19/1
Lipton, iced tea, mix, diet, all flavors	1 T	0	0	0	0/0
Lipton, iced tea, mix, To Go, all flavors	1 pkt	0	0	0	0/0
Lipton, iced tea, ready to drink, most flavors	8 oz	0	16	16	16/1
Lipton, iced tea, ready to drink, green tea with citrus	8 oz	0	21	21	21/2
Lipton, iced tea, ready to drink, diet, all flavors	8 oz	0	0	0	0/0
Monster Milk, powder	2 scps	5	4	18	4/1
Muscle Milk, powder, all flavors	2 scps	5	4	16	4/1
Muscle Milk, ready to drink, all flavors	14 oz	2	3	14	3/1
Muscle Milk Light, powder, all flavors	2 scps	1	2	11	2/1
Muscle Milk Light, ready to drink, cafe latte	14 oz	5	0	11	0/1
Muscle Milk Light, ready to drink, chocolate	14 oz	5	0	12	0/1
Muscle Milk Light, ready to drink, vanilla crème	14 oz	5	0	10	0/1
Muscle Milk Naturals, powder, all flavors	2 scps	0	6	12	6/1
Muscle Milk Protein H2O, all flavors	16 oz	5	0	6	0/1
Nesquik, powder, chocolate	2 T	0	13	14	13/1
Nesquik, powder, chocolate, no sugar added	2 T	1	3	7	3/1
Nesquik, powder, strawberry	2 T	0	15	15	15/1
Nestea, bottle, green tea	20 oz	0	55	56	55/3
Nestea, bottle, green tea, diet	20 oz	0	0	0	0/0
Nestea, bottle, red tea, pomegranate & passion fruit	20 oz	0	36	36	36/2
Nestea, bottle/can, iced tea	8 oz	0	22	23	22/2
Nestea, bottle/can, iced tea, diet	8 oz	0	0	0	0/0
Nestea, carton, green tea, diet	8 oz	0	0	0	0/0
Nestea, carton, green tea, sweetened	8 oz	0	19	20	19/1
Nestea, carton, lemon iced tea, diet	8 oz	0	0	0	0/0
Nestea, carton, lemon iced tea, sweetened	8 oz	0	22	23	22/2
Nestea, carton, natural brewed iced tea, sweetened	8 oz	0	21	21	21/2
Nestea, carton, natural brewed iced tea, unsweetened	8 oz	0	0	0	0/0
Nestea, mix, lemonade tea	1⅓ T	0	14	15	14/1
Nestea, mix, sweet tea mix	1⅓ T	0	15	15	15/1
Nestea, mix, UnSweetened	2 t	0	0	0	0/0
Ocean Spray On the Go, mix, all flavors	1 pkt	0	0	0	0/0

FOOD	Svg Size	Fbr	Sgr	Cbs	S/C Val
Powerade, all flavors	8 oz	0	14	14	14/1
Powerade Zero, all flavors	8 oz	0	0	0	0/0
Slim-Fast!, cappuccino delight	1 can	5	18	25	18/2
Slim-Fast!, creamy chocolate, low carb	1 can	4	1	6	1/1
Slim-Fast!, creamy milk chocolate	1 can	5	18	25	18/2
Slim-Fast!, extra creamy chocolate, high protein	1 can	5	13	24	13/2
Slim-Fast!, French vanilla	1 can	5	18	23	18/2
Slim-Fast!, rich chocolate royale	1 can	5	18	24	18/2
Slim-Fast!, strawberries n' cream	1 can	5	18	23	18/2
Slim-Fast!, vanilla cream, low carb	1 can	0	1	4	1/0
Slim-Fast!, mix, chocolate royale, as prepared	8 oz	4	22	30	22/2
Slim-Fast!, mix, creamy chocolate, high protein, as prepared	8 oz	4	18	25	18/2
Slim-Fast!, mix, creamy vanilla, high protein, as prepared	8 oz	4	18	25	18/2
Slim-Fast!, mix, French vanilla, as prepared	8 oz	4	24	30	24/2
Slim-Fast!, mix, milk chocolate, as prepared	8 oz	5	18	30	18/2
Slim-Fast!, mix, strawberry supreme, as prepared	8 oz	4	24	30	24/2
Snapple, acai blackberry	8 oz	0	27	27	27/2
Snapple, acai mixed berry red tea	8 oz	0	9	10	9/1
Snapple, apple plum white tea	8 oz	0	21	21	21/2
Snapple, cranberry raspberry	8 oz	0	26	26	26/2
Snapple, cranberry raspberry, diet	8 oz	0	2	2	2/0
Snapple, Earl Grey black tea	8 oz	0	8	8	8/1
Snapple, English breakfast black tea	8 oz	0	10	10	10/1
Snapple, fruit punch	8 oz	0	27	27	27/2
Snapple, grapeade	8 oz	0	26	26	26/2
Snapple, green tea	8 oz	0	15	15	15/1
Snapple, green tea, diet	8 oz	0	0	0	0/0
Snapple, kiwi pear	8 oz	0	1	2	1/0
Snapple, kiwi strawberry	8 oz	0	26	27	26/2
Snapple, lemonade	8 oz	0	23	24	23/2
Snapple, lemonade iced tea	8 oz	0	25	26	25/2
Snapple, lemonade iced tea, diet	8 oz	0	2	2	2/0
Snapple, lemon tea	8 oz	0	21	21	21/2
Snapple, lemon tea, diet	8 oz	0	2	2	2/0
Snapple, lime green tea, diet	8 oz	0	0	0	0/0
Snapple, mango green tea	8 oz	0	15	15	15/1
Snapple, mango green tea, diet	8 oz	0	0	0	0/0
Snapple, mango madness	8 oz	0	25	26	25/2
Snapple, mint tea	8 oz	0	17	17	17/1
Snapple, noni berry	8 oz	0	1	2	1/0
Snapple, peach green tea	8 oz	0	21	21	21/2
Snapple, peach green tea, diet	8 oz	0	0	0	0/0
Snapple, peach pomegranate red tea	8 oz	0	10	10	10/1
Snapple, peach tea	8 oz	0	23	23	23/2

FOOD	Svg Size	Fbr	Sgr	Cbs	S/C Val
Snapple, peach tea, diet	8 oz	0	0	0	0/0
Snapple, pink lemonade	8 oz	20	25	25	25/2
Snapple, pomegranate raspberry	8 oz	0	27	27	27/2
Snapple, pomegranate raspberry red tea	8 oz	0	21	21	21/2
Snapple, raspberry peach	8 oz	0	25	27	25/2
Snapple, raspberry tea	8 oz	0	21	21	21/2
Snapple, raspberry tea, diet	8 oz	0	0	0	0/0
Snapple, Snapple apple	8 oz	0	27	27	27/2
Snapple Antioxidant Water, Awaken, dragonfruit	8 oz	0	12	12	12/1
Snapple Antioxidant Water, Awaken, strawberry acai	8 oz	0	13	13	13/1
Snapple Antioxidant Water, Defy, grape pomegranate	8 oz	0	13	13	13/1
Snapple Antioxidant Water, Protect, orange starfruit	8 oz	0	12	13	12/1
Snapple Antioxidant Water, Restore, agave melon	8 oz	0	13	13	13/1
Snapple 100% Juiced!, fruit punch	11.5 oz	0	40	42	40/3
Snapple 100% Juiced!, grape	11.5 oz	0	41	43	41/3
Snapple 100% Juiced!, green apple	11.5 oz	0	39	41	39/3
Snapple 100% Juiced!, melon berry	11.5 oz	0	39	42	39/3
Snapple 100% Juiced!, orange mango	11.5 oz	0	40	41	40/3
Snapple 100% Juiced!, strawberry lime	11.5 oz	0	39	42	39/3
SoBe, black & blue berry brew	20 oz	0	75	76	75/4
SoBe, green tea	20 oz	0	61	61	61/4
SoBe, Elixir, cranberry grapefruit	20 oz	0	63	64	63/4
SoBe, Elixir, orange carrot	20 oz	0	56	57	56/3
SoBe, Energy, citrus	20 oz	0	66	67	66/4
SoBe, Lizard Fuel, strawberry banana	20 oz	0	73	74	73/4
SoBe, Lizard Lava, strawberry daiquiri	20 oz	0	75	77	75/4
SoBe, Liz Blizz, piña colada	20 oz	0	77	80	77/4
SoBe, Nirvana, mango melon	20 oz	0	71	72	71/4
SoBe, Power, fruit punch	20 oz	0	66	67	66/4
SoBe, Tsunami, orange cream	20 oz	0	60	61	60/4
SoBe Lifewater, Bliss, strawberry kiwi	20 oz	0	25	42	25/3
SoBe Lifewater, C-boost, mango melon	20 oz	0	0	13	0/1
SoBe Lifewater, D-fense, orange tangerine	20 oz	0	24	41	24/3
SoBe Lifewater, Electrify, agave lemonade	20 oz	0	24	41	24/3
SoBe Lifewater, Enlighten, blackberry grape	20 oz	0	23	40	23/2
SoBe Lifewater, Forti-fight, black & blue berry	20 oz	0	0	15	0/1
SoBe Lifewater, Go-ji, goji melon	20 oz	0	24	42	24/3
SoBe Lifewater, Lean Machine, cherimoya punch	20 oz	0	0	15	0/1
SoBe Lifewater, Lean Machine, fuji apple pear	20 oz	0	0	15	0/1
SoBe Lifewater, Lean Machine, strawberry dragonfruit	20 oz	0	0	16	0/1
SoBe Lifewater, N-dure, acai fruit punch	20 oz	0	0	16	0/1
SoBe Lifewater, Zingseng, pomegranate cherry	20 oz	0	24	42	24/3
Tang, mix, orange	2 T	0	23	23	23/2
Tang, mix, orange, sugar free	2 T	0	0	0	0/0

FOOD	Svg Size	Fbr	Sgr	Cbs	S/C Val
Tea, unflavored & unsweetened, hot or iced, most varieties	any	0	0	0	0/0
Ultima Replenisher, most flavors	1 pkt	0	0	3	0/0
Ultima Replenisher, grape	1 pkt	0	0	4	0/0
Vitaminwater, all flavors	8 oz	0	13	13	13/1
Vitaminwater Zero, all flavors	8 oz	0	0	4	0/0
Water, all varieties	any	0	0	0	0/0
Water, seltzer	8 oz	0	0	0	0/0
Water, tonic	8 oz	0	22	22	22/2
Water, tonic, Canada Dry	10 oz	0	29	30	29/2
Water, tonic, Schweppes	10 oz	0	27	29	27/2

FRUIT & VEGETABLE JUICES

FOOD	Svg Size	Fbr	Sgr	Cbs	S/C Val
Acerola	8 oz	1	11	12	11/1
Apple, unsweetened	8 oz	1	24	29	24/2
Apple, Florida's Natural, 100% juice	8 oz	0	28	28	28/2
Apple, Hansen's, 100% juice, organic	8 oz	0	23	28	23/2
Apple, Juicy Juice, 100% juice	8 oz	0	26	28	26/2
Apple, Juicy Juice, sparkling	1 can	0	20	21	20/2
Apple, Kern's, nectar	1 can	2	37	51	37/3
Apple, Martinelli's, cider	8 oz	0	31	35	31/2
Apple, Martinelli's, cider, sparkling	8 oz	0	31	35	31/2
Apple, Martinelli's, 100% juice	10 oz	0	39	43	39/3
Apple, Martinelli's, 100% juice, unfiltered	8 oz	0	31	35	31/2
Apple, Minute Maid, 100% juice, bottle	8 oz	0	26	28	26/2
Apple, Minute Maid, 100% juice, frozen, as prepared	8 oz	0	27	28	27/2
Apple, Minute Maid Kids+, 100% juice	8 oz	0	26	28	26/2
Apple, Mott's, 100% juice	8 oz	0	29	29	29/2
Apple, Mott's for Tots, 40% less sugar	8 oz	0	15	15	15/1
Apple, Mott's Plus, light	8 oz	0	14	15	14/1
Apple, Naked, chai spiced cider	8 oz	0	29	30	29/2
Apple, Tropicana, 100% juice	8 oz	0	25	27	25/2
Apple, Welch's, 100% juice	8 oz	0	28	29	28/2
Apricot, Kern's, nectar	1 can	0	45	50	45/3
Blackberry	8 oz	0	19	20	19/1
Blueberry, Ocean Spray, cocktail	8 oz	0	28	28	28/2
Blueberry, Ocean Spray, diet	8 oz	0	2	2	2/0
Blueberry, Odwalla, Blueberry B Monster	8 oz	0	23	34	23/2
Carrot	8 oz	2	9	22	9/2
Carrot, Odwalla, 100% juice	8 oz	1	13	15	13/1
Cherry, Juicy Juice, 100% juice	8 oz	0	27	29	27/2
Coconut water	8 oz	3	6	9	6/1
Cranberry, unsweetened	8 oz	0	31	31	31/2
Cranberry, Cascadian Farm, organic, frozen, as prepared	8 oz	0	37	38	37/2
Cranberry, Ocean Spray, cocktail	8 oz	0	30	30	30/2
Cranberry, Ocean Spray, diet	8 oz	0	2	2	2/0

FOOD	Svg Size	Fbr	Sgr	Cbs	S/C Val
Cranberry, Tropicana, 100% juice	8 oz	0	32	35	32/2
Cranberry, white, Ocean Spray	8 oz	0	27	27	27/2
Cranberry, white, Ocean Spray, light	8 oz	0	10	10	10/1
Grape, unsweetened	8 oz	1	36	38	36/2
Grape, Cascadian Farm, organic, frozen, as prepared	8 oz	0	31	32	31/2
Grape, Hansen's	8 oz	0	39	40	39/2
Grape, Minute Maid, 100% juice	8 oz	0	27	28	27/2
Grape, Tropicana, 100% juice	8 oz	0	38	38	38/2
Grape, Welch's, light	8 oz	0	12	13	12/1
Grape, Welch's, 100% juice	8 oz	0	40	42	40/3
Grape, Welch's, 100% juice, organic	10 oz	0	52	53	52/3
Grape, Welch's, sparkling	8 oz	0	38	40	38/2
Grape, white, Hansen's	8 oz	0	36	36	36/2
Grape, white, Juicy Juice, 100% juice	8 oz	0	34	38	34/2
Grape, white, Welch's, 100% juice	8 oz	0	37	39	37/2
Grapefruit, Minute Maid, frozen can, as prepared	8 oz	0	20	25	20/2
Grapefruit, pink, Ocean Spray, 100% juice	8 oz	0	23	23	23/2
Grapefruit, ruby red, Florida's Natural	8 oz	0	20	22	20/2
Grapefruit, ruby red, Minute Maid	8 oz	2	32	34	32/2
Grapefruit, ruby red, Ocean Spray, cocktail	8 oz	0	28	28	28/2
Grapefruit, ruby red, Ocean Spray, light	8 oz	0	10	10	10/1
Grapefruit, ruby red, Ocean Spray, 100% juice	8 oz	0	26	26	26/2
Grapefruit, ruby red, Tropicana	8 oz	0	30	30	30/2
Grapefruit, ruby red, Tropicana, 100% juice	10 oz	0	37	42	37/3
Grapefruit, white, unsweetened	8 oz	0	22	23	22/2
Grapefruit, white, Ocean Spray, 100% juice	8 oz	0	17	21	17/2
Grapefruit, white, Tropicana, 100% juice	8 oz	0	17	22	17/2
Guava, Kern's, nectar	8 oz	0	33	37	33/2
Lemonade, Cascadian Farm, organic, frozen, as prepared	8 oz	0	26	28	26/2
Lemonade, Country Time, mix	2 T	0	16	16	16/1
Lemonade, Florida's Natural	8 oz	0	27	28	27/2
Lemonade, Minute Maid, bottle	8 oz	0	27	28	27/2
Lemonade, Minute Maid, bottle, light	8 oz	0	0	1	0/0
Lemonade, Minute Maid, can	12 oz	0	40	42	40/3
Lemonade, Minute Maid, can, light	12 oz	0	0	2	0/0
Lemonade, Minute Maid, carton	8 oz	0	29	31	29/2
Lemonade, Minute Maid, carton, light	8 oz	0	2	4	2/0
Lemonade, Minute Maid, frozen, as prepared	8 oz	0	27	29	27/2
Lemonade, Odwalla	8 oz	0	28	30	28/2
Lemonade, Odwalla, light	8 oz	0	12	14	12/1
Lemonade, Simply Lemonade	8 oz	0	28	30	28/2
Lemonade, Tropicana, light	8 oz	0	2	2	2/0
Lemonade, pink, Country Time, mix	2 T	0	16	16	16/1
Lemonade, pink, Minute Maid, bottle	8 oz	0	27	28	27/2

FOOD	Svg Size	Fbr	Sgr	Cbs	S/C Val
Lemonade, pink, Minute Maid, carton	8 oz	0	29	29	29/2
Lemonade, pink, Minute Maid, frozen, as prepared	8 oz	0	27	29	27/2
Limeade, Minute Maid, carton	8 oz	0	31	33	31/2
Limeade, Minute Maid, carton, light	8 oz	0	2	4	2/0
Limeade, Minute Maid, frozen, as prepared	8 oz	0	23	25	23/2
Limeade, Odwalla, light	8 oz	0	12	14	12/1
Limeade, Odwalla, Summertime Lime	8 oz	0	27	29	27/2
Mango, Kern's, nectar	1 can	0	44	52	44/3
Mango, Odwalla, Mango Tango	8 oz	0	30	34	30/2
Orange	8 oz	1	21	26	21/2
Orange, Dole, w/ or w/o pulp	8 oz	0	23	27	23/2
Orange, Florida's Natural, w/ or w/o pulp	8 oz	0	22	26	22/2
Orange, Juicy Juice, sparkling	1 can	0	20	21	20/2
Orange, Minute Maid, w/ or w/o pulp	8 oz	0	24	27	24/2
Orange, Minute Maid, light, low pulp	8 oz	0	10	13	10/1
Orange, Naked, 100% juice	8 oz	0	22	27	22/2
Orange, Odwalla, 100% juice	8 oz	0	24	25	24/2
Orange, Simply Orange, w/ or w/o pulp	8 oz	0	22	26	22/2
Orange, Tropicana, w/ or w/o pulp	8 oz	0	22	26	22/2
Orange, Tropicana Trop 50, w/ or w/o pulp	8 oz	0	10	13	10/1
Papaya, Kern's, nectar	1 can	0	47	52	47/3
Passionfruit, purple	8 oz	1	33	34	33/2
Passionfruit, yellow	8 oz	1	35	36	35/2
Peach, Kern's, nectar	1 can	0	42	46	42/3
Pear, Kern's, nectar	1 can	4	35	55	35/3
Pineapple, unsweetened	8 oz	1	25	32	25/2
Pineapple, Dole	8 oz	0	26	30	26/2
Pineapple, Dole, frozen	12 oz	0	25	30	25/2
Pomegranate	8 oz	0	32	33	32/2
Prune	8 oz	3	42	45	42/3
Raspberry, Cascadian Farm, frozen, as prepared	8 oz	0	30	31	30/2
Strawberry, Kern's, nectar	1 can	0	46	52	46/3
Tangerine	8 oz	1	24	25	24/2
Tomato	8 oz	1	9	10	9/1
Tomato, Campbell's	8 oz	2	7	10	7/1
Tomato, Campbell's, healthy request	8 oz	2	9	10	9/1
Tomato, Del Monte, can	8 oz	1	7	10	7/1
FRUIT & VEGETABLE JUICE BLENDS					
Fruit, Dole, piña colada	8 oz	0	24	29	24/2
Fruit, Dole, strawberry kiwi	8 oz	0	26	31	26/2
Fruit, Juicy Juice, berry	8 oz	0	27	29	27/2
Fruit, Juicy Juice, berry, sparkling	1 can	0	20	21	20/2
Fruit, Juicy Juice, strawberry banana	8 oz	0	27	29	27/2
Fruit, Juicy Juice, strawberry kiwi	8 oz	0	25	29	25/2

FOOD	Svg Size	Fbr	Sgr	Cbs	S/C Val
Fruit, Juicy Juice, tropical	8 oz	0	24	25	24/2
Fruit, Kern's, strawberry banana	1 can	0	46	52	46/3
Fruit, Kern's, strawberry kiwi	1 can	0	47	50	47/3
Fruit, Minute Maid, strawberry kiwi	8 oz	0	18	20	18/1
Fruit, Naked, Blue Machine	8 oz	7	29	40	29/2
Fruit, Naked, Green Machine	8 oz	0	28	33	28/2
Fruit, Naked, Power-C Machine	8 oz	0	23	29	23/2
Fruit, Ocean Spray, CranApple	8 oz	0	32	32	32/2
Fruit, Ocean Spray, CranApple, light	8 oz	0	10	10	10/1
Fruit, Ocean Spray, CranCherry	8 oz	0	30	30	30/2
Fruit, Ocean Spray, CranGrape	8 oz	0	31	31	31/2
Fruit, Ocean Spray, CranGrape, light	8 oz	0	10	10	10/1
Fruit, Ocean Spray, CranRaspberry	8 oz	0	28	28	28/2
Fruit, Ocean Spray, CranRaspberry, light	8 oz	0	10	10	10/1
Fruit, Odwalla, strawberry banana	8 oz	1	26	31	26/2
Fruit, Tropicana, berry blend, light	8 oz	0	2	2	2/0
Fruit, Tropicana, fruit punch	8 oz	0	32	32	32/2
Fruit, Tropicana, fruit punch, light	8 oz	0	2	2	2/0
Fruit, Tropicana, strawberry kiwi, 100% juice	8 oz	0	25	30	25/2
Fruit, Tropicana Pure, pomegranate blueberry	8 oz	0	28	32	28/2
Fruit, Tropicana Pure, raspberry acai	8 oz	0	26	31	26/2
Fruit, Tropicana Trop50, pineapple mango	8 oz	0	11	14	11/1
Fruit, Tropicana Trop50, pomegranate blueberry	8 oz	0	11	14	11/1
Fruit, V8 Splash, berry blend	8 oz	0	18	18	18/1
Fruit, V8 Splash, berry blend, diet	8 oz	0	1	3	1/0
Fruit, V8 Splash, fruit medley	8 oz	0	18	18	18/1
Fruit, V8 Splash, strawberry kiwi	8 oz	0	16	18	16/1
Fruit, V8 Splash, tropical blend	8 oz	0	16	18	16/1
Fruit, V8 Splash, tropical blend, diet	8 oz	0	1	3	1/0
Fruit, V8 Splash Smoothies, strawberry banana	8 oz	0	18	20	18/1
Fruit, V8 Splash Smoothies, tropical colada	8 oz	1	18	21	18/2
Fruit, Welch's, fruit punch, 100% juice	8 oz	0	28	30	28/2
Fruit, Welch's, fruit punch drink	8 oz	0	30	31	30/2
Fruit, Welch's, mountain berry, 100% juice	11.5 oz	0	47	49	47/3
Fruit, Welch's, mountain berry cocktail	11.5 oz	0	33	34	33/2
Fruit/Vegetable, Mott's Medleys, apple	8 oz	0	22	25	22/2
Fruit/Vegetable, Mott's Medleys, grape	8 oz	0	30	33	30/2
Fruit/Vegetable, Mott's Medleys, tropical	8 oz	0	29	32	29/2
Fruit/Vegetable, Naked, orange carrot	8 oz	1	26	29	26/2
Fruit/Vegetable, Ocean Spray Fruit & Veggie, cranberry strawberry banana	8 oz	0	27	31	27/2
Fruit/Vegetable, Ocean Spray Fruit & Veggie, cranberry strawberry banana, light	8 oz	0	11	15	11/1
Fruit/Vegetable, Ocean Spray Fruit & Veggie, tropical citrus	8 oz	0	27	32	27/2
Fruit/Vegetable, Ocean Spray Fruit & Veggie, tropical citrus, light	8 oz	0	11	15	11/1
Fruit/Vegetable, V8 V-Fusion, acai mixed berry	8 oz	0	26	27	26/2

FOOD	Svg Size	Fbr	Sgr	Cbs	S/C Val
Fruit/Vegetable, V8 V-Fusion, acai mixed berry, light	8 oz	0	10	13	10/1
Fruit/Vegetable, V8 V-Fusion, peach mango	8 oz	0	26	28	26/2
Fruit/Vegetable, V8 V-Fusion, peach mango, light	8 oz	0	10	13	10/1
Fruit/Vegetable, V8 V-Fusion, pomegranate blueberry	8 oz	0	23	25	23/2
Fruit/Vegetable, V8 V-Fusion, pomegranate blueberry, light	8 oz	1	5	7	5/1
Fruit/Vegetable, V8 V-Fusion, strawberry banana	8 oz	0	25	28	25/2
Fruit/Vegetable, V8 V-Fusion, strawberry banana, light	8 oz	0	12	12	12/1
Vegetable, R.W. Knudsen Very Veggie, low sodium	8 oz	2	6	11	6/1
Vegetable, R.W. Knudsen Very Veggie, organic	8 oz	2	8	14	8/1
Vegetable, R.W. Knudsen Very Veggie, organic low sodium	8 oz	2	8	14	8/1
Vegetable, R.W. Knudsen Very Veggie, original	8 oz	2	7	11	7/1
Vegetable, R.W. Knudsen Very Veggie, untomato	8 oz	2	12	16	12/1
Vegetable, V8, essential antioxidants	8 oz	2	6	11	6/1
Vegetable, V8, high fiber	8 oz	5	8	13	8/1
Vegetable, V8, original	8 oz	2	8	10	8/1
Vegetable, V8 V-Lite	8 oz	1	5	7	5/1

SODA & ENERGY DRINKS

FOOD	Svg Size	Fbr	Sgr	Cbs	S/C Val
Coca-Cola	12 oz	0	39	39	39/2
Coca-Cola, caffeine free	12 oz	0	39	39	39/2
Coca-Cola, cherry	12 oz	0	42	42	42/3
Coca-Cola Zero	12 oz	0	0	0	0/0
Diet Coke	12 oz	0	0	0	0/0
Dr Pepper	8 oz	0	27	27	27/2
Dr Pepper, cherry	8 oz	0	28	29	28/2
Dr Pepper, cherry vanilla	8 oz	0	25	26	25/2
Dr Pepper, diet	8 oz	0	0	0	0/0
Fanta, grape	12 oz	0	48	48	48/3
Fanta, orange	12 oz	0	44	44	44/3
Fanta, pineapple	12 oz	0	48	48	48/3
Fanta, strawberry	12 oz	0	48	48	48/3
5-Hour Energy, all flavors	2 oz	0	0	0	0/0
Ginger ale, Canada Dry	12 oz	0	32	32	32/2
Ginger ale, Hansen's	8 oz	0	24	24	24/2
Ginger ale, Hansen's, diet	12 oz	0	0	0	0/0
Ginger ale, Schweppes	8 oz	0	22	23	22/2
Ginger ale, Seagram's	12 oz	0	35	35	35/2
Monster, energy shooter, Hitman	1	0	6	7	6/1
Monster, energy shooter, Lobo	1	0	3	3	3/0
Monster, energy shooter, Sniper	1	0	3	5	3/1
Monster, Java Monster, Chai Hai	8 oz	0	13	14	13/1
Monster, Java Monster, Irish Blend	8 oz	0	14	15	14/1
Monster, Java Monster, Lo-Ball	8 oz	0	4	6	4/1
Monster, Java Monster, Loca Moca	8 oz	0	16	17	16/1
Monster, Java Monster, Mean Bean	8 oz	0	16	17	16/1

FOOD	Svg Size	Fbr	Sgr	Cbs	S/C Val
Monster, Java Monster, Nut-Up	8 oz	0	16	17	16/1
Monster, Java Monster, Originale	8 oz	0	16	17	16/1
Monster, Java Monster, Russian	8 oz	0	16	17	16/1
Monster, Nitrous Monster Energy, Anti-Gravity	12 oz	0	35	39	35/2
Monster, Nitrous Monster Energy, Killer B	12 oz	0	36	38	36/2
Monster, Nitrous Monster Energy, Super Dry	12 oz	0	38	39	38/2
Monster, X-presso Monster, Hammer	6.75 oz	0	12	14	12/1
Monster Energy	8 oz	0	27	27	27/2
Monster Energy, Assault	8 oz	0	27	27	27/2
Monster Energy, Heavy Metal	8 oz	0	22	23	22/2
Monster Energy, Import	8 oz	0	21	22	21/2
Monster Energy, Khaos	8 oz	0	17	17	17/1
Monster Energy, Lo-Carb	8 oz	0	3	3	3/0
Monster Energy, M-80	8 oz	0	23	23	23/2
Monster Energy, Mixxd	8 oz	0	27	27	27/2
Mountain Dew	12 oz	0	46	46	46/3
Pepsi	12 oz	0	41	41	41/3
Pepsi, diet	12 oz	0	0	0	0/0
Pepsi Max	12 oz	0	0	0	0/0
Pibb Xtra	8 oz	0	26	26	26/2
Red Bull	8.3 oz	0	27	28	27/2
Red Bull, sugarfree	12 oz	0	0	4	0/0
Red Bull Cola	12 oz	0	31	31	31/2
Red Bull Energy Shot	2 oz	0	6	6	6/1
Red Bull Sugarfree Shot	2 oz	0	0	0	0/0
Rockstar	8 oz	0	31	31	31/2
Rockstar, sugar free	8 oz	0	0	0	0/0
Rockstar, zero carb	16 oz	0	0	0	0/0
Rockstar Energy Cola	8 oz	0	33	33	33/2
Rockstar Energy Shot, tropical punch	2.5 oz	0	0	0	0/0
Rockstar Energy Shot, wild berry	2.5 oz	0	0	0	0/0
Rockstar Juiced, guava	8 oz	0	35	35	35/2
Rockstar Juiced, mango	8 oz	0	35	35	35/2
Rockstar Juiced, pomegranate	8 oz	0	35	35	35/2
Rockstar Punched	16 oz	0	31	31	31/2
Rockstar Punched, citrus	16 oz	0	31	32	31/2
Rockstar Recovery	8 oz	0	1	1	1/0
Rockstar Roasted, espresso	8 oz	0	16	17	16/1
Rockstar Roasted, latte	8 oz	0	17	18	17/1
Rockstar Roasted, light vanilla	8 oz	0	7	7	7/1
Rockstar Roasted, mocha	8 oz	0	17	18	17/1
Root beer, A&W	8 oz	0	31	31	31/2
Root beer, Barq's	12 oz	0	45	45	45/3
Root beer, Barq's, diet	12 oz	0	0	0	0/0

FOOD	Svg Size	Fbr	Sgr	Cbs	S/C Val
Root beer, Hansen's	12 oz	0	43	43	43/3
Root beer, Hansen's, diet	12 oz	0	0	0	0/0
Root beer, Mug	12 oz	0	43	43	43/3
7UP	8 oz	0	25	26	25/2
7UP, cherry, antioxidant	8 oz	0	25	26	25/2
7UP, cherry, antioxidant, diet	8 oz	0	0	0	0/0
7UP Plus, all flavors	8 oz	0	1	2	1/0
Sierra Mist	12 oz	0	39	39	39/2
Slice, grape	12 oz	0	50	50	50/3
Slice, orange	12 oz	0	48	48	48/3
Slice, orange, diet	12 oz	0	0	0	0/0
Slice, peach	12 oz	0	50	51	50/3
Slice, strawberry	12 oz	0	43	43	43/3
Sprite	12 oz	0	38	38	38/2
Sprite Zero	12 oz	0	0	0	0/0
Sunkist, orange	12 oz	0	50	52	50/3
Sunkist, sparkling lemonade	12 oz	0	43	44	43/3
Zevia, black cherry	12 oz	0	0	13	0/1
Zevia, cola	12 oz	0	0	12	0/1
Zevia, Dr. Zevia	12 oz	0	0	15	0/1
Zevia, ginger ale	12 oz	0	0	13	0/1
Zevia, orange	12 oz	0	0	11	0/1
Zevia, root beer	12 oz	0	0	10	0/1
Zevia, twist	12 oz	0	0	11	0/1
ALCOHOL & ALCOHOL MIXERS					
Bartles & Jaymes, blue Hawaiian	12 oz	0	28	31	28/2
Bartles & Jaymes, fuzzy navel	12 oz	0	38	43	38/3
Bartles & Jaymes, margarita	12 oz	0	42	46	42/3
Bartles & Jaymes, mojito	12 oz	0	42	46	42/3
Bartles & Jaymes, original	12 oz	0	26	29	26/2
Bartles & Jaymes, piña colada	12 oz	0	45	48	45/3
Bartles & Jaymes, strawberry daiquiri	12 oz	0	33	38	33/2
Beer	12 oz	0	0	13	0/1
Beer, light	12 oz	0	0	6	0/1
Beer, Amstel Light	12 oz	0	0	5	0/1
Beer, Asahi	12 oz	0	0	11	0/1
Beer, Bass	12 oz	0	0	13	0/1
Beer, Beck's	12 oz	0	0	20	0/1
Beer, Beck's Dark	12 oz	0	0	10	0/1
Beer, Beck's Premier Light	12 oz	0	0	4	0/0
Beer, Blue Moon	12 oz	0	0	13	0/1
Beer, Bud Light	12 oz	0	0	7	0/1
Beer, Budweiser	12 oz	0	0	11	0/1
Beer, Budweiser Select	12 oz	0	0	3	0/0

FOOD	Svg Size	Fbr	Sgr	Cbs	S/C Val
Beer, Coors	12 oz	0	0	14	0/1
Beer, Coors Light	12 oz	0	0	5	0/1
Beer, Corona	12 oz	0	0	13	0/1
Beer, Corona Light	12 oz	0	0	5	0/1
Beer, Fosters	12 oz	0	0	11	0/1
Beer, Guinness	12 oz	0	0	10	0/1
Beer, Heineken	12 oz	0	0	12	0/1
Beer, Keystone Ice	12 oz	0	0	7	0/1
Beer, Keystone Light	12 oz	0	0	5	0/1
Beer, Kirin Ichiban	12 oz	0	0	12	0/1
Beer, Kirin Light	12 oz	0	0	8	0/1
Beer, MGD	12 oz	0	0	13	0/1
Beer, Michelob Light	12 oz	0	0	9	0/1
Beer, Michelob Ultra	12 oz	0	0	3	0/0
Beer, Miller Lite	12 oz	0	0	3	0/0
Beer, Newcastle	12 oz	0	0	13	0/1
Beer, O'Doul's, nonalcoholic	12 oz	0	0	13	0/1
Beer, Pabst Blue Ribbon	12 oz	0	0	12	0/1
Beer, Pabst Light	12 oz	0	0	8	0/1
Beer, Red Stripe	12 oz	0	0	14	0/1
Beer, Rolling Rock	12 oz	0	0	10	0/1
Beer, Sam Adams Light	12 oz	0	0	10	0/1
Beer, Samuel Adams Boston Lager	12 oz	0	0	18	0/1
Beer, Sapporo	12 oz	0	0	10	0/1
Beer, Tecate	12 oz	0	0	12	0/1
Blue curacao	1 oz	0	12	13	12/1
Bourbon	1 oz	0	0	0	0/0
Brandy	1 oz	0	0	0	0/0
Chambord	1 oz	0	11	11	11/1
Cognac	1 oz	0	0	0	0/0
Gin	1 oz	0	0	0	0/0
Madeira	1 oz	0	2	4	2/0
Midori	1 oz	0	8	8	8/1
Mike's, The Classic Margarita, all flavors	11 oz	0	32	34	32/2
Mike's Hard Lemonade, all flavors	11 oz	0	32	33	32/2
Mike's Hard Lemonade, light, all flavors	11 oz	0	0	6	0/1
Mixer, bloody Mary, Mr & Mrs T, bold & spicy	4 oz	1	5	7	5/1
Mixer, bloody Mary, Mr & Mrs T, original	5 oz	1	4	7	4/1
Mixer, bloody Mary, Mr & Mrs T, premium	4 oz	0	7	9	7/1
Mixer, bloody Mary, Tabasco	8 oz	2	7	13	7/1
Mixer, margarita, Bacardi, frozen	2 oz	0	23	25	23/2
Mixer, margarita, Jose Cuervo	4 oz	0	24	24	24/2
Mixer, margarita, Mr & Mrs T	4 oz	0	24	26	24/2
Mixer, margarita, Sauza	6 oz	0	18	18	18/2

The Belly Fat Cure Sugar & Carb Counter 133

BEVERAGES & POWDERED DRINK MIXES, cont'd.

FOOD	Svg Size	Fbr	Sgr	Cbs	S/C Val
Mixer, mojito, Bacardi, frozen	2 oz	0	29	30	29/2
Mixer, piña colada, Bacardi, frozen	2 oz	0	34	36	34/2
Mixer, piña colada, Mr & Mrs T	4 oz	0	42	43	42/3
Mixer, strawberry daiquiri, Bacardi, frozen	2 oz	0	30	32	30/2
Mixer, strawberry daiquiri-margarita, Mr & Mrs T	4 oz	0	44	46	44/3
Mixer, strawberry margarita, Jose Cuervo	4 oz	0	24	24	24/2
Port	4 oz	0	0	0	0/0
Rum	1 oz	0	0	0	0/0
Sake	3 oz	0	0	6	0/1
Scotch	1 oz	0	0	0	0/0
Sherry	4 oz	0	0	14	0/1
Soju	2 oz	0	0	0	0/0
Sweet & sour, Finest Call	4 oz	0	25	27	25/2
Sweet & sour, Mr & Mrs T	4 oz	0	22	23	22/2
Tequila	1 oz	0	0	0	0/0
Triple sec	1 oz	0	11	11	11/1
Vermouth, dry	3 oz	0	1	12	1/1
Vermouth, sweet	3 oz	0	8	14	8/1
Vodka	1 oz	0	0	0	0/0
Whiskey	1 oz	0	0	0	0/0
Wine, dessert, dry	3 oz	0	1	12	1/1
Wine, dessert, sweet	3 oz	0	7	12	7/1
Wine, red	5 oz	0	1	4	1/0
Wine, white	5 oz	0	1	4	1/0

SAUCES, SYRUPS & SALAD DRESSING

FOOD	Svg Size	Fbr	Sgr	Cbs	S/C Val
SAUCES					
Alfredo sauce, Bertolli	¼ c	0	0	2	0/0
Alfredo sauce, Bertolli, four cheese rosa	¼ c	0	2	4	2/0
Alfredo sauce, Bertolli, garlic	¼ c	0	0	2	0/0
Alfredo sauce, Bertolli, mushroom	¼ c	0	0	2	0/0
Alfredo sauce, Buitoni	¼ c	0	2	4	2/0
Alfredo sauce, Buitoni, light	¼ c	0	1	5	1/1
Alfredo sauce, Classico, creamy	¼ c	0	1	3	1/0
Alfredo sauce, Classico, four cheese	¼ c	0	1	4	1/0
Alfredo sauce, Classico, mushroom	¼ c	2	0	3	0/0
Alfredo sauce, Classico, roasted garlic	¼ c	1	1	3	1/0
Alfredo sauce, Ragú, classic	¼ c	0	1	3	1/0
Alfredo sauce, Ragú, light Parmesan	¼ c	0	0	2	0/0
Barbecue sauce, Annie's Naturals, original, organic	2 T	0	7	9	7/1
Barbecue sauce, Hunt's, honey hickory	2 T	0	9	12	9/1
Barbecue sauce, Hunt's, original	2 T	0	9	12	9/1

FOOD	Svg Size	Fbr	Sgr	Cbs	S/C Val
Barbecue sauce, Jack Daniel's, original no. 7 recipe	2 T	0	8	12	8/1
Barbecue sauce, KC Masterpiece, original	2 T	0	12	15	12/1
Barbecue sauce, Kraft, honey	2 T	0	14	16	14/1
Barbecue sauce, Kraft, honey mustard	2 T	0	12	14	12/1
Barbecue sauce, Kraft, hot	2 T	0	9	10	9/1
Barbecue sauce, Kraft, original	2 T	0	13	15	13/1
Barbecue sauce, Kraft, original, light	2 T	0	3	5	3/1
Barbecue sauce, Kraft, original, Thick n Spicy	2 T	0	13	16	13/1
Barbecue sauce, Scott's	2 T	0	0	2	0/0
Barbecue sauce, Sweet Baby Ray's	2 T	0	16	17	16/1
Barbecue sauce, World Harbors, Bar-B	2 T	0	14	16	14/1
Black bean sauce, Kikkoman, w/ garlic	1 T	1	2	3	2/0
Black bean sauce, Lee Kum Kee, w/ garlic	1 T	1	3	4	3/0
Enchilada sauce, La Victoria, green, mild	¼ c	0	0	2	0/0
Enchilada sauce, La Victoria, red, hot	¼ c	0	0	2	0/0
Enchilada sauce, La Victoria, red, mild	¼ c	0	0	2	0/0
Enchilada sauce, Old El Paso	¼ c	0	1	3	1/0
Enchilada sauce, Old El Paso, green, mild	¼ c	0	1	4	1/0
Enchilada sauce, Ortega	¼ c	0	0	3	0/0
Gravy	1 c	0	0	11	0/1
Gravy, Campbell's, beef	¼ c	0	0	3	0/0
Gravy, Campbell's, brown w/ onions	¼ c	0	2	4	2/0
Gravy, Campbell's, chicken	¼ c	0	1	3	1/0
Gravy, Campbell's, country style cream	¼ c	0	1	3	1/0
Gravy, Campbell's, country style sausage	¼ c	0	1	4	1/0
Gravy, Campbell's, mushroom	¼ c	0	1	3	1/0
Gravy, Campbell's, turkey	¼ c	0	1	3	1/0
Gravy, Franco-American, beef	¼ c	0	0	3	0/0
Gravy, Franco-American, chicken	¼ c	0	0	3	0/0
Gravy, Franco-American, turkey	¼ c	0	0	4	0/0
Gravy, Heinz, classic chicken, fat free	¼ c	0	0	4	0/0
Gravy, Heinz, roasted turkey, fat free	¼ c	0	0	4	0/0
Gravy, Heinz, savory beef, fat free	¼ c	0	0	4	0/0
Gravy, Heinz HomeStyle, brown w/ onions	¼ c	0	0	3	0/0
Gravy, Heinz HomeStyle, classic chicken	¼ c	0	0	4	0/0
Gravy, Heinz HomeStyle, pork	¼ c	0	0	3	0/0
Gravy, Heinz HomeStyle, rich mushroom	¼ c	0	0	3	0/0
Gravy, Heinz HomeStyle, roasted turkey	¼ c	0	0	3	0/0
Gravy, Heinz HomeStyle, sausage	¼ c	0	1	6	1/1
Gravy, Heinz HomeStyle, savory beef	¼ c	0	0	4	0/0
Gravy, Tofurky, vegan, mushroom & "giblet"	¼ c	2	2	5	2/1
Hoisin sauce	2 T	1	9	14	9/1
Hoisin sauce, Dynasty	2 T	0	9	9	9/1
Hoisin sauce, Kikkoman	2 T	0	16	17	16/1

FOOD	Svg Size	Fbr	Sgr	Cbs	S/C Val
Hoisin sauce, Lee Kum Kee	2 T	0	21	22	21/2
Hoisin sauce, Lee Kum Kee, Panda Brand	2 T	0	18	20	18/1
Oyster sauce	1 T	0	0	2	0/0
Oyster sauce, Dynasty	1 T	0	5	5	5/1
Oyster sauce, Lee Kum Kee, Panda Brand	1 T	0	4	6	4/1
Oyster sauce, Lee Kum Kee, Panda Brand, Green Label	1 T	0	4	5	4/1
Pasta sauce, Amy's, family marinara	½ c	3	5	10	5/1
Pasta sauce, Amy's, marinara, low sodium	½ c	1	5	7	5/1
Pasta sauce, Amy's, tomato basil	½ c	3	6	11	6/1
Pasta sauce, Amy's, tomato basil, light in sodium	½ c	2	6	11	6/1
Pasta sauce, Bertolli, five cheese	½ c	0	13	14	13/1
Pasta sauce, Bertolli, marinara	½ c	1	12	14	12/1
Pasta sauce, Bertolli, tomato & basil	½ c	3	12	13	12/1
Pasta sauce, Bertolli, tomato & basil, organic	½ c	2	7	11	7/1
Pasta sauce, Bertolli, vodka	½ c	2	8	11	8/1
Pasta sauce, Buitoni, marinara	½ c	2	7	10	7/1
Pasta sauce, Buitoni, vodka	½ c	1	4	7	4/1
Pasta sauce, Classico, cabernet marinara w/ herbs	½ c	2	6	11	6/1
Pasta sauce, Classico, four cheese	½ c	3	5	12	5/1
Pasta sauce, Classico, marinara w/ plum tomatoes & olive oil	½ c	10	6	10	6/1
Pasta sauce, Classico, roasted garlic	½ c	2	5	9	5/1
Pasta sauce, Classico, tomato & basil	½ c	2	6	11	6/1
Pasta sauce, Classico, vodka	½ c	2	7	12	7/1
Pasta sauce, DeLallo, roasted garlic	½ c	1	1	10	1/1
Pasta sauce, Muir Glen, cabernet marinara	½ c	2	4	11	4/1
Pasta sauce, Muir Glen, four cheese	½ c	2	3	11	3/1
Pasta sauce, Muir Glen, tomato basil	½ c	2	4	12	4/1
Pasta sauce, Ragú, margherita, Old World Style	½ c	2	6	10	6/1
Pasta sauce, Ragú, marinara, Old World Style	½ c	2	7	11	7/1
Pasta sauce, Ragú, Parmesan & Romano, Robusto!	½ c	2	8	10	8/1
Pasta sauce, Ragú, sundried tomato & sweet basil, Chunky	½ c	2	13	18	13/1
Pasta sauce, Ragú, sweet tomato & basil, Old World Style	½ c	3	6	10	6/1
Pasta sauce, Ragú, tomato & basil, light	½ c	2	8	10	8/1
Pasta sauce, Ragú, tomato & basil, no sugar added	½ c	3	0	6	0/1
Pasta sauce, Ragú, tomato, garlic & onion, Chunky	½ c	2	13	18	13/1
Pasta sauce, Ragú, traditional, Old World Style	½ c	2	6	8	6/1
Pasta sauce, Ragú, traditional, organic	½ c	0	8	11	8/1
Pasta sauce, Seeds of Change, arrabiatta di Roma	½ c	2	0	6	0/1
Pasta sauce, Seeds of Change, marinara di Venezia	½ c	2	0	6	0/1
Pasta sauce, Seeds of Change, Romagna three cheese	½ c	2	0	9	0/1
Pasta sauce, Seeds of Change, tomato basil Genovese	½ c	2	0	9	0/1
Pasta sauce, Seeds of Change, Tuscan tomato & garlic	½ c	2	3	7	3/1
Pasta sauce, Seeds of Change, vodka Americano	½ c	2	1	8	1/1
Pesto, Buitoni, basil	¼ c	2	4	6	4/1

FOOD	Svg Size	Fbr	Sgr	Cbs	S/C Val
Pesto, Buitoni, basil, reduced fat	¼ c	2	5	9	5/1
Pesto, Classico, sun-dried tomato	¼ c	1	5	8	5/1
Pesto, Classico, traditional basil	¼ c	1	2	6	2/1
Pesto, DeLallo	1 T	0	0	0	0/0
Pizza sauce, Boboli, original	½ c	1	8	10	8/1
Pizza sauce, Contadina, four cheese	¼ c	1	2	6	2/1
Pizza sauce, Contadina, original	¼ c	1	2	6	2/1
Pizza sauce, Muir Glen, organic	¼ c	2	3	6	3/1
Pizza sauce, Ragú, homemade style	¼ c	1	3	4	3/0
Pizza sauce, Ragú PizzaQuick, traditional	¼ c	1	3	4	3/0
Sloppy Joe sauce, Del Monte	¼ c	0	9	11	9/1
Sloppy Joe sauce, Del Monte, hickory flavor	¼ c	0	11	14	11/1
Sloppy Joe sauce, Manwich	¼ c	2	10	15	10/1
Stir-fry sauce, Dynasty, Chinese	2 T	0	2	3	2/0
Stir-fry sauce, Kikkoman	1 T	0	3	4	3/0
Sweet & sour, Dynasty	2 T	0	14	14	14/1
Sweet & sour, Kikkoman	2 T	0	13	14	13/1
Sweet & sour, La Choy	2 T	0	11	14	11/1
Sweet & sour, Lee Kum Kee	1 T	0	10	12	10/1
Sweet & sour, Lee Kum Kee, Panda Brand	1 T	0	12	16	12/1
Sweet & sour, World Harbors	2 T	0	12	14	12/1
Teriyaki sauce, Kikkoman	1 T	0	2	2	2/0
Teriyaki sauce, Kikkoman, Takumi collection	1 T	0	6	6	6/1
Teriyaki sauce, La Choy	1 T	0	8	10	8/1
Teriyaki sauce, Lee Kum Kee, Panda Brand	1 T	0	6	7	6/1
Teriyaki sauce, San-J	1 T	0	3	4	3/0
Teriyaki sauce, Veri Veri Teriyaki, Soy Vey	1 T	0	5	6	5/1
Teriyaki sauce, World Harbors	2 T	0	15	17	15/1
Teriyaki sauce, World Harbors, cheriyaki	2 T	0	12	14	12/1
Teriyaki sauce, World Harbors, hot	2 T	0	15	17	15/1
Teriyaki sauce, World Harbors Angostura	1 T	0	4	4	4/0

SYRUPS

FOOD	Svg Size	Fbr	Sgr	Cbs	S/C Val
Blackberry, Smucker's	¼ c	0	44	51	44/3
Blueberry, Smucker's	¼ c	0	44	51	44/3
Blueberry, Smucker's, sugar free	¼ c	0	0	8	0/1
Boysenberry, Smucker's	¼ c	0	44	51	44/3
Butterscotch, Smucker's Sundae Syrup	2 T	0	20	25	20/2
Caramel, Hershey's	2 T	0	21	27	21/2
Caramel, Smucker's Sundae Syrup	2 T	0	20	25	20/2
Caramel, Smucker's Sundae Syrup, sugar free	2 T	0	0	24	0/2
Chocolate, Hershey's	2 T	1	20	24	20/2
Chocolate, Hershey's, lite	2 T	0	10	11	10/1
Chocolate, Hershey's, special dark	2 T	1	20	24	20/2
Chocolate, Hershey's, sugar free	2 T	0	0	5	0/1

FOOD	Svg Size	Fbr	Sgr	Cbs	S/C Val
Chocolate, Nesquik	1 T	0	12	13	12/1
Chocolate, Smucker's Sundae Syrup	2 T	1	19	24	19/2
Chocolate, Smucker's Sundae Syrup, sugar free	2 T	1	0	23	0/2
Maple	2 T	0	24	27	24/2
Maple, Aunt Jemima, lite	¼ c	1	25	26	25/2
Maple, Aunt Jemima, original	¼ c	0	32	52	32/3
Maple, Joseph's, sugar free	¼ c	0	0	9	0/1
Maple, Log Cabin, original	¼ c	0	32	50	32/3
Maple, Log Cabin, sugar free	¼ c	0	0	12	0/1
Maple, Maple Grove, sugar free	¼ c	0	0	11	0/1
Maple, Mrs. Butterworth's, lite	¼ c	0	24	25	24/2
Maple, Mrs. Butterworth's, original	¼ c	0	38	53	38/3
Maple, Mrs. Butterworth's, sugar free	¼ c	0	0	12	0/1
Maple, Nature's Hollow, sugar free	¼ c	0	0	12	0/1
Maple, Spring Tree, sugar free	¼ c	0	0	12	0/1
Raspberry, Nature's Hollow, sugar free	¼ c	0	0	12	0/1
Raspberry, Smucker's	¼ c	0	44	51	44/3
Strawberry, Hershey's	2 T	0	24	26	24/2
Strawberry, Hershey's, sugar free	2 T	0	0	4	0/0
Strawberry, Nesquik	1 T	0	13	13	13/1
Strawberry, Smucker's	¼ c	0	44	51	44/3
Strawberry, Smucker's Sundae Syrup	2 T	0	23	26	23/2
SALAD DRESSING					
Blue cheese	2 T	0	1	1	1/0
Buttermilk	2 T	0	1	6	1/1
Caesar	2 T	0	1	1	1/0
French	2 T	0	5	5	5/1
Italian	2 T	0	2	3	2/0
Peppercorn	2 T	0	1	1	1/0
Ranch	2 T	0	1	2	1/0
Russian	2 T	0	5	10	5/1
Sesame seed	2 T	0	3	3	3/0
Thousand Island	2 T	0	5	4	5/0
Annie's Naturals, artichoke Parmesan	2 T	0	0	0	0/0
Annie's Naturals, Asian sesame, organic	2 T	0	3	4	3/0
Annie's Naturals, balsamic vinaigrette	2 T	0	2	2	2/0
Annie's Naturals, balsamic vinaigrette, organic	2 T	0	3	3	3/0
Annie's Naturals, buttermilk, organic	2 T	0	1	1	1/0
Annie's Naturals, Caesar, organic	2 T	0	1	1	1/0
Annie's Naturals, cowgirl ranch	2 T	0	2	3	2/0
Annie's Naturals, cowgirl ranch, organic	2 T	0	2	3	2/0
Annie's Naturals, creamy Asiago cheese, organic	2 T	0	0	0	0/0
Annie's Naturals, French, organic	2 T	0	3	3	3/0
Annie's Naturals, gingerly vinaigrette, lite	2 T	0	2	3	2/0

FOOD	Svg Size	Fbr	Sgr	Cbs	S/C Val
Annie's Naturals, goddess	2 T	0	0	2	0/0
Annie's Naturals, goddess, organic	2 T	0	0	0	0/0
Annie's Naturals, green garlic, organic	2 T	0	0	0	0/0
Annie's Naturals, green goddess, organic	2 T	0	1	2	1/0
Annie's Naturals, herb balsamic, lite	2 T	0	2	2	2/0
Annie's Naturals, honey mustard vinaigrette, lite	2 T	0	3	5	3/1
Annie's Naturals, lemon & chive	2 T	0	0	0	0/0
Annie's Naturals, mango, fat free	2 T	0	5	5	5/1
Annie's Naturals, oil & vinegar, organic	2 T	0	0	1	0/0
Annie's Naturals, papaya poppy seed, organic	2 T	0	4	4	4/0
Annie's Naturals, pomegranate vinaigrette, organic	2 T	0	1	2	1/0
Annie's Naturals, raspberry balsamic, fat free	2 T	0	7	7	7/1
Annie's Naturals, raspberry vinaigrette, lite	2 T	0	4	4	4/0
Annie's Naturals, red wine & olive oil vinaigrette, organic	2 T	0	0	0	0/0
Annie's Naturals, roasted garlic vinaigrette, organic	2 T	0	2	3	2/0
Annie's Naturals, roasted red pepper vinaigrette	2 T	0	2	3	2/0
Annie's Naturals, sesame ginger vinaigrette, organic	2 T	0	3	4	3/0
Annie's Naturals, shiitake & sesame vinaigrette	2 T	0	0	1	0/0
Annie's Naturals, shiitake & sesame vinaigrette, organic	2 T	0	0	1	0/0
Annie's Naturals, Thousand Island, organic	2 T	0	3	4	3/0
Annie's Naturals, Tuscany Italian	2 T	0	4	5	4/1
Annie's Naturals, Woodstock	2 T	0	0	1	0/0
Bernstein's, balsamic Italian	2 T	0	1	2	1/0
Bernstein's, basil Parmesan	2 T	0	1	2	1/0
Bernstein's, cheese & garlic Italian	2 T	0	1	2	1/0
Bernstein's, cheese & garlic Italian, fat free	2 T	0	1	2	1/0
Bernstein's, Cheese Fantastico!	2 T	0	0	2	0/0
Bernstein's, Cheese Fantastico!, Light Fantastic	2 T	0	1	3	1/0
Bernstein's, chunky blue cheese	2 T	0	1	2	1/0
Bernstein's, creamy Caesar	2 T	0	0	1	0/0
Bernstein's, herb garden French	2 T	0	6	6	6/1
Bernstein's, Italian	2 T	0	1	1	1/0
Bernstein's, Parmesan garlic, Light Fantastic	2 T	0	2	6	2/1
Bernstein's, red wine & garlic Italian	2 T	0	1	2	1/0
Bernstein's, restaurant recipe Italian	2 T	0	0	1	0/0
Bernstein's, roasted garlic balsamic, Light Fantastic	2 T	0	2	3	2/0
Bernstein's, sweet herb Italian	2 T	0	5	8	5/1
Hidden Valley, coleslaw	2 T	0	4	5	4/1
Hidden Valley, ranch, bacon	2 T	0	1	1	1/0
Hidden Valley, ranch, buttermilk	2 T	0	1	2	1/0
Hidden Valley, ranch, fat free	2 T	0	3	6	3/1
Hidden Valley, ranch, Italian	2 T	0	1	2	1/0
Hidden Valley, ranch, light	2 T	0	2	3	2/0
Hidden Valley, ranch, light with sour cream	2 T	0	2	4	2/0

FOOD	Svg Size	Fbr	Sgr	Cbs	S/C Val
Hidden Valley, ranch, original	2 T	0	1	2	1/0
Ken's, Asian sesame w/ ginger & soy, lite	2 T	0	7	8	7/1
Ken's, balsamic & basil vinaigrette	2 T	0	2	2	2/0
Ken's, balsamic & basil vinaigrette, lite	2 T	0	3	3	3/0
Ken's, balsamic vinaigrette, Healthy Options	2 T	0	3	3	3/0
Ken's, blue cheese w/ Gorgonzola, Chef's Reserve	2 T	0	1	1	1/0
Ken's, buttermilk ranch	2 T	0	1	1	1/0
Ken's, Caesar	2 T	0	1	1	1/0
Ken's, Caesar, lite	2 T	0	2	3	2/0
Ken's, Caesar vinaigrette, Healthy Options	2 T	0	1	2	1/0
Ken's, chunky blue cheese	2 T	0	1	1	1/0
Ken's, chunky blue cheese, lite	2 T	0	1	4	1/0
Ken's, country French w/ Vermont honey	2 T	0	9	10	9/1
Ken's, creamy balsamic	2 T	0	8	8	8/1
Ken's, creamy Caesar	2 T	0	0	0	0/0
Ken's, creamy Caesar, lite	2 T	0	1	4	1/0
Ken's, creamy Caesar w/ roasted garlic, Chef's Reserve	2 T	0	0	1	0/0
Ken's, creamy French	2 T	0	6	6	6/1
Ken's, creamy Greek, Chef's Reserve	2 T	0	1	2	1/0
Ken's, creamy Italian	2 T	0	2	3	2/0
Ken's, creamy Parmesan w/ cracker peppercorn, lite	2 T	0	2	3	2/0
Ken's, French w/ applewood smoked bacon, Chef's Reserve	2 T	0	9	9	9/1
Ken's, Greek	2 T	0	1	2	1/0
Ken's, honey dijon, Chef's Reserve	2 T	0	6	7	6/1
Ken's, honey dijon, Healthy Options	2 T	0	7	7	7/1
Ken's, honey French, Healthy Options	2 T	0	7	8	7/1
Ken's, honey mustard	2 T	0	6	7	6/1
Ken's, Italian	2 T	0	0	1	0/0
Ken's, Italian, lite	2 T	0	1	2	1/0
Ken's, Italian w/ aged Romano	2 T	0	1	2	1/0
Ken's, Italian w/ garlic & Asiago cheese, Chef's Reserve	2 T	0	0	1	0/0
Ken's, Italian w/ Romano & red pepper, Healthy Options	2 T	0	1	2	1/0
Ken's, Northern Italian w/ basil & Romano, lite	2 T	0	1	1	1/0
Ken's, olive oil & vinegar, Healthy Options	2 T	0	3	3	3/0
Ken's, olive oil vinaigrette, lite	2 T	0	2	3	2/0
Ken's, Parmesan & peppercorn, Healthy Options	2 T	0	2	3	2/0
Ken's, peppercorn ranch	2 T	0	1	1	1/0
Ken's, ranch	2 T	0	2	2	2/0
Ken's, ranch, Chef's Reserve	2 T	0	2	3	2/0
Ken's, ranch, Healthy Options	2 T	0	1	6	1/1
Ken's, ranch, lite	2 T	0	2	2	2/0
Ken's, raspberry pecan, fat free	2 T	0	10	12	10/1
Ken's, raspberry walnut, Healthy Options	2 T	0	6	6	6/1
Ken's, raspberry walnut vinaigrette, lite	2 T	0	6	7	6/1

FOOD	Svg Size	Fbr	Sgr	Cbs	S/C Val
Ken's, red wine vinegar & olive oil	2 T	0	2	2	2/0
Ken's, Russian	2 T	0	3	5	3/1
Ken's, sun-dried tomato vinaigrette, fat free	2 T	0	12	17	12/1
Ken's, sweet Vidalia onion	2 T	0	10	10	10/1
Ken's, sweet Vidalia onion, lite	2 T	0	10	11	10/1
Ken's, sweet Vidalia onion vinaigrette, Healthy Options	2 T	0	7	7	7/1
Ken's, tableside Caesar, Chef's Reserve	2 T	0	2	2	2/0
Ken's, Thousand Island	2 T	0	3	4	3/0
Ken's, three cheese Italian	2 T	0	4	4	4/0
Ken's, zesty Italian	2 T	0	4	5	4/1
Ken's, Lite Accents, Asian vinaigrette	10 spr	0	2	2	2/0
Ken's, Lite Accents, balsamic vinaigrette	10 spr	0	1	1	1/0
Ken's, Lite Accents, honey mustard vinaigrette	10 spr	0	2	2	2/0
Ken's, Lite Accents, Italian vinaigrette	10 spr	0	1	1	1/0
Ken's, Lite Accents, raspberry walnut vinaigrette	10 spr	0	2	2	2/0
Kraft, Asian toasted sesame	2 T	0	7	8	7/1
Kraft, balsamic vinaigrette	2 T	0	4	4	4/0
Kraft, buttermilk ranch	2 T	0	3	3	3/0
Kraft, Caesar, light	2 T	0	1	3	1/0
Kraft, Caesar Italian, fat free	2 T	0	2	3	2/0
Kraft, Caesar vinaigrette w/ Parmesan	2 T	0	1	3	1/0
Kraft, Caesar w/ bacon	2 T	0	1	2	1/0
Kraft, Catalina	2 T	0	7	7	7/1
Kraft, Catalina, fat free	2 T	0	7	11	7/1
Kraft, classic Caesar	2 T	0	7	11	7/1
Kraft, classic Caesar, fat free	2 T	0	3	11	3/1
Kraft, classic Italian vinaigrette	2 T	0	2	5	2/1
Kraft, creamy French	2 T	0	5	5	5/1
Kraft, creamy French style, light	2 T	0	5	11	5/1
Kraft, creamy Italian	2 T	0	2	2	2/0
Kraft, creamy poppyseed	2 T	0	8	8	8/1
Kraft, French style, fat free	2 T	0	5	11	5/1
Kraft, garlic ranch	2 T	0	2	3	2/0
Kraft, Greek vinaigrette	2 T	0	1	2	1/0
Kraft, honey dijon	2 T	0	5	6	5/1
Kraft, honey dijon, fat free	2 T	0	5	12	5/1
Kraft, honey dijon vinaigrette	2 T	0	3	6	3/1
Kraft, Italian, fat free	2 T	0	2	4	2/0
Kraft, Parmesan Romano	2 T	0	1	2	1/0
Kraft, peppercorn ranch	2 T	0	1	2	1/0
Kraft, ranch	2 T	0	2	3	2/0
Kraft, ranch, fat free	2 T	0	3	11	3/1
Kraft, ranch, light	2 T	0	2	7	2/1
Kraft, ranch w/ bacon	2 T	0	2	2	2/0

FOOD	Svg Size	Fbr	Sgr	Cbs	S/C Val
Kraft, raspberry vinaigrette, light	2 T	0	5	5	5/1
Kraft, red wine vinaigrette, light	2 T	0	2	3	2/0
Kraft, roasted red pepper Italian w/ Parmesan	2 T	0	3	5	3/1
Kraft, Roka blue cheese	2 T	0	1	1	1/0
Kraft, sweet honey Catalina	2 T	0	8	8	8/1
Kraft, tangy tomato bacon	2 T	0	9	10	9/1
Kraft, Thousand Island	2 T	0	5	5	5/1
Kraft, Thousand Island, light	2 T	0	8	11	8/1
Kraft, three cheese ranch	2 T	0	2	3	2/0
Kraft, three cheese ranch, light	2 T	0	1	2	1/0
Kraft, Tuscan house Italian	2 T	0	2	3	2/0
Kraft, Vidalia onion vinaigrette w/ roasted red pepper	2 T	0	7	8	7/1
Kraft, zesty Italian	2 T	0	2	3	2/0
Kraft, zesty Italian, fat free	2 T	0	2	3	2/0
Newman's Own, Asian, low fat, organic	2 T	0	4	5	4/1
Newman's Own, balsamic, light, organic	2 T	0	2	3	2/0
Newman's Own, balsamic vinaigrette	2 T	0	1	3	1/0
Newman's Own, balsamic vinaigrette, Lighten Up	2 T	0	2	2	2/0
Newman's Own, Caesar	2 T	0	1	1	1/0
Newman's Own, Caesar, Lighten Up	2 T	0	2	3	2/0
Newman's Own, cranberry walnut, Lighten Up	2 T	0	7	8	7/1
Newman's Own, creamy Caesar	2 T	0	0	1	0/0
Newman's Own, family recipe Italian	2 T	0	1	1	1/0
Newman's Own, Greek vinaigrette	2 T	0	1	1	1/0
Newman's Own, honey mustard, Lighten Up	2 T	0	5	7	5/1
Newman's Own, Italian, Lighten Up	2 T	0	0	1	0/0
Newman's Own, lime vinaigrette, Lighten Up	2 T	0	4	4	4/0
Newman's Own, olive oil & vinegar	2 T	0	1	1	1/0
Newman's Own, orange ginger	2 T	0	8	9	8/1
Newman's Own, Parmesan & roasted garlic	2 T	0	1	2	1/0
Newman's Own, ranch	2 T	0	1	2	1/0
Newman's Own, raspberry & walnut, Lighten Up	2 T	0	5	7	5/1
Newman's Own, red wine vinegar & olive oil, Lighten Up	2 T	0	2	2	2/0
Newman's Own, roasted garlic balsamic, Lighten Up	2 T	0	3	3	3/0
Newman's Own, sesame ginger, Lighten Up	2 T	0	4	5	4/1
Newman's Own, sun dried tomato, Lighten Up	2 T	0	3	5	3/1
Newman's Own, three cheese balsamic	2 T	0	1	2	1/0
Newman's Own, Tuscan Italian, organic	2 T	0	1	2	1/0
Wish-Bone, Asian w/ sesame & ginger vinaigrette, light	2 T	0	5	5	5/1
Wish-Bone, balsamic & basil vinaigrette, light	2 T	0	3	3	3/0
Wish-Bone, balsamic Italian vinaigrette	2 T	0	4	4	4/0
Wish-Bone, balsamic vinaigrette	2 T	0	3	3	3/0
Wish-Bone, blue cheese, light	2 T	0	2	6	2/1
Wish-Bone, blue cheese w/ gorgonzola	2 T	0	0	1	0/0

SAUCES, SYRUPS & SALAD DRESSING, cont'd.

FOOD	Svg Size	Fbr	Sgr	Cbs	S/C Val
Wish-Bone, chunky blue cheese	2 T	0	1	1	1/0
Wish-Bone, chunky blue cheese, fat free	2 T	0	1	1	1/0
Wish-Bone, country Italian, light	2 T	0	2	3	2/0
Wish-Bone, creamy Caesar	2 T	0	1	1	1/0
Wish-Bone, creamy Caesar, light	2 T	0	2	7	2/1
Wish-Bone, creamy Italian	2 T	0	2	4	2/0
Wish-Bone, deluxe French	2 T	0	5	5	5/1
Wish-Bone, deluxe French, light	2 T	0	5	5	5/1
Wish-Bone, garlic ranch	2 T	0	1	2	1/0
Wish-Bone, honey Dijon, light	2 T	0	7	8	7/1
Wish-Bone, house Italian	2 T	0	2	3	2/0
Wish-Bone, Italian	2 T	0	4	4	4/0
Wish-Bone, Italian, fat free	2 T	0	2	3	2/0
Wish-Bone, Italian, light	2 T	0	2	3	2/0
Wish-Bone, olive oil vinaigrette	2 T	0	3	4	3/0
Wish-Bone, Parmesan peppercorn ranch, light	2 T	0	2	7	2/1
Wish-Bone, ranch	2 T	0	2	2	2/0
Wish-Bone, ranch, fat free	2 T	0	3	6	3/1
Wish-Bone, ranch, light	2 T	0	2	5	2/1
Wish-Bone, raspberry hazelnut vinaigrette	2 T	0	5	8	5/1
Wish-Bone, red wine vinaigrette	2 T	0	6	7	6/1
Wish-Bone, robusto Italian	2 T	0	3	4	3/0
Wish-Bone, Romano basil vinaigrette	2 T	0	1	2	1/0
Wish-Bone, Russian	2 T	0	6	14	6/1
Wish-Bone, sweet & spicy French	2 T	0	5	6	5/1
Wish-Bone, sweet & spicy French, light	2 T	0	6	9	6/1
Wish-Bone, Thousand Island	2 T	0	5	6	5/1
Wish-Bone, Thousand Island, light	2 T	0	5	9	5/1
Wish-Bone, Salad Spritzers, Balsamic Breeze	10 spr	0	1	1	1/0
Wish-Bone, Salad Spritzers, Caesar Delight	10 spr	0	0	0	0/0
Wish-Bone, Salad Spritzers, Italian vinaigrette	10 spr	0	1	1	1/0
Wish-Bone, Salad Spritzers, ranch vinaigrette	10 spr	0	0	0	0/0
Wish-Bone, Salad Spritzers, raspberry bliss	10 spr	0	1	2	1/0

CONDIMENTS & SPICES

FOOD	Svg Size	Fbr	Sgr	Cbs	S/C Val
Allspice, ground	1 T	1	0	4	0/0
Anise seed, whole	1 T	1	0	3	0/0
Baking powder	1 t	0	0	0	0/0
Baking soda	1 t	0	0	0	0/0
Basil, dried, ground	1 T	2	0	3	0/0
Basil, dried, leaves	1 T	1	0	1	0/0
Bay leaf, crumbled	1 T	1	0	1	0/0
Capers	1 T	0	0	0	0/0

FOOD	Svg Size	Fbr	Sgr	Cbs	S/C Val
Caraway seed	1 T	3	0	3	0/0
Cardamom, ground	1 T	2	0	4	0/0
Celery seed	1 T	1	0	3	0/0
Chili powder	1 t	1	0	1	0/0
Chutney, mango	2 T	5	8	21	8/2
Chutney, mint	¼ c	1	3	3	3/0
Chutney, tomato	2 T	2	6	6	6/1
Cilantro (coriander)	1 T	0	0	1	0/0
Cinnamon, ground	1 t	1	0	2	0/0
Cinnamon, Ceylon, ground	1 t	1	0	2	0/0
Cloves, ground	1 t	1	0	1	0/0
Cocktail sauce, Del Monte	¼ c	0	22	24	22/2
Cocktail sauce, Heinz	¼ c	1	16	19	16/1
Cocktail sauce, McCormick	¼ c	1	16	19	16/1
Coriander leaves, dried	1 T	0	0	1	0/0
Coriander seed	1 T	2	0	3	0/0
Cornstarch	1 T	0	0	7	0/1
Cream of tartar	1 t	0	0	2	0/0
Cumin seed	1 T	1	0	3	0/0
Curry paste, Patak's, hot	1 T	4	1	7	1/1
Curry paste, Patak's, mild	1 T	4	1	8	1/1
Curry paste, Thai Kitchen, green	1 T	0	1	3	1/0
Curry paste, Thai Kitchen, red	1 T	0	1	3	1/0
Curry powder	1 T	2	0	4	0/0
Dill seed	1 T	1	0	4	0/0
Dill weed, dried	1 T	0	0	2	0/0
Fennel seed, whole	1 T	2	0	3	0/0
Fenugreek seed	1 T	3	0	6	0/1
Garlic powder	1 T	1	0	7	0/1
Ginger, ground	1 T	1	0	4	0/0
Ginger, pickled	0.5 oz	0	0	1	0/0
Horseradish, prepared	1 T	1	1	2	1/0
Hot sauce	1 T	0	0	1	0/0
Hot sauce, sriracha, Huy Fong Foods, Inc.	1 t	0	1	1	1/0
Hot sauce, Tabasco	1 t	0	0	0	0/0
Ketchup	1 T	0	4	3	4/0
Ketchup, Annie's Naturals	1 T	0	2	3	2/0
Ketchup, Del Monte	1 T	0	4	4	4/0
Ketchup, Heinz	1 T	0	4	4	4/0
Ketchup, Heinz, hot & spicy	1 T	0	3	4	3/0
Ketchup, Heinz, reduced sugar	1 T	0	1	1	1/0
Ketchup, Nature's Hollow, sugar free	1 T	0	0	4	0/0
Marjoram, dried	1 T	0	0	1	0/0
Mayonnaise	1 T	0	1	0	1/0

FOOD	Svg Size	Fbr	Sgr	Cbs	S/C Val
Mayonnaise, Best Foods	1 T	0	0	0	0/0
Mayonnaise, Best Foods, light	1 T	0	0	0	0/0
Mayonnaise, Best Foods, w/ olive oil	1 T	0	0	0	0/0
Mayonnaise, Hellmann's	1 T	0	0	0	0/0
Mayonnaise, Hellmann's, light	1 T	0	0	1	0/0
Mayonnaise, Kraft	1 T	0	1	0	1/0
Mayonnaise, Kraft, hot 'n spicy	1 T	0	0	0	0/0
Mayonnaise, Kraft, light	1 T	0	1	2	1/0
Mayonnaise, Kraft, w/ olive oil	1 T	0	0	2	0/0
Mayonnaise, Smart Balance	1 T	0	0	2	0/0
Mayonnaise alternative, Follow Your Heart, Vegenaise, grapeseed oil	1 T	0	0	0	0/0
Mayonnaise alternative, Follow Your Heart, Vegenaise, original	1 T	0	0	0	0/0
Mayonnaise alternative, Follow Your Heart, Vegenaise, reduced fat	1 T	0	0	1	0/0
Mayonnaise alternative, Kraft, Miracle Whip	1 T	0	1	2	1/0
Mayonnaise alternative, Kraft, Miracle Whip, light	1 T	0	2	3	2/0
Mayonnaise alternative, Nasoya, Nayonaise, fat free	1 T	0	1	2	1/0
Mayonnaise alternative, Nasoya, Nayonaise, original	1 T	0	0	1	0/0
Miso	1 T	1	1	5	1/1
Mustard, brown	1 t	0	0	0	0/0
Mustard, chipotle, Silver Springs	1 t	0	0	0	0/0
Mustard, dijon	1 t	0	0	0	0/0
Mustard, yellow	1 t	0	0	0	0/0
Mustard seed, ground	1 T	1	0	2	0/0
Nutmeg, ground	1 T	2	2	3	2/0
Onion powder	1 T	1	0	5	0/1
Oregano, dried, ground	1 T	2	0	4	0/0
Oregano, dried, leaves	1 T	1	0	2	0/0
Paprika	1 T	3	1	4	1/0
Parsley, dried	1 T	0	0	1	0/0
Pepper, black	1 t	1	0	1	0/0
Pepper, red or cayenne	1 t	1	0	1	0/0
Pepper, white	1 t	1	0	2	0/0
Poppy seed	1 t	1	0	1	0/0
Relish, dill	1 T	0	4	5	4/1
Relish, sweet	1 T	0	4	5	4/1
Relish, Del Monte, hamburger style	1 T	0	5	5	5/1
Relish, Del Monte, hotdog style	1 T	0	3	4	3/0
Relish, Del Monte, sweet	1 T	0	5	5	5/1
Relish, Heinz, dill	1 T	0	0	0	0/0
Rosemary, dried	1 T	1	0	2	0/0
Saffron	1 t	0	0	0	0/0
Sage, ground	1 T	1	0	0	0/0
Salt, all varieties	1 t	0	0	0	0/0
Savory, ground	1 T	2	0	3	0/0

FOOD	Svg Size	Fbr	Sgr	Cbs	S/C Val
Soy sauce, shoyu	1 T	0	0	1	0/0
Soy sauce, tamari	1 T	0	0	1	0/0
Soy sauce, Kikkoman	1 T	0	0	1	0/0
Soy sauce, La Choy	1 T	0	0	1	0/0
Soy sauce, La Choy, lite	1 T	0	2	2	2/0
Soy sauce, Lee Kum Kee, lite	1 T	0	1	1	1/0
Soy sauce, Lee Kum Kee, premium	1 T	0	2	3	2/0
Soy sauce, San-J, shoyu	1 T	0	0	1	0/0
Soy sauce, San-J, tamari	1 T	0	3	4	3/0
Soy sauce, World Harbors Angostura	1 T	0	1	1	1/0
Soy sauce, World Harbors Angostura, lite	1 T	0	2	2	2/0
Spearmint, dried	1 T	1	0	1	0/0
Steak sauce, A.1.	1 T	0	2	3	2/0
Steak sauce, Lea & Perrins	1 T	0	3	5	3/1
Taco sauce	1 T	0	1	2	1/0
Taco sauce, La Victoria, all flavors	1 T	0	0	1	0/0
Taco sauce, Old El Paso, hot	1 T	0	0	1	0/0
Taco sauce, Old El Paso, medium	1 T	0	0	1	0/0
Taco sauce, Old El Paso, mild	1 T	0	1	1	1/0
Taco sauce, Ortega	1 T	0	0	2	0/0
Taco sauce, Ortega, green	1 T	0	0	0	0/0
Tarragon, dried, ground	1 T	0	0	2	0/0
Tarragon, dried, leaves	1 T	0	0	1	0/0
Tartar sauce, Hellmann's	2 T	0	2	4	2/0
Tartar sauce, Kraft	2 T	0	3	4	3/0
Tartar sauce, McCormick	2 T	0	3	3	3/0
Tartar sauce, McCormick, fat free	2 T	1	5	7	5/1
Tempura sauce	1 t	0	1	1	1/0
Thyme, dried, ground	1 T	2	0	3	0/0
Thyme, dried, leaves	1 T	1	0	2	0/0
Turmeric, ground	1 T	1	0	4	0/0
Vanilla extract	1 t	0	1	1	1/0
Vanilla extract, imitation	1 t	0	1	1	1/0
Vinegar, apple cider	1 T	0	0	0	0/0
Vinegar, balsamic	1 T	0	2	3	2/0
Vinegar, balsamic, Kirkland Signature	1 T	0	2	2	2/0
Vinegar, distilled	1 T	0	0	0	0/0
Vinegar, malt	1 T	0	1	1	1/0
Vinegar, malt, Heinz	1 T	0	0	0	0/0
Vinegar, red wine	1 T	0	0	0	0/0
Vinegar, rice	1 T	0	0	0	0/0
Vinegar, seasoned rice, Nakano, all flavors	1 T	0	5	5	5/1
Vinegar, seasoned rice, Nakano, balsamic blend	1 T	0	4	4	4/0
Wasabi	1 t	0	0	1	0/0

CONDIMENTS & SPICES, cont'd.

FOOD	Svg Size	Fbr	Sgr	Cbs	S/C Val
Worcestershire sauce	1 T	0	2	3	2/0
Worcestershire sauce, Annie's Naturals, organic	1 t	0	1	1	1/0
Worcestershire sauce, French's, classic	1 t	0	0	1	0/0
Worcestershire sauce, Lea & Perrins, original	1 t	0	1	1	1/0
Worcestershire sauce, Lea & Perrins, thick	2 T	0	6	8	6/1
Worcestershire sauce, World Harbors Angostura	1 T	0	1	1	1/0
Yeast, baker's, dry	1 T	3	0	5	0/1
Yeast, baker's, dry, average	1 pkt	2	0	3	0/0

SOUPS

FOOD	Svg Size	Fbr	Sgr	Cbs	S/C Val
Bouillon, powder, beef	1 t	0	0	0	0/0
Bouillon, powder, chicken	1 t	0	0	0	0/0
Campbell's, beef noodle	1 can	0	1	8	1/1
Campbell's, chicken & dumplings	1 can	1	1	10	1/1
Campbell's, chicken gumbo, light	1 can	1	2	12	2/1
Campbell's, chicken mushroom barley, light	1 can	2	2	14	2/1
Campbell's, chicken noodle, Healthy Request	1 can	1	1	8	1/1
Campbell's, chicken rice, Healthy Request	1 can	1	1	13	1/1
Campbell's, chicken vegetable	1 can	2	3	15	3/1
Campbell's, chicken w/ white & wild rice, light	1 can	1	1	13	1/1
Campbell's, cream of chicken, Healthy Request	1 can	1	7	12	7/1
Campbell's, cream of mushroom, Healthy Request	1 can	1	2	10	2/1
Campbell's, cream of potato	1 can	2	1	15	1/1
Campbell's, homestyle chicken noodle	1 can	2	1	9	1/1
Campbell's, Italian-style wedding, light	1 can	2	2	12	2/1
Campbell's, lentil	1 can	6	2	24	2/2
Campbell's, Manhattan clam chowder	1 can	2	2	12	2/1
Campbell's, minestrone	1 can	3	3	17	3/1
Campbell's, minestrone, Healthy Request	1 can	3	4	15	4/1
Campbell's, New England clam chowder	1 can	1	1	13	1/1
Campbell's, tomato, Healthy Request	1 can	1	10	17	10/1
Campbell's, tomato bisque	1 can	1	15	23	15/2
Campbell's, vegetable	1 can	3	7	20	7/1
Campbell's, vegetable, Healthy Request	1 can	3	5	20	5/1
Campbell's, vegetable beef	1 can	3	2	15	2/1
Campbell's, vegetable orzo, light	1 can	3	3	14	3/1
Campbell's, vegetarian vegetable	1 can	2	6	18	6/1
Campbell's, Chunky, baked potato w/ steak & cheese	1 c	3	3	21	3/2
Campbell's, Chunky, creamy chicken & dumplings	1 c	3	12	19	12/1
Campbell's, Chunky, grilled chicken & sausage gumbo, Healthy Request	1 c	3	4	21	4/2
Campbell's, Chunky, hearty beef barley	1 c	4	5	26	5/2
Campbell's, Chunky, Manhattan clam chowder	1 c	3	4	19	4/1
Campbell's, Chunky, New England clam chowder	1 c	3	1	20	1/1

FOOD	Svg Size	Fbr	Sgr	Cbs	S/C Val
Campbell's, Chunky, old-fashioned vegetable beef, Healthy Request	1 c	3	5	19	5/1
Campbell's, Chunky, savory vegetable	1 c	4	6	22	6/2
Campbell's, Chunky, savory vegetable, Healthy Request	1 c	4	8	24	8/2
Campbell's, Chunky, sirloin burger w/ country vegetables, Healthy Request	1 c	3	5	19	5/1
Campbell's, Chunky, slow roasted beef w/ mushrooms	1 c	3	14	18	14/1
Campbell's, Select Harvest, Italian-style vegetable	1 c	4	4	14	4/1
Campbell's, Select Harvest, Maryland-style crab	1 c	2	6	16	6/1
Campbell's, Select Harvest, minestrone w/ whole grain pasta	1 c	4	4	14	4/1
Campbell's, Select Harvest, roasted chicken w/ Italian herbs	1 c	3	2	8	2/1
Campbell's, Select Harvest, vegetable & pasta	1 c	4	3	13	3/1
Healthy Choice, beef pot roast	1 c	3	2	18	2/1
Healthy Choice, chicken & dumplings	1 c	3	2	22	2/2
Healthy Choice, chicken noodle	1 c	2	1	12	1/1
Healthy Choice, chicken tortilla	1 c	6	3	23	3/2
Healthy Choice, chicken w/ rice	1 c	2	1	14	1/1
Healthy Choice, country vegetable	1 c	5	4	20	4/1
Healthy Choice, garden vegetable	1 c	5	4	25	4/2
Healthy Choice, Italian-style wedding	1 c	3	1	16	1/1
Healthy Choice, New England clam chowder	1 c	3	3	20	3/1
Healthy Choice, tomato basil	1 c	3	11	28	11/2
Healthy Choice, vegetable beef	1 c	4	4	21	4/2
Herb-Ox, beef bouillon cube	1	0	0	1	0/0
Herb-Ox, chicken bouillon cube	1	0	0	1	0/0
Lipton, Cup-a-Soup, chicken noodle	1 pkt	0	0	17	0/1
Lipton, Cup-a-Soup, cream of chicken	1 pkt	0	1	14	1/1
Lipton, Cup-a-Soup, tomato	1 pkt	0	8	16	8/1
Maruchan, Instant Lunch, beef	1 pkg	2	2	38	2/2
Maruchan, Instant Lunch, chicken	1 pkg	2	2	39	2/2
Maruchan, Instant Lunch, shrimp	1 pkg	2	2	38	2/2
Maruchan, Ramen, beef	1 pkg	1	2	52	2/3
Maruchan, Ramen, chicken	1 pkg	2	2	52	2/3
Maruchan, Ramen, shrimp	1 pkg	1	1	52	1/3
Nissin, Cup Noodles, beef	1 pkg	2	2	38	2/2
Nissin, Cup Noodles, chicken	1 pkg	2	2	38	2/2
Nissin, Cup Noodles, shrimp	1 pkg	1	1	38	1/2
Nissin, Top Ramen, beef	1 pkg	4	0	54	0/3
Nissin, Top Ramen, chicken	1 pkg	4	1	52	1/3
Nissin, Top Ramen, shrimp	1 pkg	2	1	52	1/3
Progresso, beef barley, 99% fat free	1 c	4	3	20	3/1
Progresso, chicken & herb dumplings	1 c	1	1	13	1/1
Progresso, chicken & wild rice	1 c	1	1	15	1/1
Progresso, chicken noodle	1 c	1	1	12	1/1
Progresso, chicken Tuscany, high fiber	1 c	7	2	20	2/1
Progresso, creamy mushroom	1 c	1	2	9	2/1

FOOD	Svg Size	Fbr	Sgr	Cbs	S/C Val
Progresso, creamy tomato basil, high fiber	1 c	7	13	26	13/2
Progresso, hearty vegetable & noodles, high fiber	1 c	7	3	18	3/1
Progresso, homestyle minestrone, high fiber	1 c	7	3	24	3/2
Progresso, lentil	1 c	5	2	30	2/2
Progresso, Manhattan clam chowder	1 c	2	4	17	4/1
Progresso, minestrone	1 c	4	3	20	3/1
Progresso, New England clam chowder	1 c	1	2	20	2/1
Progresso, potato, broccoli & cheese chowder	1 c	2	2	20	2/1
Progresso, tomato basil	1 c	2	14	29	14/2
Progresso, turkey noodle	1 c	1	1	12	1/1
Progresso, vegetable	1 c	3	4	15	4/1
Rachael Ray, Stock in a Box, beef	1 c	0	0	0	0/0
Rachael Ray, Stock in a Box, chicken	1 c	0	1	1	1/0
Swanson, broth, beef	1 c	0	0	1	0/0
Swanson, broth, chicken	1 c	0	1	1	1/0
Swanson, broth, vegetable	1 c	1	2	3	2/0
Swanson, stock, beef	1 c	0	3	3	3/0
Swanson, stock, chicken	1 c	0	1	1	1/0
Wolfgang Puck, black bean	1 c	10	6	29	6/2
Wolfgang Puck, chicken & dumplings	1 c	2	1	14	1/1
Wolfgang Puck, chicken w/ egg noodles	1 c	1	2	14	2/1
Wolfgang Puck, chicken w/ white & wild rice	1 c	1	1	13	1/1
Wolfgang Puck, classic minestrone	1 c	2	2	17	2/1
Wolfgang Puck, classic tomato w/ basil	1 c	3	13	19	13/1
Wolfgang Puck, creamy butternut squash	1 c	3	9	22	9/2
Wolfgang Puck, creamy tomato	1 c	4	12	21	12/2
Wolfgang Puck, French onion	1 c	1	6	14	6/1
Wolfgang Puck, New England clam chowder	1 c	2	1	18	1/1
Wolfgang Puck, thick hearty vegetable	1 c	4	7	19	7/1
Wolfgang Puck, thick hearty vegetable & lentil	1 c	5	3	28	3/2
Wolfgang Puck, tortilla	1 c	6	7	27	7/2
Wolfgang Puck, vegetable barley	1 c	2	4	14	4/1

FROZEN MEALS

FOOD	Svg Size	Fbr	Sgr	Cbs	S/C Val
AMY'S					
Bowls, baked ziti	1 pkg	6	8	62	8/4
Bowls, brown rice & vegetables	1 pkg	5	7	36	7/2
Bowls, brown rice, black-eyed peas & veggies	1 pkg	8	5	38	5/2
Bowls, country cheddar	1 pkg	4	3	45	3/3
Bowls, Mexican casserole	1 pkg	7	3	70	3/4
Bowls, Mexican casserole, light in sodium	1 pkg	7	4	48	4/3
Bowls, pesto tortellini	1 pkg	3	5	45	5/3

FOOD	Svg Size	Fbr	Sgr	Cbs	S/C Val
Bowls, ravioli	1 pkg	4	7	55	7/3
Bowls, Santa Fe enchilada	1 pkg	9	5	47	5/3
Bowls, stuffed pasta shells	1 pkg	5	7	30	7/2
Bowls, teriyaki	1 pkg	6	15	52	15/3
Bowls, tortilla casserole & black beans	1 pkg	7	6	41	6/3
Burrito, beans & rice, cheddar cheese	1 pkg	7	1	46	1/3
Burrito, beans & rice, cheddar cheese, light in sodium	1 pkg	7	2	51	2/3
Burrito, beans & rice, non-dairy	1 pkg	6	2	48	2/3
Burrito, beans & rice, non-dairy, light in sodium	1 pkg	7	2	51	2/3
Burrito, black beans & vegetables	1 pkg	5	3	45	3/3
Burrito, breakfast	1 pkg	5	3	38	3/2
Burrito, especial	1 pkg	4	2	50	2/3
Burrito, Southwestern	1 pkg	6	2	38	2/2
Chili & cornbread dinner	1 pkg	10	14	59	14/3
Enchilada, black bean vegetable	½ pkg	3	2	22	2/2
Enchilada, cheese	½ pkg	2	2	18	2/1
Enchilada dinner	1 pkg	9	4	53	4/3
Enchilada dinner, cheese	1 pkg	6	6	38	6/2
Enchilada dinner, verde	1 pkg	8	5	54	5/3
Indian, mattar paneer	1 pkg	6	8	54	8/3
Indian, mattar tofu	1 pkg	5	5	40	5/2
Indian, palak paneer	1 pkg	5	5	38	5/2
Indian, paneer tikka	1 pkg	5	6	36	6/2
Indian, vegetable korma	1 pkg	7	7	41	7/3
Lasagna, cheese	1 pkg	4	8	44	8/3
Lasagna, garden vegetable	1 pkg	5	7	41	7/3
Lasagna, roasted vegetable	1 pkg	4	9	47	9/3
Lasagna, roasted vegetable, light in sodium	1 pkg	4	8	41	8/3
Lasagna, tofu vegetable	1 pkg	5	6	41	6/3
Lasagna, vegetable	1 pkg	5	5	35	5/2
Macaroni & cheese	1 pkg	3	6	47	6/3
Macaroni & cheese, with rice pasta	1 pkg	1	6	47	6/3
Macaroni & soy cheeze	1 pkg	4	2	42	2/3
Macaroni w/ non-dairy cheeze, with rice pasta	1 pkg	3	0	72	0/4
Pizza, broccoli & spinach	⅓ pkg	2	2	31	2/2
Pizza, cheese	⅓ pkg	2	4	33	4/2
Pizza, cheese, rice crust	⅓ pkg	2	5	34	5/2
Pizza, cheese, single serve	1 pkg	3	4	49	4/3
Pizza, cheese & pesto, whole wheat crust	⅓ pkg	4	4	37	4/2
Pizza, 4 cheese	⅓ pkg	2	2	31	2/2
Pizza, Margherita	⅓ pkg	3	3	32	3/2
Pizza, Margherita, single serve	1 pkg	3	4	47	4/3
Pizza, mushroom & olive	⅓ pkg	2	3	33	3/2
Pizza, mushroom & olive, single serve	1 pkg	3	4	56	4/3

FOOD	Svg Size	Fbr	Sgr	Cbs	S/C Val
Pizza, non-dairy cheeze, rice crust, single serve	1 pkg	4	7	46	7/3
Pizza, pesto	⅓ pkg	2	3	39	3/2
Pizza, pesto, single serve	1 pkg	3	3	52	3/3
Pizza, roasted vegetable	⅓ pkg	2	5	42	5/3
Pizza, roasted vegetable, single serve	1 pkg	5	10	62	10/4
Pizza, roasted vegetable, single serve, rice crust	1 pkg	5	8	55	8/3
Pizza, soy cheeze	⅓ pkg	2	3	37	3/2
Pizza, spinach	⅓ pkg	2	4	38	4/2
Pizza, spinach, rice crust	⅓ pkg	4	5	34	5/2
Pizza, spinach, single serve	1 pkg	3	5	54	5/3
Pizza, 3 cheese, cornmeal crust	⅓ pkg	2	6	41	6/3
Pocket sandwich, broccoli & cheese	1 pkg	3	4	37	4/2
Pocket sandwich, cheese pizza	1 pkg	4	5	42	5/3
Pocket sandwich, spinach feta	1 pkg	3	4	34	4/2
Pocket sandwich, spinach pizza	1 pkg	3	3	37	3/2
Pocket sandwich, tofu scramble	1 pkg	0	2	23	2/2
Pocket sandwich, vegetable pie	1 pkg	3	5	45	5/3
Pot pie, broccoli	1 pkg	4	3	46	3/3
Pot pie, Mexican tamale	1 pkg	4	2	27	2/2
Pot pie, shepherd's	1 pkg	5	5	27	5/2
Pot pie, vegetable	1 pkg	4	3	54	3/3
Pot pie, vegetable, non-dairy	1 pkg	4	3	50	3/3
Southern dinner	1 pkg	8	11	51	11/3
Stir-fry, Asian noodle	1 pkg	5	16	50	16/3
Stir-fry, Thai	1 pkg	5	2	45	2/3
Tamale, roasted vegetables	1 pkg	10	4	44	4/3
Tamale verde, black bean	1 pkg	8	6	55	6/3
Tamale verde, cheese	1 pkg	5	5	45	5/3
Tofu scramble	1 pkg	4	4	19	4/1
Tofu scramble, Mexican	1 pkg	8	4	40	4/2
Veggie loaf dinner	1 pkg	10	6	47	6/3
Veggie steak & gravy	1 pkg	7	7	50	7/3
Wrap, breakfast scramble	1 pkg	4	1	30	1/2
Wrap, Indian samosa	1 pkg	4	2	35	2/2
Wrap, Indian spinach tofu	1 pkg	6	2	28	2/2
Wrap, teriyaki	1 pkg	5	6	51	6/3
BANQUET					
Beef pot pie	1 pkg	3	5	36	5/2
Boneless pork rib meal	1 pkg	5	10	42	10/3
Chicken & broccoli pot pie	1 pkg	3	3	35	3/2
Chicken fingers meal	1 pkg	5	22	56	22/3
Chicken fried beef steak meal	1 pkg	5	6	43	6/3
Chicken fried chicken meal	1 pkg	5	2	35	2/2
Chicken nugget meal	1 pkg	4	3	29	3/2

FROZEN MEALS, cont'd.

FOOD	Svg Size	Fbr	Sgr	Cbs	S/C Val
Chicken nuggets & fries	1 pkg	3	0	31	0/2
Chicken pot pie	1 pkg	3	3	35	3/2
Chicken sesame	1 pkg	4	5	40	5/2
Fettuccine Alfredo	1 pkg	3	0	35	0/2
Fish stick meal	1 pkg	4	16	44	16/3
Homestyle grilled meat patty meal	1 pkg	3	5	50	5/3
Lasagna w/ meat sauce	1 pkg	4	4	34	4/2
Macaroni & cheese meal	1 pkg	3	4	39	4/2
Meat loaf meal	1 pkg	4	2	28	2/2
Salisbury steak meal	1 pkg	4	2	25	2/2
Spaghetti & meatballs	1 pkg	5	4	42	4/3
Swedish meatballs w/ egg noodles & sauce	1 pkg	5	0	51	0/3
Sweet & sour chicken	1 pkg	3	21	56	21/3
Turkey meal	1 pkg	5	3	32	3/2
Turkey pot pie	1 pkg	3	3	36	3/2
DIGIORNO					
Cheese Stuffed Crust, five cheese	⅕ pkg	3	7	40	7/2
Cheese Stuffed Crust, four cheese	⅕ pkg	3	6	49	6/3
Cheese Stuffed Crust, pepperoni	⅕ pkg	3	7	40	7/2
Cheese Stuffed Crust, supreme	⅙ pkg	3	6	34	6/2
Cheese Stuffed Crust, three meat	⅙ pkg	2	5	34	5/2
Classic Thin Crust, four cheese	⅕ pkg	3	5	32	5/2
Classic Thin Crust, four meat	⅕ pkg	2	5	32	5/2
Classic Thin Crust, pepperoni	⅕ pkg	2	5	31	5/2
Classic Thin Crust, pepperoni, mushroom & bacon	⅕ pkg	2	5	31	5/2
Classic Thin Crust, spinach, mushroom & garlic	⅕ pkg	3	4	32	4/2
Classic Thin Crust, supreme	⅕ pkg	3	5	33	5/2
Crispy Flatbread Pizza, Italian sausage & onions	⅓ pkg	2	3	27	3/2
Crispy Flatbread Pizza, Italian three cheese	⅓ pkg	3	3	28	3/2
Crispy Flatbread Pizza, pepperoni & fire-roasted bell peppers	⅓ pkg	2	3	26	3/2
Crispy Flatbread Pizza, Tuscan style chicken	⅓ pkg	2	2	25	2/2
Flatbread Melts, chicken & bacon ranch	1 pkg	2	4	44	4/3
Flatbread Melts, chicken Parmesan	1 pkg	2	4	45	4/3
Flatbread Melts, Italian-style meatball & four cheese	1 pkg	3	5	46	5/3
Flatbread Melts, steak & fire-roasted vegetables	1 pkg	2	4	44	4/3
For One, Garlic Bread Crust, pepperoni	1 pkg	4	12	81	12/5
For One, Thin Crispy Crust, grilled chicken & vegetable	1 pkg	4	7	64	7/4
For One, Thin Crispy Crust, pepperoni	1 pkg	6	11	83	11/5
For One, Thin Crispy Crust, supreme	1 pkg	3	7	64	7/4
For One, Traditional Crust, four cheese	1 pkg	6	11	84	11/5
For One, Traditional Crust, pepperoni	1 pkg	6	11	83	11/5
For One, Traditional Crust, sausage	1 pkg	6	11	83	11/5
For One, Traditional Crust, supreme	1 pkg	6	11	85	11/5
Garlic Bread Pizza, four cheese	⅙ pkg	3	7	41	7/3

FOOD	Svg Size	Fbr	Sgr	Cbs	S/C Val
Garlic Bread Pizza, pepperoni	⅛ pkg	3	7	40	7/2
Garlic Bread Pizza, supreme	⅛ pkg	3	5	31	5/2
Rising Crust, 8", four cheese	⅓ pkg	2	6	34	6/2
Rising Crust, 8", pepperoni	⅓ pkg	2	7	35	7/2
Rising Crust, 8", supreme	⅓ pkg	3	7	35	7/2
Rising Crust, 8", three meat	⅓ pkg	2	7	25	7/2
Rising Crust, 12", chicken supreme	⅙ pkg	3	7	41	7/3
Rising Crust, 12", four cheese	⅙ pkg	2	6	40	6/2
Rising Crust, 12", Italian sausage	⅙ pkg	2	6	40	6/2
Rising Crust, 12", pepperoni	⅙ pkg	2	6	40	6/2
Rising Crust, 12", sausage & pepperoni	⅙ pkg	2	6	40	6/2
Rising Crust, 12", spinach, mushroom & garlic	⅙ pkg	2	6	41	6/3
Rising Crust, 12", supreme	⅙ pkg	3	7	41	7/3
Rising Crust, 12", three meat	⅙ pkg	2	6	41	6/3
200 Calorie Portions, cheese & tomato	½ pkg	1	3	22	3/2
200 Calorie Portions, chicken w/ peppers & onions	½ pkg	1	2	22	2/2
200 Calorie Portions, pepperoni	½ pkg	1	3	21	3/2
Ultimate Toppings, ultimate cheese	⅕ pkg	2	5	34	5/2
Ultimate Toppings, ultimate four meat	⅕ pkg	2	5	34	5/2
Ultimate Toppings, ultimate pepperoni	⅕ pkg	2	5	34	5/2
Ultimate Toppings, ultimate supreme	⅕ pkg	2	5	35	5/2

HEALTHY CHOICE

FOOD	Svg Size	Fbr	Sgr	Cbs	S/C Val
Asian potstickers	1 pkg	6	19	75	19/4
Bacon & smokey cheddar chicken	1 pkg	3	2	32	2/2
Beef bourbon dijon	1 pkg	6	11	38	11/2
Beef pot roast	1 pkg	6	22	45	22/3
Beef tips portobello	1 pkg	5	14	34	14/2
Café Steamers, balsamic garlic chicken	1 pkg	6	7	38	7/2
Café Steamers, Cajun style chicken & shrimp	1 pkg	3	3	40	3/2
Café Steamers, chicken Margherita	1 pkg	5	9	45	9/3
Café Steamers, chicken pad thai	1 pkg	5	10	40	10/2
Café Steamers, chicken pesto classico	1 pkg	4	4	39	4/2
Café Steamers, chicken red pepper Alfredo	1 pkg	4	3	30	3/2
Café Steamers, five-spice beef & vegetables	1 pkg	4	12	48	12/3
Café Steamers, General Tso's spicy chicken	1 pkg	4	12	53	12/3
Café Steamers, grilled basil chicken	1 pkg	7	4	34	4/2
Café Steamers, grilled chicken marinara	1 pkg	5	5	35	5/2
Café Steamers, grilled vegetables Mediterranean	1 pkg	7	7	42	7/3
Café Steamers, grilled whiskey steak	1 pkg	6	14	34	14/2
Café Steamers, lemon garlic chicken & shrimp	1 pkg	6	4	35	4/2
Café Steamers, roasted beef merlot	1 pkg	5	4	21	4/2
Café Steamers, roasted chicken fresca	1 pkg	6	3	29	3/2
Café Steamers, roasted chicken marsala	1 pkg	4	5	30	5/2
Café Steamers, sweet & spicy orange zest chicken	1 pkg	6	16	46	16/3

FROZEN MEALS, cont'd.

FOOD	Svg Size	Fbr	Sgr	Cbs	S/C Val
Café Steamers, sweet sesame chicken	1 pkg	6	19	50	19/3
Chicken Alfredo Florentine	1 pkg	4	1	31	1/2
Chicken balsamico	1 pkg	6	27	56	27/3
Chicken Parmigiana	1 pkg	7	17	49	17/3
Chicken pesto Alfredo	1 pkg	7	16	39	16/2
Chicken teriyaki	1 pkg	4	6	58	6/3
Classic meatloaf	1 pkg	8	22	55	22/3
Country breaded chicken	1 pkg	6	14	50	14/3
Country herb chicken	1 pkg	5	15	34	15/2
Creamy basil pesto	1 pkg	5	5	36	5/2
Fajita steak	1 pkg	7	17	56	17/3
Fire roasted tomato chicken	1 pkg	6	18	46	18/3
Golden roasted turkey breast	1 pkg	8	18	44	18/3
Homestyle Salisbury steak	1 pkg	9	17	46	17/3
Honey ginger chicken	1 pkg	3	22	53	22/3
Lemon pepper fish	1 pkg	5	15	50	15/3
Lobster cheese ravioli	1 pkg	4	8	37	8/2
Marinara manicotti formaggio	1 pkg	8	24	61	24/4
Oven roasted chicken	1 pkg	5	12	37	12/2
Pineapple chicken	1 pkg	5	30	68	30/4
Portabella marsala pasta	1 pkg	5	4	38	4/2
Portabella spinach Parmesan	1 pkg	5	2	40	2/2
Pumpkin squash ravioli	1 pkg	6	4	52	4/3
Ravioli Florentine marinara	1 pkg	6	10	38	10/2
Roasted chicken Monterey	1 pkg	7	13	48	13/3
Roasted red pepper marinara	1 pkg	5	5	43	5/3
Roasted sesame chicken	1 pkg	5	19	50	19/3
Salisbury steak	1 pkg	9	17	46	17/3
Slow roasted turkey medallions	1 pkg	8	14	25	14/2
Spicy Caribbean chicken	1 pkg	6	12	56	12/3
Spicy shrimp diavolo	1 pkg	7	17	42	17/3
Sweet & sour chicken	1 pkg	6	28	73	28/4
Sweet & tangy chicken BBQ	1 pkg	6	19	54	19/3
Tomato basil penne	1 pkg	7	6	39	6/2
Tortellini primavera Parmesan	1 pkg	6	7	35	7/2
Turkey marsala	1 pkg	5	14	36	14/2
HOT POCKETS & LEAN POCKETS					
Hot Pockets, applewood bacon, egg & cheese	1	1	6	38	6/2
Hot Pockets, barbecue recipe beef	1	2	11	44	11/3
Hot Pockets, barbecue recipe chicken	1	2	12	46	12/3
Hot Pockets, chicken & cheddar w/ broccoli	1	2	5	38	5/2
Hot Pockets, chicken melt w/ bacon	1	2	8	36	8/2
Hot Pockets, ham & cheese	1	1	4	36	4/2
Hot Pockets, meatballs & mozzarella	1	2	8	37	8/2

FOOD	Svg Size	Fbr	Sgr	Cbs	S/C Val
Hot Pockets, Philly steak & cheese	1	1	5	37	5/2
Hot Pockets, steak & cheddar	1	1	8	36	8/2
Hot Pockets, turkey & ham w/ cheese	1	1	8	36	8/2
Hot Pockets, Calzone, four meat & four cheese	½ pkg	2	6	33	6/2
Hot Pockets, Calzone, pepperoni & three cheese	½ pkg	2	6	34	6/2
Hot Pockets, Calzone, supreme calzone	½ pkg	2	6	33	6/2
Hot Pockets, Panini, bruschetta chicken	½ pkg	3	4	25	4/2
Hot Pockets, Panini, deli-style ham & Swiss	½ pkg	3	4	26	4/2
Hot Pockets, Panini, steak & cheddar	½ pkg	1	3	25	3/2
Hot Pockets, Pizzeria, four cheese pizza	1	1	9	39	9/2
Hot Pockets, Pizzeria, four meat & four cheese pizza	1	1	7	38	7/2
Hot Pockets, Pizzeria, Italian style three meat pizza	1	2	6	38	6/2
Hot Pockets, Pizzeria, pepperoni & sausage pizza	1	2	7	38	7/2
Hot Pockets, Pizzeria, pepperoni pizza	1	2	6	37	6/2
Hot Pockets, Pizzeria, supreme pizza	1	3	7	38	7/2
Hot Pockets, Pizzeria, Cheese Stuffed Crust, pepperoni pizza	½ pkg	1	4	26	4/2
Hot Pockets, Pizzeria, Cheese Stuffed Crust, three cheese pizza	½ pkg	1	4	26	4/2
Hot Pockets, Pizzeria, Deep Dish, supreme pizza	1	4	10	60	10/3
Hot Pockets, Sideshots, Buffalo style chicken	2	1	7	40	7/2
Hot Pockets, Sideshots, cheeseburgers	2	1	6	40	6/2
Hot Pockets, Soft Baked Subs, ham & three cheese	1	1	6	33	6/2
Hot Pockets, Soft Baked Subs, meatballs & mozzarella	1	3	8	34	8/2
Hot Pockets, Soft Baked Subs, Philly steak & cheese	1	1	6	34	6/2
Hot Pockets, Soft Baked Subs, spicy pepperoni pizza	1	2	8	34	8/2
Lean Pockets, applewood bacon, eggs & cheese	1	2	12	40	12/2
Lean Pockets, barbecue recipe beef	1	2	11	46	11/3
Lean Pockets, cheeseburger	1	2	9	42	9/3
Lean Pockets, chicken & cheese, Mexican style	1	2	8	35	8/2
Lean Pockets, chicken, broccoli & cheddar, whole grain	1	4	10	40	10/2
Lean Pockets, chicken fiesta, Mexican style	1	3	13	35	13/2
Lean Pockets, chicken Parmesan	1	3	10	46	10/3
Lean Pockets, ham & cheddar, whole grain	1	3	12	39	12/2
Lean Pockets, ham, egg & cheese	1	1	12	40	12/2
Lean Pockets, meatballs & mozzarella	1	3	9	40	9/2
Lean Pockets, meatballs & mozzarella, whole grain	1	4	10	32	10/2
Lean Pockets, pepperoni pizza	1	2	10	40	10/2
Lean Pockets, Philly steak & cheese	1	2	8	39	8/2
Lean Pockets, sausage, egg & cheese	1	2	11	40	11/2
Lean Pockets, steak fajita, Mexican style	1	3	12	36	12/2
Lean Pockets, three cheese & broccoli, whole grain	1	4	9	41	9/3
Lean Pockets, turkey & ham w/ cheese, whole grain	1	3	10	38	10/2
Lean Pockets, turkey, broccoli & cheese, whole grain	1	4	11	38	11/2
Lean Pockets, Culinary Creations, garlic chicken white pizza	1	3	10	38	10/2
Lean Pockets, Culinary Creations, spinach artichoke chicken	1	3	9	39	9/2

FOOD	Svg Size	Fbr	Sgr	Cbs	S/C Val
Lean Pockets, Pizzeria, four cheese pizza	1	2	10	42	10/3
Lean Pockets, Pizzeria, grilled chicken Mediterranean	1	3	6	46	6/3
Lean Pockets, Pizzeria, sausage & pepperoni pizza	1	2	10	40	10/2
Lean Pockets, Pizzeria, supreme pizza, whole grain	1	4	11	33	11/2
Lean Pockets, Soft Baked Subs, Italian style meatballs	1	3	7	35	7/2
Lean Pockets, Soft Baked Subs, pepperoni w/ red peppers	1	2	7	36	7/2
Lean Pockets, Soft Baked Subs, Philly steak & cheese	1	1	5	34	5/2
Lean Pockets, Stuffed Quesadilla, grilled chicken & three cheese	1	2	9	49	9/3
Lean Pockets, Stuffed Quesadilla, grilled chicken fajita	1	2	5	49	5/3

HUNGRY-MAN

FOOD	Svg Size	Fbr	Sgr	Cbs	S/C Val
Backyard barbeque, XXL	1 pkg	3	32	52	32/3
Beer battered chicken, Sports Grill	1 pkg	8	3	79	3/4
Boneless fried chicken	1 pkg	6	25	85	25/5
Buffalo style chicken strips	1 pkg	8	26	103	26/6
Classic fried chicken	1 pkg	3	15	62	15/4
Country fried chicken	1 pkg	5	14	53	14/3
Grilled Bourbon steak strips	1 pkg	4	32	94	32/5
Mexican style fiesta	1 pkg	10	14	87	14/5
Roasted carved turkey, XXL	1 pkg	3	3	44	3/3
Roasted carved white meat turkey	1 pkg	5	23	80	23/4
Rotisserie chicken	1 pkg	3	14	31	14/2
Salisbury steak	1 pkg	5	19	50	19/3
Southern fried boneless chicken	1 pkg	4	2	41	2/3
Sweet & sour chicken	1 pkg	4	18	101	18/6

KASHI

FOOD	Svg Size	Fbr	Sgr	Cbs	S/C Val
Black bean mango	1 pkg	7	11	58	11/3
Caribbean carnival pizza	⅓ pkg	5	5	39	5/2
Chicken Florentine	1 pkg	5	1	31	1/2
Chicken pasta pomodoro	1 pkg	6	5	38	5/2
Chicken rustico pocket bread	1 pc	4	4	41	4/3
Garden vegetable pasta	1 pkg	9	8	51	8/3
Lemongrass coconut chicken	1 pkg	7	6	38	6/2
Margherita thin crust pizza	⅓ pkg	4	4	29	4/2
Mayan harvest bake	1 pkg	8	19	58	19/3
Mediterranean pizza	⅓ pkg	5	3	37	3/2
Mexicali black bean thin crust pizza	⅓ pkg	4	2	27	2/2
Mushroom trio & spinach thin crust pizza	⅓ pkg	4	3	28	3/2
Pesto pasta primavera	1 pkg	7	4	37	4/2
Ranchero beans	1 pkg	11	5	56	5/3
Red curry chicken	1 pkg	5	10	40	10/2
Roasted vegetable thin crust pizza	⅓ pkg	4	3	28	3/2
Sicilian veggie pizza	⅓ pkg	5	4	37	4/2
Southwest style chicken	1 pkg	6	3	32	3/2

FOOD	Svg Size	Fbr	Sgr	Cbs	S/C Val
Sweet & sour chicken	1 pkg	6	25	55	25/3
Turkey fiesta pocket bread	1 pc	4	4	42	4/3
Tuscan veggie bake	1 pkg	8	8	42	8/3
Veggie chana masala	1 pkg	8	6	44	6/3
Veggie medley pocket bread	1 pc	6	6	49	6/3

KID CUISINE

FOOD	Svg Size	Fbr	Sgr	Cbs	S/C Val
All American fried chicken	1 pkg	5	18	48	18/3
All star chicken breast nuggets	1 pkg	8	15	51	15/3
Bug safari chicken breast nuggets	1 pkg	5	15	53	15/3
Carnival corn dog	1 pkg	7	20	68	20/4
Cheese blaster mac & cheese	1 pkg	6	6	69	6/4
Deep sea adventure fish sticks	1 pkg	6	14	55	14/3
Dip & dunk toasted ravioli	1 pkg	9	18	60	18/3
Fiesta chicken & cheese quesadillas	1 pkg	8	22	58	22/3
KC's campfire hot dog	1 pkg	6	15	58	15/3
KC's constructor, cheese, beef patty, bun	1 pkg	7	14	55	14/3
KC's karate chop chicken sandwich	1 pkg	8	8	56	8/3
KC's primo pepperoni double stuffed crust pizza	1 pkg	9	18	66	18/4
Magical cheese stuffed crust pizza	1 pkg	7	22	63	22/4
Pop star popcorn chicken	1 pkg	8	14	62	14/4
Twist & twirl spaghetti w/ mini meatballs	1 pkg	8	20	61	20/4

LEAN CUISINE

FOOD	Svg Size	Fbr	Sgr	Cbs	S/C Val
Alfredo pasta w/ chicken & broccoli	1 pkg	3	5	45	5/3
Angel hair pomodoro	1 pkg	4	10	42	10/3
Apple cranberry chicken	1 pkg	6	24	54	24/3
Asian-style pot stickers	1 pkg	3	9	47	9/3
Bacon Alfredo pizza, wood fire style	1 pkg	4	4	42	4/3
Baja-style chicken quesadilla	1 pkg	8	3	34	3/2
Baked chicken	1 pkg	3	5	32	5/2
Baked chicken Florentine	1 pkg	3	5	14	5/1
Balsamic glazed chicken	1 pkg	4	11	41	11/3
BBQ chicken ranch quesadilla	1 pkg	2	7	35	7/2
BBQ-recipe chicken pizza, wood fire style	1 pkg	2	11	48	11/3
Beef & broccoli	1 pkg	2	9	39	9/2
Beef chow fun	1 pkg	3	18	54	18/3
Beef portabello	1 pkg	3	18	54	18/3
Beef pot roast	1 pkg	3	3	26	3/2
Butternut squash ravioli	1 pkg	5	11	43	11/3
Cheddar potatoes w/ broccoli	1 pkg	4	6	35	6/2
Cheese lasagna & chicken	1 pkg	3	8	34	8/2
Cheese pizza, French bread	1 pkg	5	7	53	7/3
Cheese ravioli	1 pkg	3	8	33	8/2
Chicken & vegetables	1 pkg	3	5	29	5/2

FOOD	Svg Size	Fbr	Sgr	Cbs	S/C Val
Chicken carbonara	1 pkg	3	4	33	4/2
Chicken chow mein	1 pkg	3	3	41	3/3
Chicken club panini	1 pkg	4	7	46	7/3
Chicken enchilada Suiza	1 pkg	3	6	48	6/3
Chicken fettuccini, Dinnertime Cuisine	1 pkg	6	3	48	3/3
Chicken fettuccini, Simple Favorites	1 pkg	0	6	32	6/2
Chicken Florentine	1 pkg	6	13	54	13/3
Chicken Florentine lasagna	1 pkg	3	6	36	6/2
Chicken fried rice	1 pkg	4	5	41	5/3
Chicken in peanut sauce	1 pkg	5	5	33	5/2
Chicken marsala	1 pkg	2	4	29	4/2
Chicken Mediterranean	1 pkg	6	6	32	6/2
Chicken Parmesan	1 pkg	5	10	39	10/2
Chicken pecan	1 pkg	5	14	37	14/2
Chicken Philly flatbread melts	1 pkg	5	5	46	5/3
Chicken portabello	1 pkg	2	2	48	2/3
Chicken ranch club flatbread melts	1 pkg	4	7	47	7/3
Chicken, spinach & mushroom panini	1 pkg	5	4	42	4/3
Chicken teriyaki stir fry	1 pkg	6	9	46	9/3
Chicken Tuscan	1 pkg	5	7	34	7/2
Chicken w/ almonds	1 pkg	4	13	38	13/2
Chicken w/ basil cream sauce	1 pkg	2	4	31	4/2
Classic five cheese lasagna	1 pkg	4	10	51	10/3
Classic macaroni & beef	1 pkg	4	9	42	9/3
Deluxe cheddar potatoes	1 pkg	4	7	35	7/2
Deluxe pizza, French bread	1 pkg	4	6	49	6/3
Deluxe pizza, traditional	1 pkg	4	6	49	6/3
Fettuccini Alfredo	1 pkg	3	6	54	6/3
Fiesta grilled chicken	1 pkg	4	5	33	5/2
Five cheese rigatoni	1 pkg	4	8	51	8/3
Four cheese cannelloni	1 pkg	3	9	30	9/2
Four cheese pizza	1 pkg	3	6	51	6/3
Ginger garlic stir fry w/ chicken	1 pkg	5	17	42	17/3
Glazed chicken	1 pkg	0	6	29	6/2
Glazed turkey tenderloins	1 pkg	3	19	38	19/2
Grilled chicken & penne pasta	1 pkg	6	24	52	24/3
Grilled chicken Caesar	1 pkg	3	1	33	1/2
Grilled chicken primavera	1 pkg	5	6	26	6/2
Herb roasted chicken	1 pkg	3	5	20	5/1
Honey dijon grilled chicken	1 pkg	2	9	19	9/1
Hunan stir fry w/ beef	1 pkg	5	13	37	13/2
Jumbo rigatoni w/ meatballs	1 pkg	7	11	56	11/3
Lasagna w/ meat sauce	1 pkg	4	8	45	8/3
Lemon chicken	1 pkg	5	9	35	9/2

FOOD	Svg Size	Fbr	Sgr	Cbs	S/C Val
Lemon garlic shrimp	1 pkg	5	3	54	3/3
Lemongrass chicken	1 pkg	5	7	33	7/2
Lemon pepper fish	1 pkg	2	4	40	4/2
Linguine carbonara	1 pkg	2	4	43	4/3
Macaroni & cheese	1 pkg	1	7	41	7/3
Margherita pizza, wood fire style	1 pkg	2	5	43	5/3
Meatloaf w/ gravy & whipped potatoes	1 pkg	3	4	25	4/2
Mushroom pizza, traditional	1 pkg	4	5	47	5/3
Orange chicken	1 pkg	2	11	46	11/3
Orange peel chicken	1 pkg	4	16	60	16/3
Parmesan crusted fish	1 pkg	4	8	40	8/2
Pasta Romano w/ bacon	1 pkg	4	8	43	8/3
Pepperoni pizza, French bread	1 pkg	4	6	46	6/3
Pepperoni pizza, traditional	1 pkg	3	6	50	6/3
Pesto chicken w/ bow tie pasta	1 pkg	4	7	42	7/3
Philly-style steak & cheese panini	1 pkg	4	4	38	4/2
Roasted chicken w/ lemon pepper fettuccini	1 pkg	3	3	36	3/2
Roasted garlic chicken	1 pkg	0	3	10	3/1
Roasted garlic chicken pizza, wood fire style	1 pkg	4	4	42	4/3
Roasted honey chicken	1 pkg	5	18	44	18/3
Roasted turkey & vegetables	1 pkg	3	4	12	4/1
Roasted turkey breast, Comfort Cuisine	1 pkg	3	27	48	27/3
Roasted turkey breast, Dinnertime Cuisine	1 pkg	5	11	38	11/2
Roasted vegetable pizza, deep dish	1 pkg	3	6	52	6/3
Rosemary chicken	1 pkg	5	5	30	5/2
Salisbury steak	1 pkg	10	10	27	10/2
Salisbury steak w/ macaroni & cheese	1 pkg	3	4	25	4/2
Salmon w/ basil	1 pkg	5	4	26	4/2
Santa Fe-style rice & beans	1 pkg	4	8	50	8/3
Sesame chicken	1 pkg	2	14	47	14/3
Sesame stir fry w/ chicken	1 pkg	5	14	41	14/3
Shrimp Alfredo	1 pkg	3	4	32	4/2
Shrimp & angel hair pasta	1 pkg	2	5	34	5/2
Southwest-style chicken panini	1 pkg	4	7	41	7/3
Spaghetti w/ meatballs	1 pkg	3	6	38	6/2
Spaghetti w/ meat sauce	1 pkg	4	8	55	8/3
Spinach & mushroom pizza, deep dish	1 pkg	2	4	52	4/3
Spinach, artichoke & chicken panini	1 pkg	4	4	40	4/2
Steak, cheddar & mushroom panini	1 pkg	4	6	43	6/3
Steakhouse ranch flatbread melts	1 pkg	4	7	46	7/3
Steak tips dijon	1 pkg	5	11	33	11/2
Steak tips portabello	1 pkg	3	3	10	3/1
Stuffed cabbage	1 pkg	3	6	28	6/2
Sun-dried tomato basil chicken flatbread melts	1 pkg	5	8	49	8/3

FROZEN MEALS, cont'd.

FOOD	Svg Size	Fbr	Sgr	Cbs	S/C Val
Sun-dried tomato pesto chicken	1 pkg	4	10	28	10/2
Swedish meatballs	1 pkg	3	4	35	4/2
Sweet & sour chicken	1 pkg	2	20	51	20/3
Szechuan-style stir fry w/ shrimp	1 pkg	5	13	41	13/3
Thai-style chicken	1 pkg	0	9	35	9/2
Thai-style noodles w/ chicken	1 pkg	5	13	41	13/3
Three cheese chicken	1 pkg	3	5	10	5/1
Three cheese stuffed rigatoni	1 pkg	4	6	32	6/2
Three meat pizza, deep dish	1 pkg	2	6	55	6/3
Tortilla crusted fish	1 pkg	2	7	40	7/2
Vegetable eggroll	1 pkg	2	12	62	12/4

SEEDS OF CHANGE

FOOD	Svg Size	Fbr	Sgr	Cbs	S/C Val
Fettuccine Alfredo di Roma	1 pkg	4	8	45	8/3
Hanalei vegetarian chicken teriyaki	1 pkg	4	11	47	11/3
Lasagna Calabrese	1 pkg	4	5	42	5/3
Spicy Thai peanut noodles	1 pkg	4	5	51	5/3
Spinach lasagna di Parma	1 pkg	4	6	40	6/2
Turkish seven grain pilaf	1 pkg	5	7	46	7/3
Venetian penne marinara	1 pkg	4	2	40	2/2

STOUFFER'S

FOOD	Svg Size	Fbr	Sgr	Cbs	S/C Val
Baked chicken breast	1 pkg	1	2	20	2/1
Beef pot roast	1 pkg	8	9	41	9/3
Beef stroganoff	1 pkg	2	4	34	4/2
Bourbon steak tips	1 pkg	3	22	61	22/4
Cheddar potato bake	½ pkg	2	2	21	2/2
Cheese ravioli	1 pkg	5	9	47	9/3
Cheesy spaghetti bake	1 pkg	4	6	39	6/2
Chicken à la king	1 pkg	0	7	44	7/3
Chicken Alfredo, large family size	½ pkg	2	2	28	2/2
Chicken & pasta skillets	½ pkg	6	10	42	10/3
Chicken fettuccini, Classic Meals	1 pkg	5	5	55	5/3
Chicken fettuccini, Restaurant Classics	1 pkg	5	3	94	3/5
Chicken lasagna, family size	⅕ pkg	3	2	54	2/3
Chicken Parmigiana, Restaurant Classics	1 pkg	4	10	47	10/3
Corn soufflé	½ pkg	2	8	22	8/2
Creamed chipped beef	½ pkg	0	5	9	5/1
Creamed spinach	½ pkg	2	3	8	3/1
Easy Express, brocccoli & beef skillet	½ pkg	2	4	57	4/3
Easy Express, cheese manicotti, family size	⅓ pkg	5	9	33	9/2
Easy Express, cheesy meatball rigatoni skillet	½ pkg	5	5	48	5/3
Easy Express, chicken Alfredo skillet	½ pkg	6	8	48	8/3
Easy Express, chicken & dumplings skillet	½ pkg	5	5	41	5/3
Easy Express, chicken & pasta Parmesan skillet	½ pkg	4	7	60	7/3

FOOD	Svg Size	Fbr	Sgr	Cbs	S/C Val
Easy Express, garlic chicken skillet	½ pkg	6	6	42	6/3
Easy Express, garlic shrimp skillet	½ pkg	5	4	40	4/2
Easy Express, grilled chicken & vegetables skillet	½ pkg	3	8	43	8/3
Easy Express, homestyle beef skillet	½ pkg	6	5	37	5/2
Easy Express, meatball rotini, family size	¼ pkg	3	3	38	3/2
Easy Express, rigatoni w/ chicken, family size	⅙ pkg	2	1	29	1/2
Easy Express, savory chicken & rice	½ pkg	2	3	50	3/3
Easy Express, shrimp fried rice skillet	½ pkg	8	8	50	8/3
Easy Express, steak teriyaki skillet	½ pkg	6	13	49	13/3
Easy Express, sweet & sour chicken skillet	½ pkg	2	18	66	18/4
Easy Express, teriyaki chicken skillet	½ pkg	6	10	44	10/3
Easy Express, three cheese chicken skillet	½ pkg	4	5	44	5/3
Easy Express, Yankee pot roast skillet	½ pkg	4	7	38	7/2
Escalloped chicken & noodles, family size	⅕ pkg	2	2	28	2/2
Escalloped chicken & noodles, Homestyle Classics	1 pkg	5	7	43	7/3
Fettuccini Alfredo	1 pkg	5	7	57	7/3
Fish filet	1 pkg	4	7	36	7/2
Flatbread, chicken, bacon & spinach	1 pkg	2	4	57	4/3
Flatbread, margherita	1 pkg	3	4	59	4/3
Flatbread, steak fajita	1 pkg	3	5	59	5/3
Flatbread, three meat Sicilian	1 pkg	3	5	58	5/3
Flatbread melt, chicken Alfredo	1 pkg	4	4	41	4/3
Flatbread melt, chicken quesadilla	1 pkg	4	6	41	6/3
Flatbread melt, steak mushroom cheddar	1 pkg	4	4	40	4/2
French bread pizza, cheese	1	4	4	43	4/3
French bread pizza, deluxe	1	4	5	44	5/3
French bread pizza, five cheese white	1	3	3	44	3/3
French bread pizza, grilled vegetable	1	4	5	44	5/3
French bread pizza, pepperoni	1	4	5	43	5/3
French bread pizza, pepperoni & mushroom	1	4	5	44	5/3
French bread pizza, three meat	1	4	5	43	5/3
French bread pizza, white	1	4	3	44	3/3
Fried chicken breast	1 pkg	2	2	30	2/2
Garlic chicken pasta	1 pkg	5	10	37	10/2
Green pepper steak	1 pkg	3	5	32	5/2
Grilled chicken teriyaki	1 pkg	3	12	45	12/3
Grilled lemon pepper chicken	1 pkg	4	3	24	3/2
Harvest apples	½ pkg	2	33	40	33/2
Lasagna w/ meat & sauce, Homestyle Classics	1 pkg	3	7	38	7/2
Lasagna bake w/ meat sauce	1 pkg	5	11	49	11/3
Macaroni & beef	1 pkg	4	12	45	12/3
Macaroni & cheese w/ broccoli	1 pkg	5	8	52	8/3
Macaroni & cheese, Craveable Classics, large size	½ pkg	3	1	36	1/2
Macaroni & cheese, Craveable Recipes	½ pkg	3	2	33	2/2

FOOD	Svg Size	Fbr	Sgr	Cbs	S/C Val
Meatloaf, Homestyle Classics	1 pkg	2	3	20	3/1
Meatloaf, Homestyle Selects	1 pkg	5	6	45	6/3
Monterey chicken	1 pkg	5	19	54	19/3
Panini, grilled mesquite-style chicken	1 pkg	4	7	41	7/3
Panini, smoked turkey club	1 pkg	3	2	31	2/2
Panini, Southwest-style chicken	1 pkg	4	6	42	6/3
Panini, three cheese & ham	1 pkg	4	5	42	5/3
Pork cutlet	1 pkg	3	2	31	2/2
Rigatoni w/ roasted white meat chicken	1 pkg	3	2	44	2/3
Roasted chicken	1 pkg	5	5	34	5/2
Roast turkey, Homestyle Classics	1 pkg	2	2	30	2/2
Roast turkey breast, Homestyle Selects	1 pkg	5	3	51	3/3
Salisbury steak	1 pkg	3	9	48	9/3
Sesame chicken	1 pkg	6	26	87	26/5
Shrimp scampi	1 pkg	5	5	56	5/3
Spaghetti w/ meatballs	1 pkg	6	9	45	9/3
Spaghetti w/ meat sauce	1 pkg	5	8	44	8/3
Spinach soufflé	⅓ pkg	1	4	9	4/1
Stromboli, chicken broccoli cheddar	1 pkg	4	4	45	4/3
Stromboli, Italian-style supreme	1 pkg	5	3	45	3/3
Stromboli, pepperoni & provolone	1 pkg	5	4	45	4/3
Stuffed pepper, Homestyle Classics	1 pkg	3	9	23	9/2
Swedish meatballs	1 pkg	3	6	47	6/3
Toasted sub, meatball Italiano	1 pkg	4	6	42	6/3
Toasted sub, Philly-style steak & cheese	1 pkg	3	5	39	5/2
Toasted sub, roast beef & cheddar	1 pkg	3	5	40	5/2
Toasted sub, zesty Italian	1 pkg	3	5	40	5/2
Tuna noodle casserole	1 pkg	3	3	45	3/3
Turkey tetrazzini	1 pkg	2	7	38	7/2
Veal Parmigiana	1 pkg	5	10	46	10/3
Vegetable lasagna, Homestyle Classics	1 pkg	4	9	40	9/2
Welsh rarebit	¼ pkg	0	2	6	2/1
White meat chicken pot pie	1 pkg	2	14	62	14/4
White meat turkey pot pie	1 pkg	2	10	61	10/4

WEIGHT WATCHERS SMART ONES

FOOD	Svg Size	Fbr	Sgr	Cbs	S/C Val
Angel hair marinara	1 pkg	4	7	40	7/2
Broccoli & cheddar roasted potatoes	1 pkg	4	5	35	5/2
Chicken carbonara	1 pkg	2	2	32	2/2
Chicken enchiladas Monterey	1 pkg	5	4	41	4/3
Chicken enchiladas Suiza	1 pkg	3	4	49	4/3
Chicken fettucini	1 pkg	3	2	40	2/2
Chicken marsala	1 pkg	3	4	11	4/1

FOOD	Svg Size	Fbr	Sgr	Cbs	S/C Val
Chicken Oriental	1 pkg	2	5	41	5/3
Chicken Parmesan	1 pkg	4	5	35	5/2
Chicken Santa Fe	1 pkg	4	6	11	6/1
Cranberry turkey medallions	1 pkg	4	19	43	19/3
Creamy Parmesan chicken	1 pkg	4	2	24	2/2
Creamy rigatoni w/ broccoli & chicken	1 pkg	3	2	39	2/2
Dragon shrimp lo mein	1 pkg	4	5	38	5/2
Fettucini Alfredo	1 pkg	4	3	41	3/3
Home style beef pot roast	1 pkg	4	6	18	6/1
Honey mango barbeque chicken	1 pkg	3	14	32	14/2
Lasagna bake w/ meat sauce	1 pkg	3	3	43	3/3
Lasagna Florentine	1 pkg	5	12	44	12/3
Lemon herb chicken piccata	1 pkg	2	8	41	8/3
Macaroni & cheese	1 pkg	2	5	52	5/3
Meatloaf	1 pkg	3	3	22	3/2
Mini rigatoni w/ vodka cream sauce	1 pkg	5	5	48	5/3
Orange sesame chicken	1 pkg	2	12	48	12/3
Pasta primavera	1 pkg	4	4	41	4/3
Pasta w/ ricotta & spinach	1 pkg	6	7	43	7/3
Pineapple beef teriyaki	1 pkg	2	16	40	16/2
Ravioli Florentine	1 pkg	4	12	40	12/2
Roast beef w/ gravy	1 pkg	2	2	18	2/1
Roasted chicken w/ sour cream & chive mashed potatoes	1 pkg	2	0	20	0/1
Roast turkey medallions	1 pkg	3	0	38	0/2
Salisbury steak, Bistro Selections	1 pkg	4	5	12	5/1
Salisbury steak, Classic Favorites	1 pkg	3	3	33	3/2
Santa Fe style rice & beans	1 pkg	4	6	51	6/3
Shrimp marinara	1 pkg	4	5	34	5/2
Sirloin beef & Asian style vegetables	1 pkg	3	4	27	4/2
Slow roasted turkey breast	1 pkg	2	0	18	0/1
Spaghetti w/ meat sauce	1 pkg	5	9	44	9/3
Spicy Szechuan style vegetables & chicken	1 pkg	4	4	38	4/2
Stuffed turkey breast	1 pkg	4	7	39	7/2
Swedish meatballs	1 pkg	3	4	35	4/2
Sweet & sour chicken	1 pkg	2	10	31	10/2
Teriyaki chicken & vegetables	1 pkg	3	15	39	15/2
Thai style chicken & rice noodles	1 pkg	2	10	42	10/3
Three cheese macaroni	1 pkg	3	3	48	3/3
Three cheese ziti marinara	1 pkg	4	2	47	2/3
Traditional lasagna w/ meat sauce	1 pkg	5	8	43	8/3
Tuna noodle gratin	1 pkg	3	7	37	7/2
Anytime Selections, calzone Italiano	½ pkg	6	6	47	6/3
Anytime Selections, cheese pizza minis	½ pkg	5	4	38	4/2
Anytime Selections, chicken & cheese quesadilla	1 pkg	7	1	28	1/2

FOOD	Svg Size	Fbr	Sgr	Cbs	S/C Val
Anytime Selections, chicken ranchero smart mini wraps	½ pkg	7	3	30	3/2
Anytime Selections, fiesta quesadilla	1 pkg	9	0	35	0/2
Anytime Selections, mini cheeseburger	½ pkg	3	4	20	4/1
Anytime Selections, pepperoni pizza minis	½ pkg	5	5	40	5/2
Anytime Selections, vegetable pizza minis	½ pkg	6	4	41	4/3
Artisan Creations, grilled flatbread, chicken bruschetta	1 pkg	4	6	42	6/3
Artisan Creations, grilled flatbread, savory steak & ranch	1 pkg	4	6	41	6/3
Artisan Creations, grilled flatbread, Southwestern style chicken fiesta	1 pkg	4	6	43	6/3
Artisan Creations, stone-fired crust pizza, fajita chicken	1 pkg	4	8	58	8/3
Artisan Creations, stone-fired crust pizza, four cheese	1 pkg	4	7	57	7/3
Artisan Creations, stone-fired crust pizza, pepperoni	1 pkg	4	7	58	7/3
Morning Express, breakfast quesadilla	½ pkg	6	0	29	0/2
Morning Express, cheesy scramble w/ hashbrowns	1 pkg	3	1	18	1/1
Morning Express, English muffin sandwich	½ pkg	2	3	27	3/2
Morning Express, English muffin sandwich, Canadian style bacon	½ pkg	2	4	27	4/2
Morning Express, ham & cheese scramble	1 pkg	2	1	13	1/1
Morning Express, stuffed breakfast sandwich	½ pkg	3	4	30	4/2

DINING OUT

FOOD	Svg Size	Fbr	Sgr	Cbs	S/C Val
BURGER KING					
Breakfast					
Bacon, egg & cheese biscuit sandwich	1	1	5	34	5/2
Bacon, egg & cheese Croissan'wich	1	0	5	26	5/2
Cheesy bacon BK Wrapper	1	2	2	28	2/2
Cini-minis	4 pcs	2	19	52	19/3
Double Croissan'wich w/ double bacon	1	0	6	27	6/2
Double Croissan'wich w/ double ham	1	0	6	28	6/2
Double Croissan'wich w/ double sausage	1	0	4	27	4/2
Double Croissan'wich w/ ham & bacon	1	0	6	28	6/2
Double Croissan'wich w/ ham & sausage	1	0	6	28	6/2
Double Croissan'wich w/ sausage & bacon	1	0	5	28	5/2
Egg & cheese Croissan'wich	1	0	5	26	5/2
French toast sticks	3 pcs	1	8	29	8/2
Ham, egg & cheese biscuit sandwich	1	1	5	34	5/2
Ham, egg & cheese Croissan'wich	1	0	5	27	5/2
Ham omelet sandwich	1	1	7	30	7/2
Hash browns, small	1 pkt	5	0	39	0/2
Sausage & cheese Croissan'wich	1	0	3	26	3/2
Sausage biscuit	1	1	3	32	3/2
Sausage, egg & cheese biscuit sandwich	1	1	5	34	5/2
Sausage, egg & cheese Croissan'wich	1	0	5	27	5/2

FOOD	Svg Size	Fbr	Sgr	Cbs	S/C Val
General Menu					
A.1. Steakhouse XT burger	1	4	12	55	12/3
BK Big Fish	1	3	9	67	9/4
BK Big Fish w/o Tartar Sauce	1	3	6	64	6/4
BK Chicken fries	6 pcs	1	1	16	1/1
BK Double Stacker	1	1	7	29	7/2
BK fresh apple fries	1 pkt	1	5	6	5/1
BK fresh apple fries' caramel dipping sauce	1 pkt	0	5	10	5/1
BK Quad Stacker	1	1	8	31	8/2
BK Triple Stacker	1	1	7	30	7/2
BK Veggie burger	1	7	8	43	8/3
BK Veggie burger w/ cheese	1	7	8	44	8/3
Cheeseburger	1	1	6	28	6/2
Chicken tenders	4 pcs	0	0	13	0/1
Double cheeseburger	1	1	6	28	6/2
Double hamburger	1	1	5	27	5/2
Double Whopper	1	3	11	51	11/3
Double Whopper w/ cheese	1	3	12	53	12/3
French fries, small	1 pkt	4	0	44	0/3
Hamburger	1	1	5	27	5/2
Kraft macaroni & cheese, kids meal	1	1	5	22	5/2
Onion rings, small	1 pkt	3	4	36	4/2
Original chicken sandwich	1	3	4	46	4/3
Side garden salad w/o dressing	1	1	3	16	3/1
Sourdough bacon cheeseburger	1	3	4	40	4/2
Spicy Chick'n Crisp sandwich	1	2	4	34	4/2
Steakhouse XT burger	1	3	10	53	10/3
Tacos	2	5	4	18	4/1
Tendercrisp chicken sandwich	1	3	9	68	9/4
Tendercrisp garden salad w/o dressing	1	3	5	36	5/2
Tendergrill chicken sandwich	1	3	9	68	9/4
Tendergrill garden salad w/o dressing	1	0	4	18	4/1
Triple Whopper	1	3	11	51	11/3
Triple Whopper w/ cheese	1	3	11	52	11/3
Whopper	1	3	11	51	11/3
Whopper w/ cheese	1	3	11	52	11/3
Whopper Jr.	1	2	6	28	6/2
Whopper Jr. w/ cheese	1	2	6	29	6/2
Desserts & Drinks					
Apple juice, Minute Maid	6.67 oz	0	21	23	21/2
Chocolate shake, value size	12 oz	1	51	60	51/3
Chocolate shake, small	16 oz	1	67	78	67/4
Chocolate shake, medium	22 oz	2	103	119	103/6

FOOD	Svg Size	Fbr	Sgr	Cbs	S/C Val
Dutch apple pie	1	1	23	46	23/3
Funnel cake sticks, w/ icing	1 pkt	1	30	49	30/3
Hershey's sundae pie	1	1	22	31	22/2
Mocha BK Joe	1	1	55	63	55/4
Orange juice, Minute Maid	10 oz	0	30	33	30/2
Oreo BK Sundae Shake, chocolate, small	16 oz	2	89	108	89/6
Oreo BK Sundae Shake, chocolate, medium	22 oz	3	131	159	131/8
Oreo BK Sundae Shake, vanilla, small	16 oz	1	72	90	72/5
Oreo BK Sundae Shake, vanilla, medium	22 oz	1	97	124	97/7
Strawberry shake, value size	12 oz	0	51	58	51/3
Strawberry shake, small	16 oz	0	66	77	66/4
Strawberry shake, medium	22 oz	0	102	116	102/6
Vanilla shake, value size	12 oz	0	38	46	38/3
Vanilla shake, small	16 oz	0	50	60	50/3
Vanilla shake, medium	22 oz	0	69	84	69/5

DENNY'S

Breakfast

FOOD	Svg Size	Fbr	Sgr	Cbs	S/C Val
All-American Slam	1	0	1	5	1/1
Bacon	4 pcs	0	1	2	1/0
Bacon, turkey	4 pcs	0	0	0	0/0
Bacon avocado burrito	1	8	6	91	6/5
Belgian Waffle Slam	1	2	2	32	2/2
Biscuit, buttermilk	1	0	0	13	0/1
Biscuits & sausage gravy	1	0	3	57	3/3
Country-fried steak & eggs	1	3	0	29	0/2
French Toast Slam	1	4	14	68	14/4
Grand Slamwich, w/o hash browns	1	3	9	71	9/4
Granola (4 oz) w/ milk (8 oz)	1	9	53	131	53/7
Grits	12 oz	1	0	47	0/3
Ham, slice	1	0	1	1	1/0
Ham & cheddar omelette	1	0	1	4	1/0
Hash browns	5 oz	2	1	26	1/2
Heartland scramble	1	7	12	97	12/5
Lumberjack Slam	1	3	11	60	11/3
Meat lover's scramble	1	6	12	80	12/4
Moons Over My Hammy	1	2	3	50	3/3
Oatmeal	16 oz	4	20	37	20/2
Pancakes, buttermilk	2	3	18	102	18/6
Pancakes, hearty wheat	2	8	2	64	2/4
Prime rib premium sizzlin' breakfast skillet	1	6	14	77	14/4
Sausage, patties	2	0	1	0	1/0
Southwestern sizzlin' skillet	1	6	10	71	10/4
Southwestern steak burrito	1	5	4	76	4/4

FOOD	Svg Size	Fbr	Sgr	Cbs	S/C Val
T-bone steak & eggs	1	0	1	4	1/0
Two-egg breakfast	1	0	0	1	0/0
Ultimate omelette	1	2	3	8	3/1
Veggie-cheese omelette	1	2	4	10	4/1
Yogurt	6 oz	0	25	30	25/2
Appetizers					
Chicken strips, Buffalo sauce	13 oz	1	1	53	1/3
Chicken strips, sweet & tangy BBQ sauce	13 oz	2	29	83	29/5
Fried shrimp, Buffalo sauce	8 oz	4	10	37	10/2
Fried shrimp, sweet & tangy BBQ sauce	8 oz	4	37	66	37/4
Mozzarella cheese sticks	8 oz	1	5	195	5/10
Sampler	1	6	11	139	11/7
Sampler, half size	1	3	6	84	6/5
Smothered cheese fries	10 oz	7	3	74	3/4
Tsing Tsing chicken	15 oz	1	33	92	33/5
Wings	8 oz	2	2	5	2/1
Zesty nachos	22 oz	11	11	138	11/7
Lunch & Dinner					
Burger	1	3	11	50	11/3
Burger, Boca	1	8	11	57	11/3
Burger, cheeseburger	1	3	12	51	12/3
Burger, cheesy three pack	1	8	25	164	25/9
Burger, double cheeseburger	1	4	12	52	12/3
Burger, mushroom Swiss	1	4	13	55	13/3
Burger, Slamburger	1	2	10	59	10/3
Burger, Smokin' Q three pack	1	9	35	185	35/10
Burger, Western	1	4	19	79	19/4
Chicken strips	8 oz	1	2	41	2/3
Coleslaw	5 oz	3	12	15	12/1
Corn	4 oz	1	3	26	3/2
Country-fried steak w/ gravy	1	6	1	54	1/3
French fries	5 oz	5	0	50	0/3
Green beans	3 oz	2	2	4	2/0
Grilled chicken	10 oz	0	2	4	2/0
Grilled chicken sizzlin' skillet dinner	1	5	12	72	12/4
Grilled shrimp skewers	10 oz	2	2	39	2/2
Homestyle meatloaf w/ gravy	1	0	4	14	4/1
Lemon pepper grilled tilapia	1	2	3	41	3/3
Mashed potatoes	5 oz	1	1	76	1/4
Mashed potatoes, ranchero	4 oz	1	1	50	1/3
Mashed potatoes, smoked cheddar	4 oz	1	1	49	1/3
Mushroom Swiss chopped steak	1	1	4	13	4/1
Onion rings	5 oz	3	5	48	5/3

FOOD	Svg Size	Fbr	Sgr	Cbs	S/C Val
Prime rib sizzlin' skillet dinner	1	5	13	77	13/4
Salad, chicken deluxe w/ fried chicken strips, w/o dressing	1	4	7	44	7/3
Salad, chicken deluxe w/ grilled chicken, w/o dressing	1	4	8	15	8/1
Salad, cranberry pecan chicken, w/o dressing	1	1	9	11	9/1
Salad, prime rib & bleu, w/o dressing	1	1	3	6	3/1
Sandwich, bacon, lettuce & tomato	1	2	7	35	7/2
Sandwich, chicken, fried	1	4	22	98	22/5
Sandwich, chicken, grilled	1	3	23	64	23/4
Sandwich, chicken ranch melt	1	4	3	80	3/4
Sandwich, club	1	4	9	55	9/3
Sandwich, prime rib Philly melt	1	4	5	53	5/3
Sandwich, smoked chicken melt	1	3	11	72	11/4
Sandwich, spicy Buffalo chicken melt	1	5	3	82	3/5
Sandwich, The Super Bird	1	4	6	53	6/3
Soup, broccoli & cheddar	12 oz	4	7	16	7/1
Soup, chicken noodle	12 oz	1	0	19	0/1
Soup, clam chowder	12 oz	2	12	24	12/2
Soup, vegetable beef	12 oz	3	4	18	4/1
Sweet & tangy BBQ chicken	1	3	34	108	34/6
T-bone steak	1	0	0	0	0/0
T-bone steak w/ fried shrimp	1	2	5	20	5/1
T-bone steak w/ shrimp skewer	1	0	0	0	0/0
Tilapia ranchero	1	4	4	57	4/3
Vegetable rice pilaf	5 oz	1	2	37	2/2
Desserts & Drinks					
Apple pie	7 oz	3	35	72	35/4
Cappuccino, flavored	8 oz	1	24	28	24/2
Caramel apple crisp	13 oz	4	91	134	91/7
Carrot cake	8 oz	2	77	100	77/5
Coca-Cola float	16 oz	0	63	69	63/4
Coconut cream pie	7 oz	1	43	65	43/4
French silk pie	7 oz	2	38	59	38/3
Fusion Favorite, blueberry pomegranate splash	15 oz	0	37	38	37/2
Fusion Favorite, cherry cherry limeade	15 oz	0	12	45	12/3
Fusion Favorite, four berry fizz	15 oz	0	43	44	43/3
Fusion Favorite, OJ strawberry mango	15 oz	0	56	61	56/4
Fusion Favorite, strawberry mango pucker	15 oz	1	52	56	52/3
Fusion Favorite, very double berry	15 oz	0	62	69	62/4
Fusion Favorite, white peach breeze	15 oz	0	45	46	45/3
Hershey's chocolate cake	5 oz	2	55	75	55/4
Hot chocolate	8 oz	1	24	28	24/2
Hot fudge brownie à la mode	9 oz	4	95	122	95/7
Iced tea	12 oz	0	31	35	31/2
Iced tea, raspberry Nestea	16 oz	0	23	21	23/2

FOOD	Svg Size	Fbr	Sgr	Cbs	S/C Val
Lemonade	16 oz	0	31	35	31/2
Milkshake, chocolate	12 oz	0	65	76	65/4
Milkshake, strawberry	12 oz	0	65	76	65/4
Milkshake, vanilla	12 oz	0	65	76	65/4
New York style cheesecake	7 oz	0	44	58	44/3
Oreo Bender Blaster	14 oz	3	77	113	77/6
Oreo Sundae	9 oz	3	76	103	76/6
Root beer float	16 oz	0	63	69	63/4
Tea chiller, blueberry pomegranate	15 oz	0	29	30	29/2
Tea chiller, cherry lime	15 oz	0	30	31	30/2
Tea chiller, four berry	15 oz	0	35	37	35/2
Tea chiller, peach	15 oz	0	37	38	37/2
Tea chiller, straight up lemon	15 oz	0	22	26	22/2
Tea chiller, strawberry mango	15 oz	0	33	36	33/2
KFC					
BBQ baked beans (individual side)	1	9	18	39	18/2
Biscuit	1	1	2	23	2/2
Chicken, extra crispy, breast	1	0	1	16	1/1
Chicken, extra crispy, drumstick	1	0	0	5	0/1
Chicken, extra crispy, thigh	1	0	0	10	0/1
Chicken, extra crispy, wing	1	0	0	6	0/1
Chicken, grilled	1 pc	0	0	0	0/0
Chicken, original recipe, breast	1	0	0	4	0/0
Chicken, original recipe, drumstick	1	0	0	3	0/0
Chicken, original recipe, thigh	1	0	0	5	0/1
Chicken, original recipe, wing	1	0	0	4	0/0
Chicken, spicy crispy, breast	1	1	0	12	0/1
Chicken, spicy crispy, drumstick	1	0	0	5	0/1
Chicken, spicy crispy, thigh	1	1	0	13	0/1
Chicken, spicy crispy, wing	1	0	0	0	0/0
Chocolate chip cake	1 slc	1	21	47	21/3
Cole slaw (individual side)	1	2	14	19	14/1
Corn on the cob, 3"	1	2	3	16	3/1
Corn on the cob, 5.5"	1	4	5	33	5/2
Crispy strips	2	1	0	8	0/1
Crispy Twister	1	2	5	49	5/3
Crispy Twister, w/o sauce	1	2	4	48	4/3
Green beans (individual side)	1	1	1	3	1/0
KFC Famous Bowl, mashed potatoes	1	6	3	77	3/4
Little Bucket parfait, chocolate creme	1	1	22	37	22/2
Little Bucket parfait, lemon creme	1	0	47	60	47/3
Little Bucket parfait, strawberry shortcake	1	1	20	39	20/2
Macaroni & cheese (individual side)	1	2	4	20	4/1
Mashed potatoes (individual side)	1	1	0	15	0/1

FOOD	Svg Size	Fbr	Sgr	Cbs	S/C Val
Mashed potatoes, w/ gravy (individual side)	1	1	0	19	0/1
Popcorn chicken (kids size)	1	2	0	16	0/1
Popcorn chicken (individual size)	1	3	0	22	0/2
Potato wedges (individual side)	1	3	0	33	0/2
Pot pie	1	3	14	57	14/3
Salad, BLT, crispy, w/o dressing	1	3	4	14	4/1
Salad, BLT, roasted, w/o dressing	1	3	4	6	4/1
Salad, Caesar, crispy, w/o dressing or croutons	1	3	3	12	3/1
Salad, Caesar, roasted, w/o dressing or croutons	1	2	3	4	3/0
Salad, Caesar, side, w/o dressing or croutons	1	1	1	2	1/0
Salad, house, w/o dressing	1	1	2	2	2/0
Salad croutons, Parmesan garlic	1 pkt	1	1	8	1/1
Salad dressing, Heinz buttermilk ranch	1 pkt	0	1	0	1/0
Salad dressing, Hidden Valley fat-free ranch	1 pkt	0	2	8	2/1
Salad dressing, KFC creamy Parmesan Caesar	1 pkt	0	2	4	2/0
Salad dressing, Marzetti light Italian	1 pkt	0	1	2	1/0
Sandwich, double crunch	1	1	5	35	5/2
Sandwich, double crunch, w/o sauce	1	1	4	34	4/2
Sandwich, Double Down, grilled	1	0	1	3	1/0
Sandwich, Double Down, original recipe	1	1	1	11	1/1
Sandwich, honey BBQ	1	1	19	42	19/3
Sandwich, KFC Fish Snacker	1	2	5	31	5/2
Sandwich, KFC Fish Snacker, w/o sauce	1	1	4	29	4/2
Sandwich, KFC Snacker	1	2	4	28	4/2
Sandwich, KFC Snacker, Buffalo sauce	1	2	4	30	4/2
Sandwich, KFC Snacker, honey BBQ sauce	1	2	12	32	12/2
Sandwich, KFC Snacker, w/o sauce	1	2	4	27	4/2
Sandwich, Tender Roast	1	0	6	29	6/2
Sandwich, Tender Roast, w/o sauce	1	0	4	28	4/2
Wings, honey BBQ	1 pc	1	2	5	2/1
Wings, honey BBQ, boneless	1 pc	1	2	7	2/1
Wings, fiery Buffalo	1 pc	1	0	4	0/0
Wings, fiery Buffalo, boneless	1 pc	1	0	6	0/1

MCDONALD'S

Breakfast

Bacon, egg & cheese biscuit, regular biscuit	1	2	3	37	3/2
Bacon, egg & cheese biscuit, large biscuit	1	3	4	43	4/3
Bacon, egg & cheese McGriddle	1	2	15	48	15/3
Big Breakfast, w/ hotcakes & regular biscuit	1	6	17	111	17/6
Big Breakfast, w/ hotcakes & large biscuit	1	4	3	56	3/3
Big Breakfast, w/ regular biscuit	1	3	3	51	3/3
Big Breakfast, w/ large biscuit	1	4	3	56	3/3
Biscuit, regular	1	2	2	33	2/2

FOOD	Svg Size	Fbr	Sgr	Cbs	S/C Val
Biscuit, large	1	3	3	39	3/2
Egg McMuffin	1	2	3	30	3/2
Grape jam	0.5 oz	0	9	9	9/1
Hash brown	1	2	0	15	0/1
Hotcakes	5.3 oz	3	14	60	14/3
Hotcakes, w/ sausage	6.8 oz	3	14	61	14/4
McSkillet burrito w/ sausage	1	3	4	44	4/3
McSkillet burrito w/ steak	1	3	4	44	4/3
Sausage biscuit, regular biscuit	1	2	2	34	2/2
Sausage biscuit, large biscuit	1	3	3	39	3/2
Sausage biscuit w/ egg, regular biscuit	1	2	2	36	2/2
Sausage biscuit w/ egg, large biscuit	1	3	3	42	3/3
Sausage burrito	1	1	2	26	2/2
Sausage, egg & cheese McGriddle	1	2	15	48	15/3
Sausage McGriddle	1	2	15	44	15/3
Sausage McMuffin	1	2	2	29	2/2
Sausage McMuffin w/ egg	1	2	2	30	2/2
Sausage patty	1	0	0	1	0/0
Scrambled eggs	2	0	0	1	0/0
Southern style chicken biscuit, regular biscuit	1	2	3	41	3/3
Southern style chicken biscuit, large biscuit	1	3	4	46	4/3
Strawberry preserves	0.5 oz	0	9	9	9/1
Syrup	1 pkg	0	32	45	32/3
General Menu					
Angus bacon & cheese	1	4	13	63	13/4
Angus deluxe	1	4	10	61	10/4
Angus mushroom & Swiss	1	4	8	59	8/3
Big Mac	1	3	9	45	9/3
Big N' Tasty	1	3	8	37	8/2
Big N' Tasty, w/ cheese	1	3	8	38	8/2
Cheeseburger	1	2	6	33	6/2
Chicken McNuggets	4 pcs	0	0	11	0/1
Chicken McNuggets	6 pcs	0	0	16	0/1
Chicken McNuggets	10 pcs	0	0	27	0/2
Chicken Selects premium breast strips	3 pcs	0	0	23	0/2
Double cheeseburger	1	2	7	34	7/2
Double Quarter Pounder, w/ cheese	1	3	9	40	9/2
Filet-O-Fish	1	2	5	38	5/2
French fries, small	1 pkt	3	0	29	0/2
French fries, medium	1 pkt	5	0	48	0/3
Hamburger	1	2	6	31	6/2
McChicken	1	2	5	40	5/2
McDouble	1	2	7	33	7/2
McRib	1	3	11	44	11/3

FOOD	Svg Size	Fbr	Sgr	Cbs	S/C Val
Quarter Pounder	1	2	8	37	8/2
Quarter Pounder, w/ cheese	1	3	9	40	9/2
Premium crispy chicken classic sandwich	1	3	12	59	12/3
Premium crispy chicken club sandwich	1	4	13	60	13/3
Premium crispy chicken ranch BLT sandwich	1	3	13	62	13/4
Premium grilled chicken classic sandwich	1	3	11	51	11/3
Premium grilled chicken club sandwich	1	4	12	52	12/3
Premium grilled chicken ranch BLT sandwich	1	3	12	54	12/3
Salad, fruit & walnut w/ yogurt	1	2	25	31	25/2
Salad, premium bacon ranch salad w/ crispy chicken, w/o dressing	1	3	6	20	6/1
Salad, premium bacon ranch salad w/ grilled chicken, w/o dressing	1	3	5	12	5/1
Salad, premium bacon ranch salad, w/o chicken or dressing	1	3	4	10	4/1
Salad, premium Caesar salad w/ crispy chicken, w/o dressing	1	3	6	20	6/1
Salad, premium Caesar salad w/ grilled chicken, w/o dressing	1	3	5	12	5/1
Salad, premium Caesar salad, w/o chicken or dressing	1	3	4	9	4/1
Salad, premium Southwest salad w/ crispy chicken, w/o dressing	1	6	12	38	12/2
Salad, premium Southwest salad w/ grilled chicken, w/o dressing	1	6	11	30	11/2
Salad, premium Southwest salad, w/o chicken or dressing	1	6	6	20	6/1
Salad, side	1	1	2	4	2/0
Salad croutons, butter garlic	1 pkg	1	0	10	0/1
Salad dressing, Newman's Own creamy Caesar	2 oz	0	2	4	2/0
Salad dressing, Newman's Own creamy Southwest	1.5 oz	0	3	11	3/1
Salad dressing, Newman's Own low fat balsamic vinaigrette	1.5 oz	0	3	4	3/0
Salad dressing, Newman's Own low fat family recipe Italian	1.5 oz	0	1	8	1/1
Salad dressing, Newman's Own ranch	2 oz	0	4	9	4/1
Sauce, barbeque	1 pkg	0	10	12	10/1
Sauce, creamy ranch	1.3 oz	0	8	10	8/1
Sauce, hot mustard	1 pkg	0	10	12	10/1
Sauce, Southwestern chipotle barbeque	1.3 oz	1	11	15	11/1
Sauce, spicy Buffalo	1.3 oz	0	8	10	8/1
Sauce, sweet 'n sour	1 pkg	2	6	9	6/1
Sauce, tangy honey mustard	1.3 oz	0	8	10	8/1
Snack Wrap, chipotle BBQ, crispy	1	1	4	35	4/2
Snack Wrap, chipotle BBQ, grilled	1	1	5	28	5/2
Snack Wrap, honey mustard, crispy	1	1	4	34	4/2
Snack Wrap, honey mustard, grilled	1	1	4	27	4/2
Snack Wrap, Mac	1	1	3	26	3/2
Snack Wrap, ranch, crispy	1	1	2	33	2/2
Snack Wrap, ranch, grilled	1	1	2	26	2/2
Southern style crispy chicken sandwich	1	1	6	39	6/2
Desserts					
Apple dippers	1 pkg	0	8	6	8/1
Apple dippers' caramel dip	0.8 oz	0	18	24	18/2
Apple pie	1	4	13	32	13/2

FOOD	Svg Size	Fbr	Sgr	Cbs	S/C Val
Cinnamon melts	4 oz	3	32	66	32/4
Cookie, chocolate chip	1	1	15	21	15/2
Cookie, oatmeal raisin	1	1	13	22	13/2
Cookie, sugar	1	0	11	21	11/2
Fruit 'n yogurt parfait	5 oz	0	19	25	19/2
Fruit 'n yogurt parfait, w/ granola	5.3 oz	1	21	31	21/2
Ice cream cone, kiddie	1 oz	0	6	8	6/1
Ice cream cone, vanilla, reduced fat	3.2 oz	0	18	24	18/2
McFlurry, w/ M&M's	12.3 oz	1	85	96	85/5
McFlurry, w/ Oreos	11.9 oz	1	73	88	73/5
Sundae, hot caramel	6.4 oz	1	44	60	44/3
Sundae, hot fudge	6.3 oz	2	48	54	48/3
Sundae, strawberry	6.3 oz	1	45	49	45/3
Triple Thick Shake, chocolate, small	12 oz	1	63	76	63/4
Triple Thick Shake, chocolate, medium	16 oz	1	84	102	84/6
Triple Thick Shake, strawberry, small	12 oz	0	63	73	63/4
Triple Thick Shake, strawberry, medium	16 oz	0	84	97	84/5
Triple Thick Shake, vanilla, small	12 oz	0	54	72	54/4
Triple Thick Shake, vanilla, medium	16 oz	0	72	96	72/5
Drinks					
Cappuccino, small	12 oz	0	9	9	9/1
Cappuccino, medium	16 oz	0	11	11	1/1
Cappuccino, caramel, small	12 oz	0	32	32	32/2
Cappuccino, caramel, medium	16 oz	0	40	41	40/3
Cappuccino, hazelnut, small	12 oz	0	34	34	34/2
Cappuccino, hazelnut, medium	16 oz	0	42	42	42/3
Cappuccino, sugar-free vanilla, small	12 oz	0	7	15	7/1
Cappuccino, sugar-free vanilla, medium	16 oz	0	9	18	9/1
Cappuccino, vanilla, small	12 oz	0	34	34	34/2
Cappuccino, vanilla, medium	16 oz	0	42	42	42/3
Frappe, caramel, small	12 oz	0	57	61	57/4
Frappe, caramel, medium	16 oz	0	71	76	71/4
Frappe, mocha, small	12 oz	0	56	62	56/4
Frappe, mocha, medium	16 oz	0	70	78	70/4
Hot chocolate, small	12 oz	0	35	41	35/3
Hot chocolate, medium	16 oz	0	45	53	45/3
Iced coffee, small	8 oz	0	22	22	22/2
Iced coffee, medium	11.5 oz	0	30	30	30/2
Iced coffee, caramel, small	8 oz	0	20	21	20/2
Iced coffee, caramel, medium	11.5 oz	0	27	27	27/2
Iced coffee, hazelnut, small	8 oz	0	21	21	21/2
Iced coffee, hazelnut, medium	11.5 oz	0	29	29	29/2
Iced coffee, sugar-free vanilla, small	8 oz	0	1	8	1/1
Iced coffee, sugar-free vanilla, medium	11.5 oz	0	2	11	2/1

FOOD	Svg Size	Fbr	Sgr	Cbs	S/C Val
Iced coffee, vanilla, small	8 oz	0	21	21	21/2
Iced coffee, vanilla, medium	11.5 oz	0	28	29	28/2
Iced latte, small	12 oz	0	6	6	6/1
Iced latte, medium	16 oz	0	8	8	8/1
Iced latte, caramel, small	12 oz	0	29	29	29/2
Iced latte, caramel, medium	16 oz	0	31	31	31/2
Iced latte, hazelnut, small	12 oz	0	31	31	31/2
Iced latte, hazelnut, medium	16 oz	0	33	33	33/2
Iced latte, sugar-free vanilla, small	12 oz	0	4	12	4/1
Iced latte, sugar-free vanilla, medium	16 oz	0	6	14	6/1
Iced latte, vanilla, small	12 oz	0	31	31	31/2
Iced latte, vanilla, medium	16 oz	0	33	33	33/2
Iced mocha, medium	16 oz	0	35	42	35/3
Latte, small	12 oz	0	11	11	11/1
Latte, medium	16 oz	0	13	13	13/1
Latte, caramel, small	12 oz	0	35	35	35/2
Latte, caramel, medium	16 oz	0	43	43	43/3
Latte, hazelnut, small	12 oz	0	36	36	36/2
Latte, hazelnut, medium	16 oz	0	45	45	45/3
Latte, sugar-free vanilla, small	12 oz	0	7	15	7/1
Latte, sugar-free vanilla, medium	16 oz	0	9	18	9/1
Latte, vanilla, small	12 oz	0	36	36	36/2
Latte, vanilla, medium	16 oz	0	44	44	44/3
Mocha, small	12 oz	0	33	40	33/2
Mocha, medium	16 oz	0	41	48	41/3

PIZZA HUT

Pizza

FOOD	Svg Size	Fbr	Sgr	Cbs	S/C Val
Large hand-tossed style pizza (14"), cheese	⅛ pie	2	4	38	4/2
Large hand-tossed style pizza (14"), ham & pineapple	⅛ pie	2	6	39	6/2
Large hand-tossed style pizza (14"), Meat Lover's	⅛ pie	2	4	38	4/2
Large hand-tossed style pizza (14"), pepperoni	⅛ pie	2	4	37	4/2
Large hand-tossed style pizza (14"), supreme	⅛ pie	2	5	38	5/2
Large hand-tossed style pizza (14"), Veggie Lover's	⅛ pie	3	5	39	5/2
Large pan pizza (14"), cheese	⅛ pie	2	3	37	3/2
Large pan pizza (14"), ham & pineapple	⅛ pie	2	4	39	4/2
Large pan pizza (14"), Meat Lover's	⅛ pie	2	3	37	3/2
Large pan pizza (14"), pepperoni	⅛ pie	2	3	36	3/2
Large pan pizza (14"), supreme	⅛ pie	2	3	38	3/2
Large pan pizza (14"), Veggie Lover's	⅛ pie	2	4	38	4/2
Large stuffed crust pizza (14"), cheese	⅛ pie	2	5	39	5/2
Large stuffed crust pizza (14"), ham & pineapple	⅛ pie	2	6	41	6/3
Large stuffed crust pizza (14"), Meat Lover's	⅛ pie	2	5	39	5/2
Large stuffed crust pizza (14"), pepperoni	⅛ pie	2	4	38	4/2

FOOD	Svg Size	Fbr	Sgr	Cbs	S/C Val
Large stuffed crust pizza (14"), supreme	⅛ pie	2	5	40	5/2
Large stuffed crust pizza (14"), Veggie Lover's	⅛ pie	3	5	40	5/2
Large Thin 'n Crispy pizza (14"), cheese	⅛ pie	1	5	29	5/2
Large Thin 'n Crispy pizza (14"), ham & pineapple	⅛ pie	1	7	31	7/2
Large Thin 'n Crispy pizza (14"), Meat Lover's	⅛ pie	1	5	28	5/2
Large Thin 'n Crispy pizza (14"), pepperoni	⅛ pie	1	5	28	5/2
Large Thin 'n Crispy pizza (14"), supreme	⅛ pie	2	5	30	5/2
Large Thin 'n Crispy pizza (14"), Veggie Lover's	⅛ pie	2	6	30	6/2
Medium hand-tossed style pizza (12"), cheese	⅛ pie	1	3	26	3/2
Medium hand-tossed style pizza (12"), ham & pineapple	⅛ pie	1	4	27	4/2
Medium hand-tossed style pizza (12"), Meat Lover's	⅛ pie	1	3	25	3/2
Medium hand-tossed style pizza (12"), pepperoni	⅛ pie	1	3	25	3/2
Medium hand-tossed style pizza (12"), supreme	⅛ pie	2	3	26	3/2
Medium hand-tossed style pizza (12"), Veggie Lover's	⅛ pie	2	3	27	3/2
Medium pan pizza (12"), cheese	⅛ pie	1	2	27	2/2
Medium pan pizza (12"), ham & pineapple	⅛ pie	1	3	28	3/2
Medium pan pizza (12"), Meat Lover's	⅛ pie	1	2	27	2/2
Medium pan pizza (12"), pepperoni	⅛ pie	1	3	26	3/2
Medium pan pizza (12"), supreme	⅛ pie	2	2	27	2/2
Medium pan pizza (12"), Veggie Lover's	⅛ pie	2	3	28	3/2
Medium Pizza Mia pizza (12"), cheese	⅛ pie	1	2	27	2/2
Medium Pizza Mia pizza (12"), pepperoni	⅛ pie	1	2	26	2/2
Medium Thin 'n Crispy pizza (12"), cheese	⅛ pie	1	4	22	4/2
Medium Thin 'n Crispy pizza (12"), ham & pineapple	⅛ pie	1	5	23	5/2
Medium Thin 'n Crispy pizza (12"), Meat Lover's	⅛ pie	1	4	22	4/2
Medium Thin 'n Crispy pizza (12"), pepperoni	⅛ pie	1	4	21	4/2
Medium Thin 'n Crispy pizza (12"), supreme	⅛ pie	1	4	22	4/2
Medium Thin 'n Crispy pizza (12"), Veggie Lover's	⅛ pie	1	4	23	4/2
PANormous pizza (9"), cheese	1 pie	6	10	124	10/7
PANormous pizza (9"), ham & pineapple	1 pie	6	14	128	14/7
PANormous pizza (9"), Meat Lover's	1 pie	6	10	123	10/7
PANormous pizza (9"), pepperoni	1 pie	6	9	121	9/7
PANormous pizza (9"), supreme	1 pie	7	11	125	11/7
PANormous pizza (9"), Veggie Lover's	1 pie	8	12	127	12/7
Personal Pan Pizza (6"), cheese	1 pie	3	7	69	7/4
Personal Pan Pizza (6"), ham & pineapple	1 pie	3	9	71	9/4
Personal Pan Pizza (6"), Meat Lover's	1 pie	3	7	68	7/4
Personal Pan Pizza (6"), pepperoni	1 pie	3	6	67	6/4
Personal Pan Pizza (6"), supreme	1 pie	3	6	67	6/4
Personal Pan Pizza (6"), Veggie Lover's	1 pie	4	8	70	8/4
P'Zone, classic	½ pie	3	3	77	3/4
P'Zone, meaty	½ pie	2	3	76	3/4
P'Zone, pepperoni	½ pie	2	3	76	3/4

FOOD	Svg Size	Fbr	Sgr	Cbs	S/C Val
Other Menu Items					
Breadstick	1	1	2	19	2/1
Cheesestick	1	1	2	20	2/1
Cinnamon sticks	2	1	8	26	8/2
Cinnamon sticks' icing	2 oz	0	38	44	38/3
Hershey's Chocolate Dunkers	2	1	9	26	9/2
Hershey's chocolate dipping sauce	1.5 oz	1	18	24	18/2
Sauce, blue cheese	1.5 oz	0	2	2	2/0
Sauce, marinara	3 oz	2	9	12	9/1
Sauce, ranch	1.5 oz	0	1	2	1/0
Stuffed pizza roller	1	1	2	24	2/2
Tuscani pasta, creamy chicken Alfredo	½ pkg	6	10	50	10/3
Tuscani pasta, lasagna	½ pkg	5	11	43	11/3
Tuscani pasta, meaty marinara	½ pkg	6	10	50	10/3
Wings, bone-out, all-American	2	1	0	11	0/1
Wings, bone-out, Buffalo burnin' hot	2	1	2	18	2/1
Wings, bone-out, Buffalo medium	2	1	2	18	2/1
Wings, bone-out, Buffalo mild	2	1	2	18	2/1
Wings, bone-out, Cajun	2	1	6	21	6/2
Wings, bone-out, garlic Parmesan	2	1	1	11	1/1
Wings, bone-out, honey BBQ	2	1	12	27	12/2
Wings, bone-out, spicy Asian	2	1	13	24	13/2
Wings, bone-out, spicy BBQ	2	1	11	21	11/2
Wings, crispy bone-in, all-American	2	1	0	8	0/1
Wings, crispy bone-in, Buffalo burnin' hot	2	1	2	16	2/1
Wings, crispy bone-in, Buffalo medium	2	2	2	16	2/1
Wings, crispy bone-in, Buffalo mild	2	1	2	16	2/1
Wings, crispy bone-in, Cajun	2	2	6	19	6/1
Wings, crispy bone-in, garlic Parmesan	2	1	1	9	1/1
Wings, crispy bone-in, honey BBQ	2	1	12	24	12/2
Wings, crispy bone-in, spicy Asian	2	1	13	21	13/2
Wings, crispy bone-in, spicy BBQ	2	1	11	19	11/1
Wings, traditional, all-American	2	0	0	0	0/0
Wings, traditional, Buffalo burnin' hot	2	1	2	8	2/1
Wings, traditional, Buffalo medium	2	1	2	8	2/1
Wings, traditional, Buffalo mild	2	1	2	8	2/1
Wings, traditional, Cajun	2	1	6	11	6/1
Wings, traditional, garlic Parmesan	2	0	1	1	1/0
Wings, traditional, honey BBQ	2	0	12	16	12/1
Wings, traditional, spicy Asian	2	0	13	13	13/1
Wings, traditional, spicy BBQ	2	0	11	11	11/1

FOOD	Svg Size	Fbr	Sgr	Cbs	S/C Val

STARBUCKS

Coffee Drinks

FOOD	Svg Size	Fbr	Sgr	Cbs	S/C Val
Caffè Americano, tall	12 oz	0	0	2	0/0
Caffè Americano, grande	16 oz	0	0	3	0/0
Caffè latte, nonfat milk, tall	12 oz	0	14	15	14/1
Caffè latte, nonfat milk, grande	16 oz	0	18	19	18/1
Caffè latte, soy milk, tall	12 oz	0	14	18	14/1
Caffè latte, soy milk, grande	16 oz	0	17	23	17/2
Caffè latte, whole milk, tall	12 oz	0	13	14	13/1
Caffè latte, whole milk, grande	16 oz	0	16	18	16/1
Caffè misto, nonfat milk, tall	12 oz	0	8	8	8/1
Caffè misto, nonfat milk, grande	16 oz	0	10	10	10/1
Caffè misto, soy milk, tall	12 oz	0	8	10	8/1
Caffè misto, soy milk, grande	16 oz	0	10	12	10/1
Caffè misto, whole milk, tall	12 oz	0	7	7	7/1
Caffè misto, whole milk, grande	16 oz	0	9	9	9/1
Caffè mocha, nonfat milk, w/o whipped cream, tall	12 oz	0	25	32	25/2
Caffè mocha, nonfat milk, w/o whipped cream, grande	16 oz	2	32	42	32/3
Caffè mocha, nonfat milk, w/ whipped cream, tall	12 oz	0	26	34	26/2
Caffè mocha, nonfat milk, w/ whipped cream, grande	16 oz	2	34	44	34/3
Caffè mocha, soy milk, w/o whipped cream, tall	12 oz	2	25	34	25/2
Caffè mocha, soy milk, w/o whipped cream, grande	16 oz	3	32	45	32/3
Caffè mocha, soy milk, w/ whipped cream, tall	12 oz	2	26	36	26/2
Caffè mocha, soy milk, w/ whipped cream, grande	16 oz	3	34	47	34/3
Caffè mocha, whole milk, w/o whipped cream, tall	12 oz	0	24	31	24/2
Caffè mocha, whole milk, w/o whipped cream, grande	16 oz	2	31	40	31/2
Caffè mocha, whole milk, w/ whipped cream, tall	12 oz	0	25	33	25/2
Caffè mocha, whole milk, w/ whipped cream, grande	16 oz	2	32	42	32/3
Cappuccino, nonfat milk, tall	12 oz	0	8	9	8/1
Cappuccino, nonfat milk, grande	16 oz	0	10	12	10/1
Cappuccino, soy milk, tall	12 oz	0	8	11	8/1
Cappuccino, soy milk, grande	16 oz	0	10	15	10/1
Cappuccino, whole milk, tall	12 oz	0	8	9	8/1
Cappuccino, whole milk, grande	16 oz	0	9	11	9/1
Caramel macchiato, nonfat milk, tall	12 oz	0	23	25	23/2
Caramel macchiato, nonfat milk, grande	16 oz	0	32	35	32/2
Caramel macchiato, soy milk, tall	12 oz	0	23	28	23/2
Caramel macchiato, soy milk, grande	16 oz	0	32	38	32/2
Caramel macchiato, whole milk, tall	12 oz	0	22	24	22/2
Caramel macchiato, whole milk, grande	16 oz	0	31	34	31/2
Cinnamon dolce latte, nonfat milk, w/o whipped cream, tall	12 oz	0	30	31	30/2
Cinnamon dolce latte, nonfat milk, w/o whipped cream, grande	16 oz	0	39	41	39/3
Cinnamon dolce latte, nonfat milk, w/ whipped cream, tall	12 oz	0	31	33	31/2

FOOD	Svg Size	Fbr	Sgr	Cbs	S/C Val
Cinnamon dolce latte, nonfat milk, w/ whipped cream, grande	16 oz	0	40	43	40/3
Cinnamon dolce latte, soy milk, w/o whipped cream, tall	12 oz	0	30	34	30/2
Cinnamon dolce latte, soy milk, w/o whipped cream, grande	16 oz	0	39	44	39/3
Cinnamon dolce latte, soy milk, w/ whipped cream, tall	12 oz	0	31	36	31/2
Cinnamon dolce latte, soy milk, w/ whipped cream, grande	16 oz	0	40	46	40/3
Cinnamon dolce latte, whole milk, w/o whipped cream, tall	12 oz	0	29	30	29/2
Cinnamon dolce latte, whole milk, w/o whipped cream, grande	16 oz	0	37	39	37/2
Cinnamon dolce latte, whole milk, w/ whipped cream, tall	12 oz	0	30	32	30/2
Cinnamon dolce latte, whole milk, w/ whipped cream, grande	16 oz	0	39	41	39/3
Coffee, brewed, unflavored, unsweetened, all sizes	1	0	0	0	0/0
Dark cherry mocha, nonfat milk, w/o whipped cream, tall	12 oz	0	38	44	38/3
Dark cherry mocha, nonfat milk, w/o whipped cream, grande	16 oz	2	49	56	49/3
Dark cherry mocha, nonfat milk, w/ whipped cream, tall	12 oz	2	40	46	40/3
Dark cherry mocha, nonfat milk, w/ whipped cream, grande	16 oz	2	52	61	52/4
Dark cherry mocha, whole milk, w/o whipped cream, tall	12 oz	0	37	43	37/3
Dark cherry mocha, whole milk, w/o whipped cream, grande	16 oz	2	48	57	48/3
Dark cherry mocha, whole milk, w/ whipped cream, tall	12 oz	2	39	45	39/3
Dark cherry mocha, whole milk, w/ whipped cream, grande	16 oz	2	50	60	50/3
Espresso, solo (single)	1 oz	0	0	0	0/0
Espresso, doppio (double)	2 oz	0	0	2	0/0
Espresso con panna, solo (single)	1 oz	0	0	2	0/0
Espresso macchiato, nonfat milk, solo (single)	1 oz	0	0	0	0/0
Espresso macchiato, nonfat milk, doppio (double)	2 oz	0	0	2	0/0
Espresso macchiato, soy milk, solo (single)	1 oz	0	0	0	0/0
Espresso macchiato, soy milk, doppio (double)	2 oz	0	0	2	0/0
Espresso macchiato, whole milk, solo (single)	1 oz	0	0	0	0/0
Espresso macchiato, whole milk, doppio (double)	2 oz	0	0	2	0/0
Flavored latte, nonfat milk, tall	12 oz	0	27	28	27/2
Flavored latte, nonfat milk, grande	16 oz	0	35	37	35/2
Flavored latte, soy milk, tall	12 oz	0	27	31	27/2
Flavored latte, soy milk, grande	16 oz	0	35	41	35/3
Flavored latte, whole milk, tall	12 oz	0	26	27	26/2
Flavored latte, whole milk, grande	16 oz	0	33	36	33/2
Frappuccino, caffè vanilla, w/o whipped cream, tall	12 oz	0	43	49	43/3
Frappuccino, caffè vanilla, w/o whipped cream, grande	16 oz	0	58	67	58/4
Frappuccino, caffè vanilla, w/ whipped cream, tall	12 oz	0	45	52	45/3
Frappuccino, caffè vanilla, w/ whipped cream, grande	16 oz	0	60	70	60/4
Frappuccino, caffè vanilla, light, w/o whipped cream, tall	12 oz	2	23	30	23/2
Frappuccino, caffè vanilla, light, w/o whipped cream, grande	16 oz	3	32	42	32/3
Frappuccino, caramel, w/o whipped cream, tall	12 oz	0	38	44	38/3
Frappuccino, caramel, w/o whipped cream, grande	16 oz	0	45	53	45/3
Frappuccino, caramel, w/ whipped cream, tall	12 oz	0	39	46	39/3
Frappuccino, caramel, w/ whipped cream, grande	16 oz	0	48	57	48/3
Frappuccino, caramel, light, w/o whipped cream, tall	12 oz	2	18	25	18/2

FOOD	Svg Size	Fbr	Sgr	Cbs	S/C Val
Frappuccino, caramel, light, w/o whipped cream, grande	16 oz	3	21	30	21/2
Frappuccino, cinnamon dolce, w/o whipped cream, tall	12 oz	0	42	51	42/3
Frappuccino, cinnamon dolce, w/o whipped cream, grande	16 oz	0	54	64	54/4
Frappuccino, cinnamon dolce, w/ whipped cream, tall	12 oz	0	44	53	44/3
Frappuccino, cinnamon dolce, w/ whipped cream, grande	16 oz	0	56	68	56/4
Frappuccino, cinnamon dolce, light, tall	12 oz	2	17	24	17/2
Frappuccino, cinnamon dolce, light, grande	16 oz	3	21	29	21/2
Frappuccino, coffee, w/o whipped cream, tall	12 oz	0	31	37	31/2
Frappuccino, coffee, w/o whipped cream, grande	16 oz	0	40	48	40/3
Frappuccino, coffee, light, w/o whipped cream, tall	12 oz	2	12	18	12/1
Frappuccino, coffee, light, w/o whipped cream, grande	16 oz	3	16	25	16/2
Frappuccino, espresso, w/o whipped cream, tall	12 oz	0	22	27	22/2
Frappuccino, espresso, w/o whipped cream, grande	16 oz	0	31	38	31/2
Frappuccino, java chip, w/o whipped cream, tall	12 oz	0	40	50	40/3
Frappuccino, java chip, w/o whipped cream, grande	16 oz	2	52	64	52/4
Frappuccino, java chip, w/ whipped cream, tall	12 oz	0	42	52	42/3
Frappuccino, java chip, w/ whipped cream, grande	16 oz	2	55	67	55/4
Frappuccino, java chip, light, w/o whipped cream, tall	12 oz	3	20	30	20/2
Frappuccino, java chip, light, w/o whipped cream, grande	16 oz	4	24	36	24/2
Frappuccino, mocha, w/o whipped cream, tall	12 oz	0	34	41	34/3
Frappuccino, mocha, w/o whipped cream, grande	16 oz	0	45	54	45/3
Frappuccino, mocha, w/ whipped cream, tall	12 oz	0	36	43	36/3
Frappuccino, mocha, w/ whipped cream, grande	16 oz	0	47	57	47/3
Frappuccino, mocha, light, w/o whipped cream, tall	12 oz	2	15	23	15/2
Frappuccino, mocha, light, w/o whipped cream, grande	16 oz	3	19	29	19/2
Frappuccino, white chocolate mocha, w/o whipped cream, tall	12 oz	0	41	47	41/3
Frappuccino, white chocolate mocha, w/o whipped cream, grande	16 oz	0	51	59	51/3
Frappuccino, white chocolate mocha, w/ whipped cream, tall	12 oz	0	43	49	43/3
Frappuccino, white chocolate mocha, w/ whipped cream, grande	16 oz	0	54	62	54/4
Iced caffè Americano, tall	12 oz	0	0	2	0/0
Iced caffè Americano, grande	16 oz	0	0	3	0/0
Iced caffè latte, nonfat milk, tall	12 oz	0	9	10	9/1
Iced caffè latte, nonfat milk, grande	16 oz	0	11	13	11/1
Iced caffè latte, soy milk, tall	12 oz	0	9	13	9/1
Iced caffè latte, soy milk, grande	16 oz	0	12	17	12/1
Iced caffè latte, whole milk, tall	12 oz	0	8	9	8/1
Iced caffè latte, whole milk, grande	16 oz	0	10	12	10/1
Iced caffè mocha, nonfat milk, w/o whipped cream, tall	12 oz	0	20	27	20/2
Iced caffè mocha, nonfat milk, w/o whipped cream, grande	16 oz	2	26	36	26/2
Iced caffè mocha, nonfat milk, w/ whipped cream, tall	12 oz	0	22	29	22/2
Iced caffè mocha, nonfat milk, w/ whipped cream, grande	16 oz	2	29	39	29/2
Iced caffè mocha, soy milk, w/o whipped cream, tall	12 oz	2	20	28	20/2
Iced caffè mocha, soy milk, w/o whipped cream, grande	16 oz	3	26	38	26/2
Iced caffè mocha, soy milk, w/ whipped cream, tall	12 oz	2	22	31	22/2

FOOD	Svg Size	Fbr	Sgr	Cbs	S/C Val
Iced caffè mocha, soy milk, w/ whipped cream, grande	16 oz	3	29	41	29/3
Iced caffè mocha, whole milk, w/o whipped cream, tall	12 oz	0	19	26	19/2
Iced caffè mocha, whole milk, w/o whipped cream, grande	16 oz	2	25	35	25/2
Iced caffè mocha, whole milk, w/ whipped cream, tall	12 oz	0	21	28	21/2
Iced caffè mocha, whole milk, w/ whipped cream, grande	16 oz	2	28	38	28/2
Iced caramel macchiato, nonfat milk, tall	12 oz	0	23	25	23/2
Iced caramel macchiato, nonfat milk, grande	16 oz	0	31	34	31/2
Iced caramel macchiato, soy milk, tall	12 oz	0	23	28	23/2
Iced caramel macchiato, soy milk, grande	16 oz	0	32	38	32/2
Iced caramel macchiato, whole milk, tall	12 oz	0	22	24	22/2
Iced caramel macchiato, whole milk, grande	16 oz	0	30	33	30/2
Iced cinnamon dolce latte, nonfat milk, w/o whipped cream, tall	12 oz	0	25	26	25/2
Iced cinnamon dolce latte, nonfat milk, w/o whipped cream, grande	16 oz	0	33	35	33/2
Iced cinnamon dolce latte, nonfat milk, w/ whipped cream, tall	12 oz	0	27	28	27/2
Iced cinnamon dolce latte, nonfat milk, w/ whipped cream, grande	16 oz	0	36	39	36/2
Iced cinnamon dolce latte, soy milk, w/o whipped cream, tall	12 oz	0	25	28	25/2
Iced cinnamon dolce latte, soy milk, w/o whipped cream, grande	16 oz	0	33	38	33/2
Iced cinnamon dolce latte, soy milk, w/ whipped cream, tall	12 oz	0	27	31	27/2
Iced cinnamon dolce latte, soy milk, w/ whipped cream, grande	16 oz	0	36	41	36/3
Iced cinnamon dolce latte, whole milk, w/o whipped cream, tall	12 oz	0	24	25	24/2
Iced cinnamon dolce latte, whole milk, w/o whipped cream, grande	16 oz	0	32	34	32/2
Iced cinnamon dolce latte, whole milk, w/ whipped cream, tall	12 oz	0	26	28	26/2
Iced cinnamon dolce latte, whole milk, w/ whipped cream, grande	16 oz	0	34	37	34/2
Iced coffee, nonfat milk, tall	12 oz	0	18	18	18/1
Iced coffee, nonfat milk, grande	16 oz	0	24	24	24/2
Iced coffee, soy milk, tall	12 oz	0	18	19	18/1
Iced coffee, soy milk, grande	16 oz	0	24	25	24/2
Iced coffee, whole milk, tall	12 oz	0	18	18	18/1
Iced coffee, whole milk, grande	16 oz	0	24	24	24/2
Iced dark cherry mocha, nonfat milk, w/o whipped cream, tall	12 oz	0	33	39	33/2
Iced dark cherry mocha, nonfat milk, w/o whipped cream, grande	16 oz	2	43	51	43/3
Iced dark cherry mocha, nonfat milk, w/ whipped cream, tall	12 oz	2	35	42	35/3
Iced dark cherry mocha, nonfat milk, w/ whipped cream, grande	16 oz	2	46	56	46/3
Iced dark cherry mocha, whole milk, w/o whipped cream, tall	12 oz	0	32	38	32/2
Iced dark cherry mocha, whole milk, w/o whipped cream, grande	16 oz	2	42	51	42/3
Iced dark cherry mocha, whole milk, w/ whipped cream, tall	12 oz	2	35	41	35/3
Iced dark cherry mocha, whole milk, w/ whipped cream, grande	16 oz	2	45	55	45/3
Iced flavored latte, nonfat milk, tall	12 oz	0	27	28	27/2
Iced flavored latte, nonfat milk, grande	16 oz	0	35	37	35/2
Iced flavored latte, soy milk, tall	12 oz	0	27	31	27/2
Iced flavored latte, soy milk, grande	16 oz	0	35	41	35/3
Iced flavored latte, whole milk, tall	12 oz	0	26	27	26/2
Iced flavored latte, whole milk, grande	16 oz	0	33	36	33/2
Iced peppermint mocha, nonfat milk, w/o whipped cream, tall	12 oz	0	32	39	32/2

FOOD	Svg Size	Fbr	Sgr	Cbs	S/C Val
Iced peppermint mocha, nonfat milk, w/o whipped cream, grande	16 oz	2	42	52	42/3
Iced peppermint mocha, nonfat milk, w/ whipped cream, tall	12 oz	0	34	41	34/3
Iced peppermint mocha, nonfat milk, w/ whipped cream, grande	16 oz	2	45	56	45/3
Iced peppermint mocha, soy milk, w/o whipped cream, tall	12 oz	2	32	41	32/3
Iced peppermint mocha, soy milk, w/o whipped cream, grande	16 oz	2	42	54	42/3
Iced peppermint mocha, soy milk, w/ whipped cream, tall	12 oz	2	34	43	34/3
Iced peppermint mocha, soy milk, w/ whipped cream, grande	16 oz	2	45	57	45/3
Iced peppermint mocha, whole milk, w/o whipped cream, tall	12 oz	0	31	38	31/2
Iced peppermint mocha, whole milk, w/o whipped cream, grande	16 oz	2	42	52	42/3
Iced peppermint mocha, whole milk, w/ whipped cream, tall	12 oz	0	33	41	33/3
Iced peppermint mocha, whole milk, w/ whipped cream, grande	16 oz	2	44	55	44/3
Iced skinny flavored latte, nonfat milk, tall	12 oz	0	8	9	8/1
Iced skinny flavored latte, nonfat milk, grande	16 oz	0	10	12	10/1
Iced skinny flavored latte, 2% milk, tall	12 oz	0	7	9	7/1
Iced skinny flavored latte, 2% milk, grande	16 oz	0	9	12	9/1
Iced white chocolate mocha, nonfat milk, w/o whipped cream, tall	12 oz	0	40	42	40/3
Iced white chocolate mocha, nonfat milk, w/o whipped cream, grande	16 oz	0	52	55	52/3
Iced white chocolate mocha, nonfat milk, w/ whipped cream, tall	12 oz	0	41	44	41/3
Iced white chocolate mocha, nonfat milk, w/ whipped cream, grande	16 oz	0	55	59	55/3
Iced white chocolate mocha, soy milk, w/o whipped cream, tall	12 oz	0	40	43	40/3
Iced white chocolate mocha, soy milk, w/o whipped cream, grande	16 oz	0	53	58	53/3
Iced white chocolate mocha, soy milk, w/ whipped cream, tall	12 oz	0	42	46	42/3
Iced white chocolate mocha, soy milk, w/ whipped cream, grande	16 oz	0	55	61	55/4
Iced white chocolate mocha, whole milk, w/o whipped cream, tall	12 oz	0	41	43	41/3
Iced white chocolate mocha, whole milk, w/o whipped cream, grande	16 oz	0	52	55	52/3
Iced white chocolate mocha, whole milk, w/ whipped cream, tall	12 oz	0	41	43	41/3
Iced white chocolate mocha, whole milk, w/ whipped cream, grande	16 oz	0	54	58	54/3
Peppermint mocha, nonfat milk, w/o whipped cream, tall	12 oz	0	37	44	37/3
Peppermint mocha, nonfat milk, w/o whipped cream, grande	16 oz	2	49	59	49/3
Peppermint mocha, nonfat milk, w/ whipped cream, tall	12 oz	0	38	46	38/3
Peppermint mocha, nonfat milk, w/ whipped cream, grande	16 oz	2	50	61	50/4
Peppermint mocha, soy milk, w/o whipped cream, tall	12 oz	2	37	47	37/3
Peppermint mocha, soy milk, w/o whipped cream, grande	16 oz	3	49	62	49/4
Peppermint mocha, soy milk, w/ whipped cream, tall	12 oz	2	38	48	38/3
Peppermint mocha, soy milk, w/ whipped cream, grande	16 oz	3	50	64	50/4
Peppermint mocha, whole milk, w/o whipped cream, tall	12 oz	0	36	43	36/3
Peppermint mocha, whole milk, w/o whipped cream, grande	16 oz	2	47	58	47/3
Peppermint mocha, whole milk, w/ whipped cream, tall	12 oz	0	38	45	38/3
Peppermint mocha, whole milk, w/ whipped cream, grande	16 oz	2	49	60	49/3
Skinny cinnamon dolce latte, nonfat milk, tall	12 oz	0	12	14	12/1
Skinny cinnamon dolce latte, nonfat milk, grande	16 oz	0	17	19	17/1
Skinny cinnamon dolce latte, 2% milk, tall	12 oz	0	12	14	12/1
Skinny cinnamon dolce latte, 2% milk, grande	16 oz	0	15	18	15/1
Skinny flavored latte, nonfat milk, tall	12 oz	0	8	9	8/1

FOOD	Svg Size	Fbr	Sgr	Cbs	S/C Val
Skinny flavored latte, nonfat milk, grande	16 oz	0	10	12	10/1
Skinny flavored latte, 2% milk, tall	12 oz	0	7	9	7/1
Skinny flavored latte, 2% milk, grande	16 oz	0	9	12	9/1
White chocolate mocha, nonfat milk, w/o whipped cream, tall	12 oz	0	45	47	45/3
White chocolate mocha, nonfat milk, w/o whipped cream, grande	16 oz	0	58	61	58/4
White chocolate mocha, nonfat milk, w/ whipped cream, tall	12 oz	0	46	48	46/3
White chocolate mocha, nonfat milk, w/ whipped cream, grande	16 oz	0	60	64	60/4
White chocolate mocha, soy milk, w/o whipped cream, tall	12 oz	0	45	49	45/3
White chocolate mocha, soy milk, w/o whipped cream, grande	16 oz	0	58	65	58/4
White chocolate mocha, soy milk, w/ whipped cream, tall	12 oz	0	46	51	46/3
White chocolate mocha, soy milk, w/ whipped cream, grande	16 oz	0	60	67	60/4
White chocolate mocha, whole milk, w/o whipped cream, tall	12 oz	0	44	46	44/3
White chocolate mocha, whole milk, w/o whipped cream, grande	16 oz	0	57	60	57/3
White chocolate mocha, whole milk, w/ whipped cream, tall	12 oz	0	45	47	45/3
White chocolate mocha, whole milk, w/ whipped cream, grande	16 oz	0	59	62	59/4

Noncoffee Drinks

FOOD	Svg Size	Fbr	Sgr	Cbs	S/C Val
Caramel apple spice, w/o whipped cream, tall	12 oz	0	51	57	51/3
Caramel apple spice, w/o whipped cream, grande	16 oz	0	66	74	66/4
Caramel apple spice, w/ whipped cream, tall	12 oz	0	52	59	52/3
Caramel apple spice, w/ whipped cream, grande	16 oz	0	68	76	68/4
Frappuccino, chai, w/ whipped cream, tall	12 oz	0	33	34	33/2
Frappuccino, chai, w/ whipped cream, grande	16 oz	0	48	50	48/3
Frappuccino, cinnamon dolce, w/o whipped cream, tall	12 oz	0	42	51	42/3
Frappuccino, cinnamon dolce, w/o whipped cream, grande	16 oz	0	54	64	54/4
Frappuccino, cinnamon dolce, w/ whipped cream, tall	12 oz	0	44	53	44/3
Frappuccino, cinnamon dolce, w/ whipped cream, grande	16 oz	0	56	68	56/4
Frappuccino, double chocolaty chip, w/o whipped cream, tall	12 oz	2	43	57	43/3
Frappuccino, double chocolaty chip, w/o whipped cream, grande	16 oz	2	57	75	57/4
Frappuccino, double chocolaty chip, w/ whipped cream, tall	12 oz	2	45	59	45/3
Frappuccino, double chocolaty chip, w/ whipped cream, grande	16 oz	2	59	78	59/4
Frappuccino, green tea, w/o whipped cream, tall	12 oz	0	46	47	46/3
Frappuccino, green tea, w/o whipped cream, grande	16 oz	0	65	66	65/4
Frappuccino, green tea, w/ whipped cream, tall	12 oz	0	48	49	48/3
Frappuccino, green tea, w/ whipped cream, grande	16 oz	0	67	70	67/4
Frappuccino, strawberries & crème, w/o whipped cream, tall	12 oz	0	42	51	42/3
Frappuccino, strawberries & crème, w/o whipped cream, grande	16 oz	0	54	64	54/4
Frappuccino, strawberries & crème, w/ whipped cream, tall	12 oz	0	44	53	44/3
Frappuccino, strawberries & crème, w/ whipped cream, grande	16 oz	0	56	68	56/4
Frappuccino, vanilla bean, w/o whipped cream, tall	12 oz	2	43	57	43/3
Frappuccino, vanilla bean, w/o whipped cream, grande	16 oz	2	57	75	57/4
Frappuccino, vanilla bean, w/ whipped cream, tall	12 oz	2	45	59	45/3
Frappuccino, vanilla bean, w/ whipped cream, grande	16 oz	2	59	78	59/4
Frappuccino, white chocolate, w/o whipped cream, tall	12 oz	0	51	60	51/3
Frappuccino, white chocolate, w/o whipped cream, grande	16 oz	1	67	78	67/4

FOOD	Svg Size	Fbr	Sgr	Cbs	S/C Val
Frappuccino, white chocolate, w/ whipped cream, tall	12 oz	0	56	65	56/4
Frappuccino, white chocolate, w/ whipped cream, grande	16 oz	0	79	92	79/5
Hot chocolate, nonfat milk, w/o whipped cream, tall	12 oz	0	31	37	31/2
Hot chocolate, nonfat milk, w/o whipped cream, grande	16 oz	2	40	48	40/3
Hot chocolate, nonfat milk, w/ whipped cream, tall	12 oz	0	33	39	33/2
Hot chocolate, nonfat milk, w/ whipped cream, grande	16 oz	0	41	50	41/3
Hot chocolate, soy milk, w/o whipped cream, tall	12 oz	2	31	40	31/2
Hot chocolate, soy milk, w/o whipped cream, grande	16 oz	3	40	52	40/3
Hot chocolate, soy milk, w/ whipped cream, tall	12 oz	2	33	42	33/3
Hot chocolate, soy milk, w/ whipped cream, grande	16 oz	3	41	54	41/3
Hot chocolate, whole milk, w/o whipped cream, tall	12 oz	0	30	36	30/2
Hot chocolate, whole milk, w/o whipped cream, grande	16 oz	2	38	46	38/3
Hot chocolate, whole milk, w/ whipped cream, tall	12 oz	0	32	38	32/2
Hot chocolate, whole milk, w/ whipped cream, grande	16 oz	2	40	49	40/3
Tazo, brewed tea, all flavors, all sizes	1	0	0	0	0/0
Tazo, iced latte, Awake, nonfat milk, grande	16 oz	0	34	35	34/2
Tazo, iced latte, Awake, soy milk, grande	16 oz	0	34	38	34/2
Tazo, iced latte, Awake, whole milk, grande	16 oz	0	33	34	33/2
Tazo, iced latte, chai, nonfat milk, tall	12 oz	0	31	33	31/2
Tazo, iced latte, chai, nonfat milk, grande	16 oz	0	42	44	42/3
Tazo, iced latte, chai, soy milk, tall	12 oz	0	32	35	32/2
Tazo, iced latte, chai, soy milk, grande	16 oz	0	43	47	43/3
Tazo, iced latte, chai, whole milk, tall	12 oz	0	31	32	31/2
Tazo, iced latte, chai, whole milk, grande	16 oz	0	41	44	41/3
Tazo, iced latte, green tea, nonfat milk, tall	12 oz	0	31	32	31/2
Tazo, iced latte, green tea, nonfat milk, grande	16 oz	0	43	45	43/3
Tazo, iced latte, green tea, soy milk, tall	12 oz	0	31	35	31/2
Tazo, iced latte, green tea, soy milk, grande	16 oz	2	44	48	44/3
Tazo, iced latte, green tea, whole milk, tall	12 oz	0	30	31	30/2
Tazo, iced latte, green tea, whole milk, grande	16 oz	0	42	44	42/3
Tazo, latte, Awake, nonfat milk, tall	12 oz	0	24	24	24/2
Tazo, latte, Awake, nonfat milk, grande	16 oz	0	32	32	32/2
Tazo, latte, Awake, soy milk, tall	12 oz	0	25	27	25/2
Tazo, latte, Awake, soy milk, grande	16 oz	0	33	35	33/2
Tazo, latte, Awake, whole milk, tall	12 oz	0	23	23	23/2
Tazo, latte, Awake, whole milk, grande	16 oz	0	31	31	31/2
Tazo, latte, chai, nonfat milk, tall	12 oz	0	32	33	32/2
Tazo, latte, chai, nonfat milk, grande	16 oz	0	42	44	42/3
Tazo, latte, chai, soy milk, tall	12 oz	0	32	35	32/3
Tazo, latte, chai, soy milk, grande	16 oz	0	42	47	42/3
Tazo, latte, chai, whole milk, tall	12 oz	0	31	33	31/2
Tazo, latte, chai, whole milk, grande	16 oz	0	41	43	41/3
Tazo, latte, Earl Grey, nonfat milk, tall	12 oz	0	24	24	24/2
Tazo, latte, Earl Grey, nonfat milk, grande	16 oz	0	32	32	32/2

FOOD	Svg Size	Fbr	Sgr	Cbs	S/C Val
Tazo, latte, Earl Grey, soy milk, tall	12 oz	0	25	27	25/2
Tazo, latte, Earl Grey, soy milk, grande	16 oz	0	33	35	33/2
Tazo, latte, Earl Grey, whole milk, tall	12 oz	0	23	23	23/2
Tazo, latte, Earl Grey, whole milk, grande	16 oz	0	31	31	31/2
Tazo, latte, green tea, nonfat milk, tall	12 oz	0	41	42	41/3
Tazo, latte, green tea, nonfat milk, grande	16 oz	0	56	57	56/3
Tazo, latte, green tea, soy milk, tall	12 oz	2	42	46	42/3
Tazo, latte, green tea, soy milk, grande	16 oz	3	57	63	57/4
Tazo, latte, green tea, whole milk, tall	12 oz	0	40	41	40/3
Tazo, latte, green tea, whole milk, grande	16 oz	0	54	56	54/3
Tazo, latte, vanilla rooibos, nonfat milk, tall	12 oz	0	24	24	24/2
Tazo, latte, vanilla rooibos, nonfat milk, grande	16 oz	0	32	32	32/2
Tazo, latte, vanilla rooibos, soy milk, tall	12 oz	0	25	27	25/2
Tazo, latte, vanilla rooibos, soy milk, grande	16 oz	0	33	35	33/2
Tazo, latte, vanilla rooibos, whole milk, tall	12 oz	0	23	23	23/2
Tazo, latte, vanilla rooibos, whole milk, grande	16 oz	0	31	31	31/2
Tazo, shaken iced tea, black, tall	12 oz	0	15	16	15/1
Tazo, shaken iced tea, black, grande	16 oz	0	20	21	20/2
Tazo, shaken iced tea, green, tall	12 oz	0	15	16	15/1
Tazo, shaken iced tea, green, grande	16 oz	0	20	21	20/2
Tazo, shaken iced tea, passion, tall	12 oz	0	15	16	15/1
Tazo, shaken iced tea, passion, grande	16 oz	0	20	21	20/2
Tazo, shaken iced tea lemonade, black, tall	12 oz	0	25	25	25/2
Tazo, shaken iced tea lemonade, black, grande	16 oz	0	33	33	33/2
Tazo, shaken iced tea lemonade, green, tall	12 oz	0	25	25	25/2
Tazo, shaken iced tea lemonade, green, grande	16 oz	0	33	33	33/2
Tazo, shaken iced tea lemonade, passion, tall	12 oz	0	25	25	25/2
Tazo, shaken iced tea lemonade, passion, grande	16 oz	0	33	33	33/2
Vivanno smoothie, chocolate, nonfat or 2% milk, grande	16 oz	6	30	48	30/3
Vivanno smoothie, chocolate, soy milk, grande	16 oz	7	30	50	30/3
Vivanno smoothie, orange mango, nonfat or 2% milk, grande	16 oz	5	34	51	34/3
Vivanno smoothie, orange mango, soy milk, grande	16 oz	5	34	51	34/3
Vivanno smoothie, strawberry, nonfat or 2% milk, grande	16 oz	7	41	56	41/3
Vivanno smoothie, strawberry, soy milk, grande	16 oz	6	39	54	39/3
White hot chocolate, nonfat milk, w/o whipped cream, tall	12 oz	0	46	47	46/3
White hot chocolate, nonfat milk, w/o whipped cream, grande	16 oz	0	61	62	61/4
White hot chocolate, nonfat milk, w/ whipped cream, tall	12 oz	0	47	49	47/3
White hot chocolate, nonfat milk, w/ whipped cream, grande	16 oz	0	62	64	62/4
White hot chocolate, soy milk, w/o whipped cream, tall	12 oz	0	46	50	46/3
White hot chocolate, soy milk, w/o whipped cream, grande	16 oz	0	61	66	61/4
White hot chocolate, soy milk, w/ whipped cream, tall	12 oz	0	47	52	47/3
White hot chocolate, soy milk, w/ whipped cream, grande	16 oz	0	62	68	62/4
White hot chocolate, whole milk, w/o whipped cream, tall	12 oz	0	45	46	45/3
White hot chocolate, whole milk, w/o whipped cream, grande	16 oz	0	59	61	59/4

FOOD	Svg Size	Fbr	Sgr	Cbs	S/C Val
White hot chocolate, whole milk, w/ whipped cream, tall	12 oz	0	46	47	46/3
White hot chocolate, whole milk, w/ whipped cream, grande	16 oz	0	61	63	61/4
Food					
Bagel, Asiago	1	2	5	54	5/3
Bagel, Chonga	1	3	5	52	5/3
Bagel, Hawaiian	1	2	17	60	17/3
Bagel, multigrain	1	4	8	62	8/4
Bagel, plain	1	2	8	64	8/4
Bar, blueberry oat	1	5	19	47	19/3
Bar, marshmallow dream	1	0	15	43	15/3
Bar, rich toffee pecan	1	0	17	42	17/3
Bread, Mallorca sweet	1 slc	0	12	42	12/3
Bread, pumpkin	1 slc	2	38	60	38/3
Breakfast sandwich, bacon, Gouda cheese & egg frittata	1	0	0	31	0/2
Breakfast sandwich, black forest ham, Parmesan frittata & cheddar	1	0	0	32	0/2
Breakfast sandwich, reduced-fat turkey bacon w/ egg whites	1	3	6	47	6/3
Breakfast sandwich, sausage, egg & cheese	1	2	3	42	3/3
Brownie, double chocolate	1	3	30	46	30/3
Bun, morning	1	2	19	45	19/3
Cake, banana chocolate chip coffee, reduced fat	1 slc	3	51	79	51/4
Cake, cinnamon swirl coffee, reduced fat	1 slc	2	39	62	39/4
Cake, classic coffee	1 slc	0	36	63	36/4
Cake, iced lemon pound	1 slc	0	47	68	47/4
Cake, marble pound	1 slc	0	34	53	34/3
Cake, very berry coffee, reduced fat	1 slc	4	30	58	30/3
Cookie, chocolate chunk	1	2	31	50	31/3
Cookie, indulgent chocolate	1	3	31	40	31/2
Cookie, outrageous oatmeal	1	3	36	56	36/3
Croissant, butter	1	0	4	32	4/2
Croissant, chocolate	1	2	10	34	10/2
Cupcake, chocolate bloom	1	0	32	42	32/3
Danish, cheese	1	0	16	39	16/2
Doughnut, chocolate mini sparkle	1	0	10	16	10/1
Doughnut, chocolate old-fashioned	1	2	35	57	35/3
Doughnut, old-fashioned glazed	1	0	34	57	34/3
Doughnut, vanilla mini sparkle	1	0	10	16	10/1
Fritter, apple	1	0	27	59	27/3
Muffin, apple bran	1	7	34	64	34/4
Muffin, blueberry streusel	1	2	33	59	33/3
Muffin, red raspberry, low fat	1	2	37	65	37/4
Muffin, zucchini walnut	1	2	28	52	28/3
Oatmeal, Starbucks perfect	1	4	0	25	0/2
Oatmeal, Starbucks perfect, w/ brown sugar topping	1	4	13	38	13/2
Oatmeal, Starbucks perfect, w/ dried fruit topping	1	6	20	49	20/3

FOOD	Svg Size	Fbr	Sgr	Cbs	S/C Val
Oatmeal, Starbucks perfect, w/ nut medley topping	1	4	0	27	0/2
Parfait, dark cherry yogurt	1	3	39	61	39/4
Parfait, Greek yogurt honey	1	30	32	43	32/3
Parfait, strawberry & blueberry yogurt	1	3	39	60	39/3
Plate, fruit & cheese	1	3	24	37	24/2
Plate, protein	1	5	17	39	17/2
Roll, double iced cinnamon	1	3	34	70	34/4
Roll, 8-grain	1	5	17	67	17/4
Salad, deluxe fruit blend	1	2	19	23	19/2
Salad, picnic pasta	1	3	3	53	3/3
Sandwich, chicken Santa Fe flatbread	1	2	2	47	2/3
Sandwich, egg salad	1	3	10	54	10/3
Sandwich, ham & Swiss	1	2	0	43	0/3
Sandwich, Roma tomato & mozzarella	1	2	0	40	0/2
Sandwich, tarragon chicken salad	1	3	15	62	15/4
Sandwich, tuna melt panini	1	3	2	49	2/3
Sandwich, turkey & Swiss	1	2	5	36	5/2
Scone, blueberry	1	2	17	61	17/4
Scone, cinnamon chip	1	3	34	70	34/4
Scone, cranberry orange	1	2	34	73	34/4
Scone, maple oat pecan	1	3	24	59	24/3
Scone, petite vanilla bean	1	0	10	21	10/2
Scone, pumpkin	1	2	43	78	43/4
Scone, raspberry	1	2	18	59	18/3
Wrap, chicken & vegetables	1	4	3	36	3/2
Wrap, egg white, spinach & feta	1	6	4	33	4/2
Wrap, huevos rancheros	1	8	4	35	4/2

SUBWAY

**6" Sandwiches (on 9-grain wheat bread
w/ lettuce, tomatoes, onions, green peppers & cucumbers)**

Big Philly Cheesesteak	1	6	7	54	7/3
Black forest ham	1	5	7	48	7/3
BLT	1	5	5	45	5/3
Chicken & bacon ranch	1	6	7	49	7/3
Cold cut combo	1	5	6	48	6/3
The Feast	1	6	8	51	8/3
Italian BMT	1	5	7	48	7/3
Meatball marinara	1	9	17	71	17/4
Oven roasted chicken	1	5	7	49	7/3
Roast beef	1	5	6	46	6/3
Spicy Italian	1	6	7	48	7/3
Subway Club	1	5	6	48	6/3
Subway Melt	1	5	7	49	7/3

FOOD	Svg Size	Fbr	Sgr	Cbs	S/C Val
Sweet onion chicken teriyaki	1	5	17	60	17/3
Tuna	1	5	6	46	6/3
Turkey breast	1	5	6	48	6/3
Turkey breast & black forest ham	1	5	7	48	7/3
Veggie Delite	1	5	5	45	5/3

Flatbread Sandwiches (w/ lettuce, tomatoes, onions, green peppers & cucumbers)

Black forest ham	1	3	4	47	4/3
Oven roasted chicken	1	3	5	49	5/3
Roast beef	1	3	3	46	3/3
Subway Club	1	3	4	47	4/3
Sweet onion chicken teriyaki	1	3	15	60	15/3
Turkey breast	1	3	3	47	3/3
Turkey breast & black forest ham	1	3	4	48	4/3
Veggie Delite	1	3	3	45	3/3

Kids' Meal Sandwiches (on 9-grain mini wheat bread w/ lettuce, tomatoes, onions, green peppers & cucumbers)

Black forest ham	1	3	3	30	3/2
Roast beef	1	4	4	30	4/2
Turkey breast	1	3	4	31	4/2
Veggie Delite	1	3	3	30	3/2

Sandwich Bread Options

Bread, hearty Italian, 6"	1	2	5	41	5/3
Bread, honey oat, 6"	1	5	8	49	8/3
Bread, Italian, mini	1	1	3	26	3/2
Bread, Italian herbs & cheese, 6"	1	2	7	45	7/3
Bread, Italian white, 6"	1	1	5	38	5/2
Bread, Monterey cheddar, 6"	1	1	5	39	5/2
Bread, 9-grain wheat, 6"	1	4	3	41	3/3
Bread, Parmesan oregano, 6"	1	2	5	41	5/3
Bread, roasted garlic, 6"	1	2	7	45	7/3
Bread, wheat, mini	1	3	2	28	2/2
English muffin, light wheat	1	5	0	16	0/1
Flatbread	1	2	0	41	0/3
Wrap	1	1	0	51	0/3

Sandwich Options and Condiments (amount on a 6" sub, flatbread, or salad)

Bacon	2 slcs	0	0	0	0/0
Banana peppers	3 slcs	0	0	0	0/0
Cheese, American, processed	0.4 oz	0	0	1	0/0
Cheese, cheddar	0.5 oz	0	0	0	0/0
Cheese, Monterey cheddar, shredded	0.5 oz	0	0	1	0/0

FOOD	Svg Size	Fbr	Sgr	Cbs	S/C Val
Cheese, mozzarella, shredded	0.5 oz	0	0	0	0/0
Cheese, pepper-jack	0.5 oz	0	0	0	0/0
Cheese, provolone	0.5 oz	0	0	0	0/0
Cheese, Swiss	0.5 oz	0	0	0	0/0
Chicken patty, roasted	2.5 oz	0	2	4	2/0
Chicken strips	2.5 oz	0	0	0	0/0
Cucumbers	3 slcs	0	0	0	0/0
Dressing, ranch	0.75 oz	0	1	1	1/0
Egg patty, regular or whites	1	1	0	3	0/0
Green peppers	3 slcs	0	0	0	0/0
Ham	2 oz	0	2	2	2/0
Jalapeño peppers	3 slcs	0	0	0	0/0
Lettuce	0.75 oz	0	0	0	0/0
Mayonnaise	1 T	0	0	0	0/0
Mayonnaise, light	1 T	0	0	0	0/0
Meatballs	7 oz	4	11	25	11/2
Meats, cold cut combo	2.5 oz	0	1	2	1/0
Meats, Italian BMT	2.25 oz	0	2	2	2/0
Meats, spicy Italian	2 oz	0	1	7	1/1
Meats, Subway Club	2.75 oz	0	1	2	1/0
Mustard	1 t	0	0	0	0/0
Olives	3 slcs	0	0	0	0/0
Onions	0.5 oz	0	0	1	0/0
Pickles	3 slcs	0	0	1	0/0
Roast beef	2.5 oz	0	1	1	1/0
Sauce, chipotle Southwest	0.75 oz	0	0	1	0/0
Sauce, honey mustard, fat free	0.75 oz	0	6	7	6/1
Sauce, sweet onion, fat free	0.75 oz	0	8	9	8/1
Seafood Sensation	2.5 oz	0	1	7	1/1
Steak	2.5 oz	0	1	4	1/0
Tomatoes	3 slcs	0	0	2	0/0
Tuna	2.5 oz	0	0	0	0/0
Turkey breast	2 oz	0	1	2	1/0
Veggie patty	1	3	2	12	2/1
Vinaigrette, red wine, fat free	0.75 oz	0	3	6	3/1
Vinegar	1 t	0	0	0	0/0
Breakfast Egg Muffin Melts (on light-wheat English muffin)					
Black forest ham, egg & cheese	1	5	1	18	1/1
Black forest ham, egg & cheese, w/ egg whites	1	5	1	18	1/1
Double bacon, egg & cheese	1	5	0	18	1/1
Double bacon, egg & cheese, w/ egg whites	1	5	0	18	0/1
Egg & cheese	1	5	0	18	0/1
Egg & cheese, w/ egg whites	1	5	0	18	0/1
Mega	1	5	0	18	0/1

FOOD	Svg Size	Fbr	Sgr	Cbs	S/C Val
Mega, w/ egg whites	1	5	0	18	0/1
Sausage, egg & cheese	1	5	0	18	0/1
Sausage, egg & cheese, w/ egg whites	1	5	0	18	0/1
Steak, egg & cheese	1	6	1	19	1/1
Steak, egg & cheese, w/ egg whites	1	5	0	19	0/1
Western egg w/ cheese	1	6	1	19	1/1
Western egg w/ cheese, w/ egg whites	1	5	1	19	1/1
Breakfast Egg Omelet Sandwiches (on 9-grain wheat bread)					
Black forest ham, egg & cheese	1	5	5	47	5/3
Black forest ham, egg & cheese, w/ egg whites	1	4	4	46	4/3
Double bacon, egg & cheese	1	5	4	47	4/3
Double bacon, egg & cheese, w/ egg whites	1	4	4	46	4/3
Egg & cheese	1	5	4	46	4/3
Egg & cheese, w/ egg whites	1	4	3	45	3/3
Mega	1	5	4	47	4/3
Mega, w/ egg whites	1	4	4	46	4/3
Sausage, egg & cheese	1	5	4	46	4/3
Sausage, egg & cheese, w/ egg whites	1	4	4	45	4/3
Steak, egg & cheese	1	5	5	48	5/3
Steak, egg & cheese, w/ egg whites	1	4	4	47	4/3
Western egg w/ cheese	1	5	5	47	5/3
Western egg w/ cheese, w/ egg whites	1	4	5	47	5/3
Other Menu Items					
Apple slices	1 pkg	2	7	9	7/1
Cookie, chocolate chip	1	1	18	30	18/2
Cookie, chocolate chunk	1	0	17	30	17/2
Cookie, double chocolate chip	1	1	20	30	20/2
Cookie, M&M	1	0	18	32	18/2
Cookie, oatmeal raisin	1	1	17	30	17/2
Cookie, peanut butter	1	1	16	26	16/2
Cookie, sugar	1	0	14	28	14/2
Cookie, white chip macadamia nut	1	1	18	29	18/2
Hash browns	4 pcs	2	0	17	0/1
Salad, black forest ham, w/o dressing	1	4	6	12	6/1
Salad, oven roasted chicken strips, w/o dressing	1	4	4	10	4/1
Salad, roast beef, w/o dressing	1	4	5	10	5/1
Salad, Subway Club, w/o dressing	1	4	6	12	6/1
Salad, turkey breast, w/o dressing	1	4	5	12	5/1
Salad, turkey breast & ham, w/o dressing	1	4	6	12	6/1
Salad, Veggie Delite, w/o dressing	1	4	4	10	4/1
Salad dressing, Italian, fat free	2 oz	0	4	7	4/1
Salad dressing, ranch	2 oz	0	3	3	3/0
Soup, chicken & dumpling	10 oz	2	2	23	2/2

FOOD	Svg Size	Fbr	Sgr	Cbs	S/C Val
Soup, chicken tortilla	10 oz	3	4	11	4/1
Soup, chili con carne	10 oz	10	7	35	7/2
Soup, chipotle chicken corn chowder	10 oz	2	4	22	4/2
Soup, cream of potato w/ bacon	10 oz	3	3	26	3/2
Soup, fire-roasted tomato orzo	10 oz	2	4	24	4/2
Soup, golden broccoli & cheese	10 oz	4	3	16	3/1
Soup, minestrone	10 oz	3	4	17	4/1
Soup, New England style clam chowder	10 oz	4	2	20	2/1
Soup, roasted chicken noodle	10 oz	1	2	12	2/1
Soup, rosemary chicken & dumpling	10 oz	1	3	14	3/1
Soup, Spanish style chicken & rice w/ pork	10 oz	1	1	16	1/1
Soup, tomato garden vegetable w/ rotini	10 oz	3	8	20	8/1
Soup, vegetable beef	10 oz	3	5	17	5/1
Soup, wild rice w/ chicken	10 oz	1	3	26	3/2
TACO BELL					
Burrito, bean, fresco	1	11	4	56	4/3
Burrito, bean, regular	1	11	3	55	3/3
Burrito, beefy 5-layer	1	9	6	69	6/4
Burrito, chicken, grilled stuft	1	9	5	77	5/4
Burrito, chicken, regular	1	3	3	48	3/3
Burrito, chicken, supreme	1	3	3	48	3/3
Burrito, chicken, supreme, fresco	1	8	4	50	4/3
Burrito, ground beef, grilled stuft	1	12	6	79	6/4
Burrito, ground beef, supreme	1	9	5	52	5/3
Burrito, ground beef, volcano	1	8	6	81	6/5
Burrito, ½ pound cheesy potato	1	7	5	57	5/3
Burrito, ½ pound combo	1	10	3	52	3/3
Burrito, ½ pound nacho crunch	1	6	5	54	5/3
Burrito, 7-layer	1	12	5	68	5/4
Burrito, steak, grilled stuft	1	9	6	76	6/4
Burrito, steak, supreme	1	7	5	51	5/3
Burrito, steak, supreme, fresco	1	8	4	50	4/3
Chalupa, chicken, Baja	1	3	4	29	4/2
Chalupa, chicken, nacho cheese	1	3	4	30	4/2
Chalupa, chicken, supreme	1	3	4	30	4/2
Chalupa, ground beef, Baja	1	5	4	31	4/2
Chalupa, ground beef, nacho cheese	1	4	4	31	4/2
Chalupa, ground beef, supreme	1	5	4	31	4/2
Chalupa, steak, Baja	1	3	4	29	4/2
Chalupa, steak, nacho cheese	1	3	4	30	4/2
Chalupa, steak, supreme	1	3	4	29	4/2
Cinnamon twists	1 pkt	1	10	26	10/2
Crunchwrap supreme	1	6	7	71	7/4
Empanada, caramel apple	1	2	13	39	13/2

FOOD	Svg Size	Fbr	Sgr	Cbs	S/C Val
Enchirito, chicken	1	7	2	31	2/2
Enchirito, ground beef	1	6	2	35	2/2
Enchirito, steak	1	7	2	33	2/2
Gordita, chicken, Baja	1	3	6	29	6/2
Gordita, chicken, nacho cheese	1	2	6	30	6/2
Gordita, chicken, supreme	1	2	6	29	6/2
Gordita, ground beef, Baja	1	4	6	30	6/2
Gordita, ground beef, nacho cheese	1	4	6	31	6/2
Gordita, ground beef, supreme	1	4	6	31	6/2
Gordita, steak, Baja	1	4	6	30	6/2
Gordita, steak, nacho cheese	1	4	6	31	6/2
Gordita, steak, supreme	1	2	6	29	6/2
Guacamole, side order	1	1	0	2	0/0
Mexican pizza	1	8	2	47	2/3
Meximelt, chicken	1	4	2	23	2/2
Meximelt, ground beef	1	4	2	23	2/2
Meximelt, steak	1	4	2	23	2/2
Nachos	1	2	2	31	2/2
Nachos, BellGrande	1	15	5	78	5/4
Nachos, supreme	1	8	3	42	3/3
Nachos, triple layer	1	7	2	39	2/2
Nachos, volcano	1	16	6	89	6/5
Pintos 'n cheese	1	9	1	19	1/1
Potatoes, cheesy fiesta	1	3	2	28	2/2
Quesadilla, chicken	1	4	3	41	3/3
Quesadilla, steak	1	4	3	40	3/2
Rice, Mexican	1	1	1	21	1/2
Roll-up, cheese	1	2	1	19	1/1
Salad, chicken, fiesta taco	1	12	8	75	8/4
Salad, chicken, ranch taco	1	9	6	71	6/4
Salad, ground beef, fiesta taco	1	12	8	75	8/4
Salad, ground beef, fiesta taco, w/o shell	1	11	7	41	7/3
Salad, steak, chipotle taco	1	8	7	70	7/4
Salsa, side order	1	0	1	1	1/0
Soft taco, chicken ranchero	1	2	2	21	2/2
Soft taco, chicken ranchero, fresco	1	2	3	22	3/2
Soft taco, ground beef, fresco	1	3	2	22	2/2
Soft taco, ground beef, regular	1	3	2	21	2/2
Soft taco, ground beef, supreme	1	2	2	21	2/2
Soft taco, potato, crispy	1	3	2	31	2/2
Soft taco, steak, fresco	1	3	2	22	2/2
Soft taco, steak, regular	1	2	2	20	2/1
Sour cream, reduced fat, side order	1	0	1	2	1/0
Taco, ground beef, double decker	1	8	2	38	2/2

FOOD	Svg Size	Fbr	Sgr	Cbs	S/C Val
Taco, ground beef, fresco	1	3	1	13	1/1
Taco, ground beef, regular	1	3	1	12	1/1
Taco, ground beef, supreme	1	3	2	15	2/1
Taco, ground beef, volcano	1	3	1	14	1/1
Taquitos, chicken	1	2	2	37	2/2
Taquitos, steak	1	2	3	37	3/2
Tortada, bacon ranch	1	4	5	57	5/3
Tortada, salsa roja	1	4	5	60	5/3

For more information on products, visit the Websites listed below:

Almond Breeze Almond Milk: **bluediamond.com**
Amazing Grass SuperFood Drink Mixes: **amazinggrass.com**
Arrowhead Mills Flours & Baking Mixes: **arrowheadmills.com**
Barlean's Omega Swirl: **barleans.com**
Bob's Red Mill: **bobsredmill.com**
Cascadian Farm: **cascadianfarm.com**
Clemmy's Ice Cream: **clemmysicecream.com**
DeLallo Pesto & Pasta Sauce: **delallo.com**
El Burrito Soy Products: **elburrito.com**
Ener-G Foods Light Brown Rice Loaf & Egg Replacer: **ener-g.com**
FAGE Yogurt: **fageusa.com**
Follow Your Heart Vegan Products: **followyourheart.com**
Food for Life Ezekiel 4:9 Products: **foodforlife.com**
Jay Robb Whey Protein: **jayrobb.com**
Jennies Unsweetened Coconut Macaroons: **macaroonking.com**
Joseph's Sugar-Free Products: **josephslitecookies.com**
Judy's Candy Company Sugar-Free Caramels & Peanut Brittle: **judyscandy.com**
La Tortilla Factory: **latortillafactory.com**
LowCarb Specialties, Inc. ChocoPerfection: **lowcarbspecialties.com**
Morningstar Farms Vegetarian Products: **morningstarfarms.com**
Nature's Hollow Sugar-Free Products: **probstfarms.com**
Perfectly Sweet Sugar-Free Licorice & Cinna Cubs: **perfectlysweet.com**
Pirate's Booty: **piratesbooty.com**
PureVia: **purevia.com**
Scott's Barbecue Sauce: **scottsbarbecuesauce.com**
Seeds of Change Organic Food: **seedsofchangefoods.com**
Simply Potatoes: **simplypotatoes.com**
Stevia SweetLeaf Sweetener: **sweetleaf.com**
Truvia: **truvia.com**
Tumaro's Gourmet Tortillas: **tumaros.com**
Ultima Replenisher Drink Mixes: **ultimareplenisher.com**
U.S. Mills Cereal: **usmillsinc.com**
Vitalicious VitaMuffins and VitaTops: **vitalicious.com**
Wholly Guacamole: **eatwholly.com**
Xlear, Inc. Xylitol Products (such as Spry gum): **xlear.com**
Zevia Soda: **zevia.com**

Acknowledgments

To Heather, Parker, and Owen, thank you for your love and support.

To Robbie McMillin, Jared Davis, Oliver Stephenson, and Michelle McGowen—my core content team—your hard work and incredible talents were invaluable to this project. I can't thank you enough for your dedication and commitment to creating truly outstanding content.

A huge thank-you to Lorraine E. Fisher for your invaluable research on this project. I couldn't have done it without you.

To Reid Tracy and Louise Hay, thank you for standing behind my work.

Finally, to my clients, thank you—your support and feedback in refining this program has truly been a gift. You are a critical part of creating the change our world needs . . . it all starts with you!

• • • •

About the Author

JORGE CRUISE used to be 40 pounds overweight. Today, he is internationally recognized as the leading health expert for busy people and is the author of four consecutive *New York Times* best-selling series, with more than five million books in print in over 15 languages, including *The Belly Fat Cure, 8 Minutes in the Morning, The 3-Hour Diet, The 12-Second Sequence,* and *Body at Home.* He is also a contributing editor for *USA WEEKEND Magazine, The Costco Connection* magazine, *First for Women* magazine, and *Extra* TV. He has appeared on *The Oprah Winfrey Show,* CNN, *Good Morning America,* the *Today* show, *Dateline NBC, The View, The Tyra Banks Show,* and VH1.

Jorge received his bachelor's degree from the University of California, San Diego (UCSD); and has fitness credentials from the Cooper Institute for Aerobics Research, the American College of Sports Medicine (ACSM), and the American Council on Exercise (ACE).

• • • •